Pediatric Fluid, Electrolyte, and Acid-Base Disorders

A CASE-BASED APPROACH

Pediatric Fluid, Electrolyte, and Acid-Base Disorders

A CASE-BASED APPROACH

Editor

Farahnak Assadi, MD
Emeritus Professor of Pediatrics
Division of Nephrology
Rush University Medical Center
Chicago, Illinois, USA

ELSEVIER

Elsevier
1600 John F. Kennedy Blvd.
Ste 1800
Philadelphia, PA 19103-2899

PEDIATRIC FLUID, ELECTROLYTE, AND ACID-BASE DISORDERS:
A CASE-BASED APPROACH

ISBN: 978-0-443-11113-6

Notice

Practitioners and researchers must always rely on their own experience and knowledge in evaluating and using any information, methods, compounds or experiments described herein. Because of rapid advances in the medical sciences, in particular, independent verification of diagnoses and drug dosages should be made. To the fullest extent of the law, no responsibility is assumed by Elsevier, authors, editors, or contributors for any injury and/or damage to persons or property as a matter of products liability, negligence or otherwise, or from any use or operation of any methods, products, instructions, or ideas contained in the material herein.

Executive Content Strategist: Nancy Duffy
Senior Content Development Specialist: Vasowati Shome
Publishing Services Manager: Shereen Jameel
Project Manager: Gayathri S
Design Direction: Renee Duenow

Printed in India

Last digit is the print number: 9 8 7 6 5 4 3 2 1

Working together
to grow libraries in
developing countries

www.elsevier.com • www.bookaid.org

To my families,
to my students, residents, fellows,
and to all my patients for whom I have cared,
who always taught me so much.

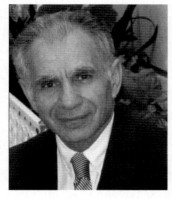

Dr. Farahnak Assadi is a Distinguished Emeritus Professor of Pediatrics and Chief of Pediatric Nephrology at Rush University Medical Center. He received his medical degree from Tehran University, where he completed his dissertation with distinction. He completed his residency training in pediatrics at Thomas Jefferson University Medical College and furthered his specialty training with a fellowship in nephrology at the University of Pennsylvania Children's Hospital of Philadelphia.

Dr. Assadi served as Professor of Pediatrics and Chief of Pediatric Nephrology at Thomas Jefferson University Hospital and DuPont Hospital for Children from 1990 to 2000 prior to joining the faculty of Rush University Medical Center. During his tenure he was instrumental in establishing a world-class Pediatric Nephrology Program at Dupont Hospital for Children, which became the national model for organ transplantation in the state of Delaware.

Dr. Assadi is an internationally recognized leader in the field of pediatric nephrology, and he has led a distinguished career as a clinician and researcher on the health and welfare of pediatric communities and the influence of culture in patient-provider communication worldwide.

Dr. Assadi has an impressive record of scholarly activity. He has authored over 150 peer-reviewed articles, textbooks, and book chapters. He has received numerous research grants and is an internationally renowned author and speaker. He is an expert on renal physiology and fluid-electrolytes and acid-base disorders. His research interests are in aspects of newborn developmental renal physiology, hypertension, and chronic renal failure. Dr. Assadi is a competent clinician, outstanding teacher, and a gifted scientist. As a testament to his excellence, he received over 25 teaching, mentoring, and patients' care awards.

An officer of numerous national and international scholarly societies, Dr. Assadi has served as a senior elected member for the Society for Pediatric Research, American Society of Pediatric Nephrology, American Society of Nephrology, National Kidney Foundation, North American Renal Transplant Society, and the International Society of Pediatric Nephrology.

Learning medicine is a challenging, evolving, and life-long endeavor. A case-based approach in medicine helps medical students, residents, and practicing physicians begin this process by engaging them in reflection on cases that resonate with the experiences of life in medicine.

The primary purpose of writing the Case-Based Approach to the Pediatric Fluid, Electrolyte, and Acid-Base Disorders book is to provide a comprehensive, state-of-the-art review and understanding of pediatric fluid, electrolyte, and acid-base disorders in a concise and reliable format that are frequently encountered in real world clinical decision making. The book is specifically useful for renal fellows, nephrologists, and other practicing physicians seeking to undertake certification and recertification board examinations.

This book is the product of author's nearly half a century of teaching in leading university hospitals in America, including University of Illinois School of Medicine, University of Pennsylvania, Children's Hospital of Philadelphia, Thomas Jefferson University, duPont Hospital for Children, and Rush University Medical Center.

This book presents 215 real cases frequently seen by medical students, residents, practicing physicians, and other health care provides during their routine daily clinical practice. The 215 cases were selected not only from the author's publications but also from publications of other authors with expertise in the practice of clinical nephrology.

The 215 cases are divided into 12 chapters and each chapter contains extensive discussions of clinical characteristics, differential diagnosis, and treatments of relevant renal electrolyte disorders. Each case study begins with a succinct summary of patient's history, signs and symptoms, examination, and initial investigation followed by questions and answers. The answers provide a detailed discussion on each topic, with further cross-references and discussions where appropriate. These true-to-life cases will help students, residents, and practicing physicians to recognize important clinical symptoms and signs and to develop the diagnostic and management skills needed for the cases they will encounter on their routine daily clinical practice. Ideal for students, residents, and fellows rotating on nephrology subspecialty services, the material is also useful as a first-line resource for other practicing physicians who need quick access to current scientific and clinical information on managing pediatric fluid, electrolyte, and acid-base disorders.

Farahnak Assadi, MD
Emeritus Professor of Pediatrics
Division of Nephrology
Rush University Medical Center
Chicago, Illinois, USA

*Disease is an abnormal state of the body which primarily and independently produces
a disturbance in the normal functions of the body. It may be an abnormality of temperature
or from structure. Symptoms are a manifestation of some abnormal state in the body. It may
be harmful as a colic pain or harmless as flushing of cheeks in peri-pneumonia.*

*Anyone wishing to study medicine must master the science of interaction between natures,
the body in health and the body in diseases. Illnesses do not come upon us out of blue. They
are developed from small daily sins against nature. In treating every patient, a conscientious
physician must declare the past, diagnose the present, and foretell the future. He or she must
make a habit of two things—to improve, or at least to do no harm to the patient*

AVICENNA

Many of the individuals to whom I am most indebted are only indirect contributors to this book. They are the people who saw some glimmer of hope in the author early in his career and nurtured him in what has been the most rewarding life in pediatrics and nephrology. During my fellowship training at the University of Pennsylvania, Children's Hospital of Philadelphia, Professors David Cornfeld and Michael E. Norman established the groundwork for my subsequent career in nephrology. They provided an intellectual environment and I have always been grateful for their efforts on my behalf. In the beginning of my career at the University of Illinois, one could hardly have had a better mentor than Professor Ira Rosenthal. After moving to Thomas Jefferson University Medical College, I received extraordinary help from Professor Robert Brent. He supported my efforts to establish the core of an outstanding nephrology program at duPont Hospital for Children in Wilmington DE. Leading the Division of Nephrology at Rush University Medical Center has been one of the greatest fortunes of my life. Professor Samuel Gotoff made it enjoyable to come to work each and every day for several years.

This book would not have been possible without the help of many student, residents, fellows, and colleagues in nephrology and related discipline at the leading national and international universities around the world. I am grateful to all of them for their exemplary contributions.

Farahnak Assadi, MD
Emeritus Professor of Pediatrics
Division of Nephrology
Rush University Medical Center
Chicago, Illinois, USA

ABG	Arterial blood gas
ACE	Angiotensin-converting enzyme
ACEI	Angiotensin-converting enzyme inhibition
ACTH	Adrenocorticotropic hormone
AD	Autosomal dominant
ADH	Antidiuretic hormone
ADTKD	Autosomal dominant tubulointerstitial kidney disease
AG	Anion gap
AKI	Acute kidney injury
AME	Apparent mineralocorticoid excess
AR	Autosomal recessive
ARB	Angiotensin receptor blockade
ARF	Acute renal failure
ASD	Aldosterone synthase deficiency
ATP	Adenosine triphosphate
BP	Blood pressure
BUN	Blood urea nitrogen
C	Complement
CAH	Congenital adrenal hyperplasia
cGMP	Cyclic guanosine monophosphate
CKD	Chronic kidney disease
Cl	Chloride
Cr	Creatinine
CRA	Chronic respiratory alkalosis
CRH	Corticotrophin-releasing hormone
CRRT	Continuous renal replacement therapy
CSW	Cerebral salt wasting
CT	Computed tomography
CTLA-4	Cytotoxic T lymphocyte antigen 4
DI	Diabetes insipidus
DOC	Deoxycorticosterone
dRTA	Distal renal tubular acidosis
DTPA	Diethylene triamino pentaacetic acid
ECF	Extracellular fluid
ECV	Extracellular volume
EEG	Electrocardiogram
eGFR	Estimated glomerular filtration rate
ENaC	Epithelial sodium channel
ESRD	End-stage-renal disease
FEK	Fractional excretion potassium
FENa	Fractional excretion sodium
FEPO$_4$	Fractional excretion phosphate
FEU	Fractional excretion urate
FHPP	Familial hypokalemic periodic paralysis
FIH	Familial isolated hypoparathyroidism

FS	Fanconi syndrome
GFR	Glomerular filtration rate
GN	Glomerulonephritis
HCT	Hydrochlorothiazide
HD	Hemodialysis
HHS	Hyponatremic hypertensive syndrome
HVDRR	Hereditary vitamin D-resistant rickets
ICU	Intensive care unit
IgA	Immunoglobulin A
IgG	immunoglobulin G
JGA	Juxta glomerular apparatus
INR	International normalized ratio
IVP	Intravenous pyelogram
K	Potassium
KCl	Potassium chloride
MAG 3	Tc-mercaptoacetyltriglycine
MMF	Mycophenolate mofetil
MRI	Magnetic resonance imaging
MSK	Medullary sponge kidney
MSH	Melanocyte stimulating hormone
Na	Sodium
NAGMA	Normal anion gap metabolic acidosis
NH$_3$	Ammonia
NH$_4$	Ammonium
NSAID	Non-steroidal anti-inflammatory drug
PAC	Plasma aldosterone concentration
PD	Peritoneal dialysis
PD-1	Programmed cell death protein
PHA	Pseudohypoaldosteronism
PICU	Pediatric intensive care unit
PLA2R	Phospholipase A2 receptor antibody
PNa	Plasma sodium
PRA	Plasma renin activity
PTH	Parathyroid hormone
PTHrP	Parathyroid hormone-related peptide
PTT	Partial thromboplastin time
RAS	Renin-angiotensin system
RRT	Renal replacement therapy
RTA	Renal tubular acidosis
SGLT2	Sodium-glucose cotransporter 2
SIADH	Syndrome inappropriate antidiuretic hormone
SLE	Systemic lupus erythematous
TBNa	Total body sodium
TBW	Total body water
TJGA	Tumor juxtaglomerular apparatus
TNF-α	Tumor necrosis factor-α
TNSALP	Tissue non-specific alkaline phosphatase
TPN	Total parenteral nutrition

TRP	Tubular reabsorption of phosphate
TSH	Thyroid stimulating hormone
TTKG	Transtubular potassium gradient
UAG	Urine anion gap
UTI	Urinary tract infection
UVJ	Ureterovesical junction
VCUG	Voiding cystoureterography
VUR	Vesicoureteral reflux

CONTENTS

CHAPTER 1

Hyponatremia

Case Study 1

A 12-year-old male with a history of Hodgkin lymphoma and hypertension presented to the hospital with a 2-week duration of weakness and fatigue. He also reported a poor appetite and decreased oral intake but no weight loss. He denied shortness of breath, syncope, nausea, vomiting, or diarrhea. He also denied headache, confusion, polyuria, or polydipsia.

Home medications included amlodipine 10 mg once a day, lisinopril 10 mg once a day, and pembrolizumab 200 mg intravenously every 3 weeks. The latter was started 3 months prior to admission, and he had recently completed three cycles of therapy.

On admission, he was clinically euvolemic, blood pressure was 118/78 mmHg, and heart rate 62 beats/min. Initial work-up was notable for hyponatremia with serum sodium level of 120 mmol/L and metabolic acidosis with total bicarbonate of 16 mmol/L. Other laboratory results were: serum sodium 120 mmol/L, potassium 3.5 mmol/L, chloride 90 mmol/L, creatinine 0.6 mg/dL, BUN 8 mg/dL, phosphorous 2.6 mg/dL, aldosterone 5 ng/dL (reference: 7.4 to 29.8), thyroid-stimulating hormone (TSH) 1.04 mIU/L (reference: 0.44 to 3.98), adrenocorticotropic hormone (ACTH) 5.1 pg/mL (reference: 7.2 to 63.3), and cortisol level measured in the morning 1.0 μg/dL (reference: 2.5 to 20.0).

A spot urinary protein-creatinine ratio was 0.12 mg/mg, and urine pH was 6.0. Urine analysis did not show any microscopic hematuria or pyuria. There was no glycosuria. Urinary sodium was 52 mmol/L, potassium 19 mmol/L, chloride 63 mmol/L, and osmolality 299 mOsm/kg.

Computed tomography scan of the abdomen was normal. Other laboratory studies including titers of serum antinuclear antibody, anti-neutrophil cytoplasmic antibody, and anti-SSA/SSB; tests for hepatitis B and C virus; and levels of C3 and C4 were all unrevealing.

What are the MOST likely causes of this patient's hyponatremia and metabolic acidosis? (Select all that apply)

    A. Syndrome inappropriate antidiuretic hormone (SIADH) and distal renal tubular acidosis (dRTA) secondary to immune checkpoint inhibitor therapy
    B. SIADH and proximal RTA secondary to immune checkpoint inhibitor therapy
    C. Immune-mediated central adrenal insufficiency causing SIADH and dRTA
    D. SIADH and dRTA secondary to immune checkpoint inhibitor therapy

The correct answers are A and C
Comment: This patient had hypophysitis, which precipitated adrenal insufficiency. Low levels of ACTH and cortisol support this conclusion.

The laboratory work-up for this patient (inappropriate high urine osmolality in the presence of serum hypoosmolality, normal renal function, and absence of clinical features of dehydration or volume overload) is highly suggestive of SIADH.[1–3]

Hyponatremia caused by SIADH is common in cancer patients receiving immune checkpoint inhibitors, and acute hyponatremia secondary to pembrolizumab has been reported.[1-3] This patient also had normal anion gap metabolic acidosis with positive urine anion gap and low positive urine osmolar gap (< 150 mOsm/kg), which is highly suggestive of dRTA.[4] Although dRTA is usually associated with hypokalemia, simultaneous adrenal insufficiency could have offset this finding.

Diagnosis of the etiology of hyponatremia is necessary in order to provide appropriate treatment. Laboratory assessments, including measurements of plasma osmolality, urine osmolality, and urine sodium, and clinical assessment of extracellular volume status are critical to the differential diagnosis of hyponatremia.

There are various causes of SIADH in a cancer patient: it may be a result of ectopic vasopressin production by tumor cells or a consequence of stimulation of vasopressin secretion or potentiation of vasopressin effects by anticancer drugs or palliative medications.[5] There are many traditional chemotherapeutic treatments that can cause hyponatremia. Recently, immune checkpoint inhibitors have revolutionized the treatment of various solid tumors.[6,7] There are adverse kidney effects associated with the development of hyponatremia and possibly SIADH.

dRTA is a tubulopathy characterized by dysfunction of distal urinary acidification, which subsequently can lead to a normal anion gap metabolic acidosis. Common causes include autoimmune diseases, drugs, genetic diseases, and tubulointerstitial diseases; however, in many cases a cause is not identified.[7]

In this patient, the dRTA is likely secondary to a renal immunotherapy-related adverse event. There has been extensive literature characterizing the various endocrinopathies associated with immune checkpoint inhibitors, including primary adrenal insufficiency, hypothyroidism, hyperthyroidism, and hypophysitis. Although the risk of immune checkpoint inhibitor–associated adrenal insufficiency is less than 1%, it is still associated with significant morbidity and mortality.[1-3]

The combination of hyponatremia, dRTA, and adrenal insufficiency in this patient is highly suggestive that his hyponatremia was secondary to adrenal insufficiency, which in turn we considered as an immunotherapy-related adverse event.

The patient was started on hydrocortisone 40 mg daily. This was accompanied by improvement in serum sodium and bicarbonate levels. Two days later, the patient's hyponatremia and metabolic acidosis had resolved. He was eventually discharged on a tapering dose of steroids. Rapid resolution of both conditions upon initiation of steroids suggests that they are both immune-mediated adverse effects associated with pembrolizumab.

Case Study 2

A 12-year-old girl with no significant medical history presented with 4 hours of acute left leg swelling. Venous ultrasonography of the affected limb showed acute deep vein thrombosis involving the left femoral vein with extension to the external iliac vein and inferior vena cava. The patient was started on treatment with noxaparin and warfarin. Despite anticoagulation therapy, she developed small bilateral pulmonary emboli, and an inferior vena cava filter was placed. Hypercoagulable work-up was positive for lupus anticoagulant, high titers of anticardiolipin antibodies, and moderately elevated titers of anti-2 glycoprotein antibodies suggestive of antiphospholipid syndrome. On the third day of hospitalization, the patient developed acute hyponatremia with a sodium level that decreased from 137 to 115 mmol/L and normal anion gap metabolic acidosis. At that time patient's serum potassium was 4.8 mmol/L, chloride 90 mmol/L, bicarbonate 19 mmol/L, BUN 20 mg/dL, creatinine 0.7 mg/dL. Serum osmolality was 242 mOsm/kg, urine osmolality 290 mOsm/kg, and urine sodium 77 mmol/L. Serum cortisol level measured in the morning was 0.3 µg/dL (reference: 5 to 20 µg/dL). Arterial blood gas showed pH 7.31, PCO$_2$ 37 mmHg, PO$_2$ 80 mmHg, and bicarbonate 20 mmol/L.

Throughout this time, the patient was asymptomatic. On physical examination, pulse rate was 90 beats/min and blood pressure was 120/75 mmHg, with no orthostatic changes. Cardiovascular examination showed normal heart sounds, lungs were clear to auscultation, and there was no peripheral edema. Neurologic examination findings were normal.

What is the MOST likely cause of hyponatremia in this patient and how should be treated?

A. Syndrome inappropriate antidiuretic hormone (SIADH)
B. Liddle syndrome
C. Apparent mineralocorticoid excess
D. Primary adrenal insufficiency

The correct answer is D
Comment: The major causes of euvolemic hyponatremia are SIADH, hypothyroidism, glucocorticoid deficiency, and decreased urinary solute excretion, as in beer potomania or a very low-protein diet.[1] SIADH is the most frequent cause of euvolemic hyponatremia and can be seen in pulmonary diseases, malignancies, central nervous system diseases, and with certain drugs.[2]

In patients with SIADH, the non-physiologic secretion of antidiuretic hormone (ADH) leads to increased water reabsorption, resulting in dilutional hyponatremia when the intake of free water exceeds its excretory capacity.[3–5] Hyponatremia in hypothyroidism is seen primarily in severe cases or myxedema.[2] The mechanism by which hypothyroidism induces hyponatremia is incompletely understood. It is thought to be due to decreased cardiac output leading to the release of ADH through the carotid sinus baroreceptors.

Adrenal insufficiency should be ruled out before diagnosing SIADH. Glucocorticoid deficiency can cause hyponatremia in both primary and secondary adrenal insufficiency.[6–8] Solute intake has a central role as a determinant of free water excretion. Inadequate dietary solute intake with reduced urinary solute excretion limits water excretion.[5] This enables hyponatremia to develop with even modest water intake. This same mechanism is responsible for the hyponatremia seen in individuals who drink large quantities of beer (known as beer potomania) because beer has a low sodium content and these individuals often have limited overall dietary intake. This disturbance also can be observed in individuals with restricted protein or salt intake in combination with generous water intake.

The first step in the evaluation of euvolemic hyponatremia is to check for thyroid or adrenal abnormalities.

Our patient did not have hypertension and her thyroid-stimulating hormone level was normal. However, a random cortisol level was very low at 0.3 μg/dL, measured at 6 AM (reference: 5 to 24 μg/dL). Corticotrophin level was elevated, and a cosyntropin stimulation test confirmed the diagnosis of primary adrenal insufficiency. Computed tomography of the abdomen showed bilateral adrenal enlargement with no contrast enhancement suggestive of hemorrhagic necrosis, possibly due to adrenal vein thrombosis from antiphospholipid syndrome. The patient's sodium level corrected within 60 hours after giving 3% saline solutions in addition to intravenous steroid replacement with hydrocortisone. The patient was discharged on a regimen of warfarin and low-dose aspirin with oral steroid replacement therapy, including hydrocortisone and fludrocortisone. Repeated work-up 12 weeks later confirmed the diagnosis of antiphospholipid antibody syndrome. The levels of sodium and the rest of the electrolytes were normal.

Hyponatremia is the most common electrolyte abnormality encountered in clinical practice, occurring in up to 30% of hospitalized patients.[6] Adrenal insufficiency, a rare but important endocrine disorder that results in hyponatremia, is caused by either primary adrenal failure (most commonly due to autoimmune adrenalitis) or impairment of the hypothalamic-pituitary axis (primarily pituitary disease).[7–9] Hyponatremia in adrenal insufficiency is multifactorial. Mineralocorticoid deficiency is present only in primary adrenal insufficiency and results in hypovolemia, low blood pressure, postural hypotension, and occasionally prerenal acute kidney injury. Other metabolic features of primary adrenal insufficiency include hyponatremia (90% of patients with primary adrenal insufficiency), hyperkalemia (65%), and salt craving (15%). In addition, plasma ADH is stimulated by decreased circulating blood volume, which then triggers water retention. In addition to hyponatremia and hyperkalemia, mild hyperchloremic acidosis can occur with mineralocorticoid deficiency. Hyperkalemia suppresses the production of renal ammonia, leading to reduced ammonium ion excretion and thus reduced net acid excretion.[10,11] Although the main cause of decreased ammonia production is hyperkalemia itself, aldosterone deficiency or resistance also may contribute to the decrease. Hyponatremia also can develop in secondary adrenal insufficiency due to failure to fully suppress ADH secretion in response to hypoosmolarity. ADH and corticotrophin-releasing hormone in the parvocellular neurons of the paraventricular nucleus are negatively regulated by glucocorticoids. When the negative feedback action of glucocorticoids is removed, the result is up regulation of corticotrophin-releasing hormone and ADH gene expression in the paraventricular nucleus neurons. Animal experimental studies showed that glucocorticoids also inhibit ADH gene transcription and decrease messenger RNA stability.[12] In both glucocorticoid and mineralocorticoid deficiency, the changes in hemodynamics also have a role in causing hyponatremia, separately from ADH, because they limit the delivery of tubular fluid to the diluting segment of the nephron. The pathogenesis of adrenal insufficiency in antiphospholipid syndrome is related to vascular complications, including adrenal vein thrombosis and edema of the adrenal gland, resulting in obstructed arterial supply and hemorrhagic infarction.[13,14] The adrenal glands' unique vascular anatomy, featuring a rich arterial supply but only a single vein with limited drainage, predisposes these patients to thrombosis.[13]

The primary therapy for all types of adrenal insufficiency is glucocorticoids. Although several types of glucocorticoids are available, hydrocortisone is preferred because its short half-life is the most similar to the normal circadian rhythm of cortisol. Patients with primary adrenal insufficiency also require mineralocorticoid therapy (fludrocortisone). The mineralocorticoid dose can be modified based on serum potassium level and plasma renin activity and the symptoms experienced by the patient, such as orthostatic dizziness or salt craving. Suppressed plasma renin activity can be a helpful indicator of an overdose of fludrocortisone, an overdose that may cause retention of fluid, edema, and hypertension.

Case Study 3

A 15-year-old woman is started on hydrochlorothiazide and a low-sodium diet for the treatment of hypertension. After 1 week, she complains of weakness, muscle cramps, and postural dizziness. On physical examination, the patient is found to be alert and oriented. The blood pressure is 130/86 mmHg (the pretreatment level was 150/100 mmHg). The skin turgor is decreased, and the jugular venous pressure is less than 5 cmH$_2$O. The laboratory data are serum sodium 119 mmol/L, potassium 2.1 mmol/L, chloride 71 mmol/L, bicarbonate 34 mmol/L, plasma osmolality 252 mOsm/kg, urine osmolality 540 mOsm/kg, urine sodium 4 mmol/L.

What are the MOST likely causes for this patient's hyponatremia? (Select all that apply)

    A. Hydrochlorothiazide
    B. Volume depletion
    C. Increased ADH secretion
    D. Water retention
    E. Potassium depletion

The correct answers are A, B, C, and D
Comment: All of these factors contributed to hyponatremia. Hydrochlorothiazide-induced volume depletion (physical findings plus low urine sodium concentration), which enhanced

antidiuretic hormone (ADH) release (high urine osmolality of 540 mOsm/kg), resulting in water retention and hyponatremia. The loss of potassium also played a contributory role via a transcellular K^+-Na^+ exchange.[1,2]

Therapy should include the administration of sodium and potassium in a hypertonic solution, such as 40 mmol of KCl added to each liter of isotonic saline. There is little justification for water restriction, since the patient is volume depleted. In view of the metabolic alkalosis, KCl, not potassium citrate is indicated (since citrate is metabolized into bicarbonate). Half-isotonic saline should also be avoided because it is a hypotonic solution that will further lower the plasma sodium concentration.

Case Study 4

A 17-year-old male with hypertension treated with unknown medications is admitted to the hospital in a comatose state, responding only to deep pain. On physical examination, the blood pressure is found to be 180/120 mmHg. The skin turgor is reduced, and the neck veins are flat. After appropriate studies, the diagnosis of an intracerebral hemorrhage is made. To minimize the degree of brain swelling, the patient is given a total of 25 g of mannitol. Only 100 mL of 5% dextrose in water is given. The laboratory data at this time include serum sodium 120 mmol/L, potassium 3.3 mmol/L, chloride 78 mmol/L, bicarbonate 29 mmol/L, plasma osmolality 253 mOsm/kg, urine osmolality 240 mOsm/kg, and urine sodium 45 mmol/L.

What is the MOST likely diagnosis of this patient's hyponatremia?

    A. Pseudohyponatremia due to mannitol
    B. Volume depletion
    C. SIADH
    D. Neurogenic salt wasting syndrome

The correct answer is B
Comment: Hyponatremia in this patient is due to volume depletion, probably induced by diuretic therapy for hypertension.[1,2] The physical findings suggestive of hypovolemia, hypokalemia, and high plasma bicarbonate concentration are all compatible with this diagnosis. Pseudohyponatremia due to mannitol is not present since the measured plasma osmolality is low and is similar to the calculated value [calculated plasma osmolality = $2 \times 120 + (125 \div 18) + (15 \div 2.8) = 252$ mOsml/kg]. SIADH due to stroke also cannot account for hyponatremia. Hyponatremia must have preceded the stroke, since the patient subsequently received only 100 mL of water, a quantity that is insufficient to lower the plasma sodium concentration.

Case Study 5

A 19-year-old man weighing 70 kg is admitted to the hospital with a 2-week history of progressive lethargy and obtundation. The physical examination is within normal limits except for the obtundation. The following laboratory studies are obtained: Serum sodium 105 mmol/L, potassium 4 mmol/L, chloride 72 mmol/L, bicarbonate 21 mmol/L, plasma osmolality 210 mOsm/kg, urine osmolality 604 mOsml/kg, and urine sodium 78 moml/L.

What is the most likely diagnosis and how and at what initial rate would you raise the plasma sodium concentration?

    A. Pseudohyperaldosteronism
    B. Diuretic abuse
    C. Adrenal insufficiency
    D. Syndrome of inappropriate antidiuretic secretion (SIADH)

The correct answer is D

Comment: The most likely diagnosis is SIADH.[1-3] Hypertonic saline should be given initially in view of the marked hyponatremia and neurologic symptoms.

The approximate sodium deficit that must be corrected to raise the plasma sodium concentration to a safe value of 120 mmol/L can be estimated from Na^+ deficit = 0.6 × 70 (120 to 105) or 630 mmol.

This requires approximately 1200 mL of 3% saline, which should be given at the rate of 40 mL/h over 30 hours to raise the plasma sodium concentration by 0.5 mmol/L/h. Furosemide will enhance the efficacy of this regimen by lowering urine osmolality, thereby increasing free-water excretion.

Case Study 6

A previously healthy 18-year-old girl experienced three grand mal seizures 2 days after an appendectomy. She received 10 mg of diazepam and 150 mg of phenytoin intravenously and underwent laryngeal intubation with mechanical ventilation. She had been treated with 6 L of 5% dextrose containing 37-mmol sodium/L during the first 3 days after surgery. She is stuporous and responds to pain but not to commands. She is euvolemic, her weight is 46 kg, serum sodium is 110 mmol/L, potassium is 4.1 mmol/L, uric acid is 3.1 mg/dL, and osmolality is 228 mOsm/kg H_2O. Urine osmolality is 510 mOsm/kg.

What is the appropriate initial fluid for treating this patient's hyponatremia?

    A. Infusion of 3% saline at 70 mL/h
    B. Infusion of 0.9% saline at 150 mL/h
    C. Infusion of 0.45% saline at 300 mL/h
    D. Infusion of 0.2% saline at 600 mL/h

The correct answer is A

Comment: Hypotonic hyponatremia in this patient is a result of water retention (use of hypotonic solution) caused by the impaired water excretion due to her SIADH postoperatively on the presence of hypotonic hyponatremia and concentrated urine in a euvolemic patient, the absence of a history of diuretic use, and the absence of clinical evidence of hypothyroidism or hypoadrenalism.[1]

The goal of treatment here is a rapid increase in serum sodium level to the point where mental status is improved and the risk of further seizures is decreased adequately. The infusion of 3% saline, diuretic use, and fluid restriction are management tools, which allow for these goals to be achieved.

The effect of 1 L of 3% hypertonic saline on serum sodium change is estimated by the following formula[2,3]:

$$Na^+ \text{ change mmol} / L = [\text{infusate } Na^+ \text{ mmol} / L] - [\text{serum } Na^+ \text{ mmol} / L] \div (TBW \text{ liters} + 1)$$

According to the formula, the infusion of 1 L of 3% saline will increase the serum sodium concentration by 14.4 mmol/L ([513–110] + [27 + 1] = 14.4).

Given the seriousness of the patient's symptoms the initial goal is to raise the serum sodium concentration by 4 mmol/L over the next 2 hours; thus 139 mL of 3% hypertonic saline (2 ÷ 14.4), or 70 mL/h, was required.

At the end of 2 hours, patient's mental status is substantially improved and her serum sodium concentration is 114 mmol/L. The goal of treatment now is to raise serum sodium slowly by additional 3 mmol/L over the next 3 hours, thus the infusion rate of 3% saline was reduced to 35 mL/h. Five hours after fluid therapy, the serum sodium concentration is 117 mmol/L. The patient is fully alert and oriented. The new goal of treatment is to slowly increase serum sodium concentration by 8 mmol/L over the next 24 hours. The 3% hypertonic is stopped and fluid therapy with 0.9% saline began; thus, 1.32 L of 0.9% saline (154 - 117) ÷ (27 + 1) or 55 mL/h was required.

Case Study 7

A 50-kg male has SIADH due to a tumor. He appears clinically euvolemic. The serum sodium is in steady state and 127 mmol/L, and K^+ is 4.0 mmol/L. There are no symptoms attributable to hyponatremia. Patient is clinically euvolemic and consuming a usual diet.

How much water restriction would correct the hyponatremia?

   A. 2200 mL
   B. 1900 mL
   C. 1600 mL
   D. 1300 mL

The correct answer is B
Comment: Hypotonic hyponatremia in this euvolemic patient is due to water retention in the presence of normal sodium stores due to SIADH. Physiologically, in patients with SIADH, the $TBNa^+$ is normal, but the TBW is increased proportionately to the fall in plasma sodium (PNa^+) concentration, due to overproduction of ADH. The treatment plan is to remove excess water. Because $TBNa^+$ is the product of TBW and PNa^+ concentration, the excess water gain in SIADH patients can be estimated using the following equation[1-3]:

$TBNa^+$ at health = $TBNa^+$ in SIADH or (50 kg × 0.6) × 135 mmol/L = (TBW × 127mmol/L) or patient's TBW = [30 L] × 135mmol/L ÷ 127 mEq/L or 31.9 L. Patient's estimated water retention is 1.9 L (31.9 − 30).

This patient is alert and asymptomatic. The treatment plan includes water restriction and/or the intravenous administration of furosemide along with isotonic saline. Close monitoring of patient's urine output, weight, and serum sodium concentration is required.

Case Study 8

A 14-year-old female is brought to the hospital because of watery diarrhea for the past 3 days. Past medical history is significant for essential hypertension. She has been on a low-sodium diet and hydrochlorothiazide daily for the control of hypertension.

On examination she appears mildly lethargic but consolable. She weighs 45 kg, blood pressure is 96/56 mmHg, and the pulse is 100 beats/min. The jugular vein is flat, and skin turgor is decreased. The serum sodium concentration is 121 mmol/L, potassium 3.2 mmol/L, bicarbonate 26 mmol/L, BUN 46 mg/dL, creatinine 1.4 mg/dL, osmolality 232 mOsm/kg H_2O, and urine osmolality is 650 mOsm/kg H_2O.

What is the appropriate initial fluid for treating this patient's hyponatremia?

   A. 0.9% saline at 222 mL/h
   B. 0.45% saline at 444 mL/h
   C. 0.9% saline at 444 mL/h
   D. 0.45% saline at 222 mL/h

The correct answer is C

Comment: In this patient, hypotonic hyponatremia is due to sodium and water losses caused by thiazide diuretic, low-salt diet, and new onset of diarrhea. The sodium loss is greater than the water loss and that is why the patient has hyponatremia. The goal of treatment is to restore the extracellular volume depletion. Hydrochlorothiazide and water are withheld, and infusion of a 0.9% saline containing 30 mmol of KCl/L is initiated.

The effect of 1 L of 0.9% saline on serum sodium change can be estimated using the following formula[1,2]:

$$Na^+ \text{ change} = [\text{infusate } (Na^+ \text{ mmol/L} + K^+ \text{ mmol/L})] - (\text{serum } Na^+ \text{ mmol/L})$$
$$\div \text{TBW liters} + 1$$

According to formula, the infusion of 1 L of 0.9% saline containing 30 mEq KCl will increase the serum Na^+ concentration by 6.57 mmol/L [154 + 30] − [121] ÷ [27 + 1] = 2.25. The initial treatment goal is to raise the serum sodium concentration by 2.0 mmol/L over the next 2 hours. Therefore, 888 mL 0.9% saline (2 ÷ 2.25) or 444 mL/h is required. Isotonic saline is effective in correcting hyponatremia caused by volume depletion because elimination of a volume stimulus for vasopressin secretion results in a water diuresis, thus helping improving hyponatremia.

Two hours later, the blood pressure is 128/72 mmHg, the serum sodium is 123 mmol/L, and potassium is 3.9 mmol/L. Patient's mental status is substantially improved. At this point the goal of treatment is to raise serum sodium slowly by 5 mmol/L over the next 12 hours; thus 2.17 L 0.9% saline or 230 mL/h will promote the correction of hyponatremia.

Frequent monitoring of the serum sodium concentration, every 6 to 8 hours, is necessary in order to make further adjustments in the amount of fluid administered.

Case Study 9

A 7-year-old boy with chronic obstructive lung disease due to cystic fibrosis is admitted to the hospital with a 2-week history of progressive lethargy. The physical examination is within normal limits except for the lethargy. The following laboratory studies are obtained: plasma sodium 111 mmol/L, potassium 4 mEq/L, chloride 72 mEq/L, bicarbonate 21 mEq/L, urate 2.9 mg/dL, plasma osmolality 222 mOsm/L, urine Na^+ 78 mEq/L, and urine osmolality 604 mOsm/L.

What solution should be used and at what approximate hourly rate to get the patient out of danger?

    A. 0.3% saline at 70 mL/h
    B. 0.9% saline at 140 mL/h
    C. 0.45% saline at 280 mL/h
    D. 0.2% saline at 35 mL/h

The correct answer is D

Comment: In this patient, hypotonic hyponatremia is a result of water retention in the presence of normal Na^+ stores due to impaired water excretion that is associated with the syndrome inappropriate antidiuretic (SIADH). The aim of treatment should be to raise the serum sodium concentration to about 120 mmol/L in the first 12 hours.

The effect of 1 L of 3% hypertonic saline on serum Na^+ change can be estimated using the following formula[1,2]:

$$Na^+ \text{ change} = (\text{infusate } Na^+ \text{ mmol / L}) - [\text{serum } Na^+ \text{ mmol / L}] \div (\text{TBW liters} + 1)$$

According to this formula, the infusion of 1 L of 3% saline will increase the serum sodium concentration by 28.7 mEq/L (513 − 105) ÷ (13.2 + 1) = 28.7 mmol/L.

Given the seriousness of the patient's symptoms the initial goal is to raise the serum sodium concentration by 4 mEq/L over the next 2 hours; thus 70 mL of 3% hypertonic saline (2 ÷ 28.7), or 35 mL/h, is required.[3] Furosemide will enhance this effect by making the urine relatively iso-osmotic to plasma, thereby reducing free water generation by the kidney. Frequent monitoring of the serum sodium concentration, initially every 2 to 3 hours, is necessary in order to make further adjustments in the amount of fluid administered. After patient's mental status is improved and/or serum sodium concentration increased to120 mmol/L, the goal of treatment is to raise serum sodium slowly by 5 mEq/L over the next 12 hours; thus 2.39 L 0.9% saline [154 − 120] ÷ [13.2 + 1] or 199 mL/h will promote the correction of hyponatremia. Furosemide will enhance this effect by making the urine relatively hypotonic to plasma, thereby reducing free water generation by the kidney.

Case Study 10

A previously healthy 19-year-old woman was admitted to a university teaching hospital for kidney transplant donation. Past medical history was unremarkable. The physical examination was normal. Her blood pressure was 120/76 mmHg, weight 58 kg, and the preoperative tests for renal function, urinalysis, and chest radiograph were normal. The patient's intraoperative course was uneventful. The estimated blood loss during the 2-hour surgery was 150 mL. Immediately after the surgery, she complained of pain and severe nausea. She was treated with intravenous morphine for pain and Phenergan for nausea. She received a total of 5.8 L of 0.2% saline in 5% dextrose in water during the first day of surgery. On postoperative day 2, she was noted to be confused and combative and had a brief apnea spell. Her serum sodium was 114 mmol/L. The patient was transferred to the pediatric intensive care unit. Physical examination revealed blood pressure of 142/87 mmHg, heart rate 60 beats/min, nuchal rigidity, unisocoria but no other focal neurologic findings. Two hours later, serum electrolytes (mmol/L) were sodium 110, potassium 3.8, chloride 84, bicarbonate 25, blood urea nitrogen (BUN) 2.9, glucose 5.1 mmol/L, creatinine 0.5 mg/dL, uric acid 5.1 mg/dL, serum osmolality 250 mmol/kg, and urine osmolality 625 mmol/kg. Arterial blood gas analysis showed pH 7.34, PO_2 7.58 mmHg, and PCO_2 6.3 mmHg. Hemoglobin was 8.2 g/dL. The radiograph of chest showed evidence of pulmonary edema. The pulmonary wedge pressure was 8 mmHg. A computed tomography (CT) scan of the brain was ordered. En route to the CT the patient had a seizure and respiratory arrest. She was resuscitated and her pupils were dilated. Six hours later, the urine output increased to 300 mL/h, urine osmolality fell to 60 mmol/L; serum sodium rose to 162 mmol/L and she developed central diabetes insipidus. She died 12 hours later, and the autopsy showed massive cerebral edema, uncal herniation, intact basilar artery, and patent pulmonary arteries.

Why did this patient develop pulmonary edema and hypoxia?

    A. Congestive heart failure
    B. Adrenal insufficiency
    C. Hyponatremic encephalopathy
    D. Reset hyponatremia
    E. Cerebral salt-wasting syndrome

The correct answer is C
Comment: The lethal combination of being in surgery (excess vasopressin release) and use of hypotonic solution postoperatively resulted in severe hyponatremia, cerebral edema, and neurogenic pulmonary edema. Pulmonary edema may be the first manifestation of hyponatremic encephalopathy.[1–5]

Case Study 11

A 10-month-old White male was admitted to the hospital for the repair of cleft lip. His weight was 7.5 kg, temperature 37°C, pulse 140 beats/min, and respiratory rate 45 breaths/min. Physical examination was otherwise unremarkable. Laboratory data on admission included a hematocrit of 0.41%, serum sodium 121 mmol/L, potassium 4.2 mmol/L, chloride 91 mmol/L, bicarbonate 24 mmol/L, glucose 98 mg/dL, BUN 18 mg/dL, and creatinine 0.8 mg/dL. Urinalysis revealed the following: pH 5.5, specific gravity 1.019, trace protein and no cells. Urinary sodium, chloride, and potassium were 43, 34, and 18 mmol/L, respectively. Liver function studies were normal. Serum cortisol, thyroxin, and aldosterone levels were also normal. Hyponatremia was unresponsive to high sodium intake (10 mmol/kg/24 h) or administration of fludrocortisone orally at 0.05 mg/day. Serum electrolyte values (mmol/L), while receiving salt supplements and fludrocortisones, were as follows: sodium 127, potassium 4.3, chloride 98, and bicarbonate 25. Urine sodium concentrations ranged between 128 and 178 mmol/L. Urine osmolality was 689 mOsm/kg during the initial presentation and fell to an average of 56 mmol/kg after the ECF volume contraction was corrected. Computed tomography (CT) and nuclear magnetic resonance (MRI) of the brain showed no abnormality in the hypothalamic area.

What is the most likely cause for this patient's hyponatremia?

    A. Reset osmostat
    B. Syndrome inappropriate ADH secretion (SIADH)
    C. Hypoaldosteronism
    D. Primary polydipsia
    E. Hypothyroidism

The correct answer is A
Comment: In a patient with normovolemic hyponatremia, the diagnosis of reset osmostat should be considered after exclusion of the diagnosis of SIADH and other endocrine disorders.[1-5] In this type of hyponatremia, renal diluting capacity is normal, but the normal regulation of serum tonicity takes place at a lower serum osmolality threshold. The diagnosis of reset osmostat can be confirmed by challenging these patients with a water load and measuring the ability to maximally dilute the urine osmolality.[1,2] The mechanism responsible for resetting of the osmostat is not understood. Differentiation between the patients with hyponatremia resulting from reset osmostat and those with alterations in total body sodium and water content is important, because management differs according to diagnosis. The hyponatremia in patients with reset osmostat is asymptomatic and requires no specific therapy.

Case Study 12

An 18-year-old man developed polyuria following resection of recurrent craniopharyngioma. His brain tumor was first detected when he was 10 years old. Surgical resection at that time was followed by the development of panhypopituitarism and diabetes insipidus requiring chronic hormonal replacement therapy. At 18 years of age, a recurrent tumor growth led to another surgical resection 6 days ago. Five days after the surgery, he developed polyuria followed by headache and increasing lethargy and experienced a generalized tonic-clonic seizure. His medications included Synthroid (levothyroxine sodium), Carafate, hydrocortisone, and desmopressin acetate. Examination revealed an obese, adolescent male who was found to have tachycardia (pulse 102 beats/min), ECF volume depletion, and hypotension (blood pressure 94/56 mmHg). His chest was clear, and the cardiac exam was normal. He appeared to have adequate peripheral perfusion. Urinalysis showed specific gravity 1.012, pH 6, negative dipstick, and unremarkable microscopy.

Serum electrolytes (mmol/L) were sodium 123, potassium 3.4, chloride 92, and bicarbonate 25. Serum glucose was 92 mg/dL, BUN 16 mg/dL, creatinine 0.7 mg/dL, uric acid 6.1 mg/dL, and osmolality 259 mOsm/kg. Urine sodium was 224 mmol/L, potassium 22 mmol/L, chloride 261 mmol/L, creatinine 1200 mg/L, and osmolality 509 mOsm/kg. Fractional sodium excretion was 2.5%. His urine output over the last 3 days averaged 290 mL/h, exceeding his fluid intake.

Which ONE of the following is the MOST likely cause of hyponatremia in this patient?

    A. Syndrome inappropriate antidiuretic hormone (SIADH)
    B. Diabetes insipidus
    C. Hypoaldosteronism
    D. Cerebral salt-wasting syndrome
    E. Interstitial nephritis

The correct answer is D
Comment: This patient abruptly developed polyuria, hypovolemia, and symptomatic hyponatremia 5 days after intracranial surgery. Examining the urine osmolality can narrow the differential diagnosis of his polyuria. Urine osmolality less than 100 mmol/kg indicates deficiency or resistance to vasopressin, while hyperosmolar urine indicates a solute diuresis.[1-3] This patient's urine osmolality exceeded 500 mmol/L, demonstrating that desmopressin was effective enough to produce a high rate of free water absorption (high urine flow rate on postoperative days) that undoubtedly contributed to his hyponatremia. Diabetes insipidus does not appear to be a major factor in this patient's decompensations. This case may be also due to desalination hyponatremia related to ECF overexpansion with normal saline in the setting of ADH action (high urine osmolality, Na⁺, and K⁺) or SIADH. The etiology of solute diuresis can be determined by measuring urine electrolyte concentrations. The sum of this patient's urine sodium and chloride levels approximated his urine osmolality. Therefore, he was experiencing a saline diuresis that, in the presence of hypovolemia and hyponatremia, reflected inappropriate renal salt wasting. The development of excessive natriuresis and hyponatremia shortly following brain surgery is consistent with the syndrome of cerebral salt wasting. This disorder can be differentiated from the syndrome of inappropriate ADH secretion by the presence of markedly negative water and sodium balance, higher rates of urine flow and sodium excretion, as well as a normal serum uric acid level. Treatment consists of vigorous saline replacement and, possibly, pharmacologic doses of mineralocorticoids.

Case Study 13

A 5-week-old male was admitted to the hospital because of diarrhea and dehydration. His mother was a 22-year-old female who had an uncomplicated pregnancy and delivery. His birth weight was 2.4 kg. He was discharged from the premature nursery at 2 weeks of age. When seen in the emergency room, he was severely dehydrated and tremulous. His weight was 2.1 kg, temperature 27°C, pulse 140 beats/min, and respiratory rate 45 breaths/min. Physical examination was otherwise unremarkable. Laboratory data on admission included: a hematocrit of 50%, blood urea nitrogen (BUN) 28 mg/dL, creatinine 1.7 mg/dL, Na⁺ 121 mmol/L, K⁺ 3.8 mmol/L, Cl⁻ 98 mmol/L, and bicarbonate 14 mmol/L. Urinalysis revealed the following: pH 5.5, specific gravity 1.019, trace protein, and no cells. Urinary electrolytes (mmol/L) were Na⁺ 8, Cl⁻ 43, and K⁺ 11. Serum glucose concentration was 88 mg/dL, calcium 9.2 mg/dL, and phosphorus 5.1 mg/dL. Liver function studies, including serum glutamic oxaloacetic transaminase (29 IU/mL), serum glutamic pyruvic transaminase (13 kU/mL), alkaline phosphatase (197 IU/mL), and bilirubin (0.4 mg/dL) were normal. Serum cortisol (7.3 µg/dL), thyroxine (9.1 µg/dL), and aldosterone (71 pg/mL) levels were also normal.

What is the MOST likely cause of this patient's hyponatremia and how would you treat this patient?

    A. Syndrome inappropriate secretion of antidiuretic hormone (SIADH)

    B. Adrenal insufficiency

    C. Reset hyponatremia

    D. Bartter syndrome

The correct answer is C

Comment: In a patient with euvolemic hyponatremia, the diagnosis of reset osmostat should be considered after exclusion of the diagnosis of SIADH and other endocrine disorders.[1-3] The diagnosis of SIADH is excluded by the production of maximally dilute urine with volume repletion. The hyponatremia in patients with reset osmostat is asymptomatic and requires no specific therapy.[1-3]

Case Study 14

A 19-year-old adolescent male developed polyuria following resection of craniopharyngioma. Two days after the surgery, he developed hyponatremia followed by headache and increasing lethargy and experienced a generalized tonic–colonic seizure. On examination his weight was 83 kg, pulse 102 beats/min, blood pressure 108/67 mmHg. Chest was clear, and the cardiac exam was normal. The daily urine output ranged between 4.6 and 6.9 L. Urinalysis showed specific gravity 1.012, pH 6, negative dipstick, and unremarkable microscopy. Serum electrolytes (mmol/L) were sodium 123, potassium 3.4, chloride 92, bicarbonate 25, glucose 89 mg/dL, BUN 16 mg/dL, creatinine 0.9 mg/dL, uric acid 2.2 mg/dL, and osmolality 254 mOsm/kg. Urine sodium was 265 mmol/L, potassium 22 mmol/L, chloride 231 mmol/L, osmolality 509 mOsm/kg, and fractional urate excretion (FEurate) was 21%. The FEurate remained unchanged after the correction of hyponatremia.

What is the MOST likely cause of this patient's hyponatremia?

    A. Cerebral salt wasting

    B. Reset osmostat

    C. Syndrome inappropriate ADH secretion (SIADH)

    D. Adrenal insufficiency

The correct answer is A

Comment: This patient abruptly developed polyuria, hypovolemia, and symptomatic hyponatremia shortly after intracranial surgery. The sudden increase in urine output along with the increased loss of sodium and chloride that was not matched by infusion of isotonic saline induced hypovolemia that could not be assessable by usual clinical criteria. The etiology of solute diuresis can be determined by measuring urine electrolyte concentrations. The sum of this patient's urine sodium and chloride levels closely approximated his urine osmolality. Therefore, he was experiencing a saline diuresis that, in the presence of hypovolemia and hyponatremia, reflected inappropriate cerebral-renal salt wasting (C/RSW).[1] The development of excessive natriuretic and hyponatremia shortly following brain surgery is consistent with the syndrome of C/RSW.[1] This disorder can be differentiated from SIADH by the presence of markedly negative sodium balance, higher rates of urine flow, and sodium excretion.[2-4] FEurate is also elevated in patients with C/RSW (> 10%) and remains persistently elevated even after correction of hyponatremia. Treatment consists of vigorous saline replacement.

Case Study 15

A 7-month-old female infant of Armenian origin presented with difficult feeding, vomiting, and inadequate weight gain starting from the first month of life. She was born at 38 weeks of gestation with a weight of 3.3 kg. She was fed breast milk and formula. Vomiting started at 2 months of age; she refused breast milk at 5 months. At 7 months of age, she was hospitalized because of a urinary tract infection, with mild hyponatremia (129 mmol/L) and hyperkalemia (5.7 mmol/L). Her family history was unremarkable except that her father had familial Mediterranean fever (FMF) and her mother had Hashimoto thyroiditis. On examination, she appeared mildly dehydrated. The body temperature was 36.0°C, the pulse 120 beats/min, the blood pressure 95/50 mmHg (on the left lower leg), and the respiratory rate 24 breaths/min. Her body weight was 4.7 kg (−4.05 SD), and height was 61 cm (−2.64 SD). Apart from a sacral dimple, the physical examination was normal.

Laboratory workup yielded the following: leukocyte count 14.700/mm^3 with 24.9% polymorphonuclear leukocytes, hemoglobin 10.6 g/dL, platelet count 513 × 10^3/mL, blood urea nitrogen 6 mg/dL, serum creatinine 0.25 mg/dL, albumin 4.9 g/dL, sodium 129 mmol/L, potassium 5.1 mmol/L, blood gas analysis, and other biochemical findings were normal. Plasma renin, aldosterone, and cortisol levels were normal. Urinalysis revealed a pH of 6, specific gravity of 1.012, with no leucocytes or erythrocytes, but with an elevated urine sodium level (70 mmol/L). Plasma steroid profile and levels of 17-OH progesterone and cortisol were within the normal range (0.075 and 45.1 ng/mL, respectively), with an increased serum corticosterone level (20.1 ng/mL, N 0.8 to 15 ng/mL) and decreased serum aldosterone level (0.035 ng/mL, normal range: 0.044 to 0.74 ng/mL) by liquid chromatography mass spectrometry (LC-MS). Abdominal ultrasonography showed normal findings. Esophagogastroduodenoscopy was also normal, as were the biopsy results. Her urine output was 2.3 to 3.8 mL/kg/h.

Due to persistent vomiting, she received ranitidine and sodium alginate for the treatment of possible gastroesophageal reflux disease. Metabolic screening tests including lactate and pyruvate levels, and tandem mass spectroscopy were normal. Her weight gain was 1 kg over a month. Despite salt supplementation, mild hyponatremia (129 to 132 mmol/L) and hyperkalemia (5.6 to 6.6 mmol/L) persisted.

What is the MOST likely diagnosis?

A. Bartter syndrome
B. Primary aldosteronism
C. Aldosterone synthase deficiency (ASD)
D. Congenital adrenal hyperplasia

The correct answer is C
Comment: Our patient presented with severe salt wasting with signs and symptoms of dehydration, difficult feeding, and failure to thrive in early infancy. Clinical presentation along with a typical biochemical profile including hyponatremia, hyperkalemia, normal cortisol, and sex steroids and inappropriately normal aldosterone levels suggested aldosterone synthase deficiency (ASD), subsequently confirmed by the molecular analysis of the *CYP11B2* gene.[1–4] The normal blood pressure and normal plasma renin activity of our patient may possibly be related to the presence of partial aldosterone synthase activity.

Gastrointestinal causes including gastrointestinal reflux disease, milk protein intolerance, and cystic fibrosis were ruled out based on the normal findings on esophagogastroduodenoscopy and anti-reflux medications did not improve vomiting. The result of the sweat test was also unremarkable.

The ongoing hyponatremia and mild hyperkalemia led us to consider endocrinologic problems, particularly adrenal insufficiency.[1,2] Adrenal insufficiency may be primary or secondary. Destruction or dysfunction of the adrenal cortex is the cause of primary adrenal insufficiency, while secondary adrenal insufficiency is associated with pituitary or hypothalamic diseases due to adrenocorticotropic hormone (ACTH) or corticotropin-releasing hormone (CRH) deficiencies, respectively. The presence of hyperkalemia in the present case suggested mineralocorticoid deficiency, which is characteristic of primary rather than secondary adrenal insufficiency.[1] The most common cause of primary adrenal insufficiency in childhood is congenital adrenal hyperplasia due to 21-α hydroxylase deficiency.[2] Ambiguous genitalia manifest as an important finding of 21-α hydroxylase deficiency in 46, XX infants. Hyperpigmentation is a common manifestation in primary adrenal insufficiency due to high levels of serum ACTH and melanocyte-stimulating hormone (MSH). Neither ambiguous genitalia nor hyperpigmentation existed in our case. Other endocrinologic causes of hyponatremia and hyperkalemia include isolated aldosterone deficiency, due to aldosterone synthase deficiency (ASD) and pseudo-hypoaldosteronism, which results from the inability of aldosterone to exert its effect on its target tissues.[4] Aldosterone synthase deficiency is extremely rare. It is associated with mutations in the *CYP11B2* gene.[3] Cortisol deficiency and ambiguous genitalia are not present in these cases.

As our patient was a female infant with unremarkable external genitalia, the diagnosis of congenital adrenal hyperplasia (CAH) due to 21-α hydroxylase deficiency was clinically ruled out. However, the assessment of the pituitary-adrenal axis by measurement of serum cortisol and ACTH levels was required to rule out other causes of primary adrenal insufficiency, such as rare causes of impaired adrenal steroid genesis, adrenal hypoplasia, and genetic or acquired etiologies of adrenal destruction. The diagnosis of primary adrenal insufficiency could be ruled out on the basis of normal serum cortisol and ACTH levels. Inappropriately normal serum level of aldosterone in the face of a low serum sodium level suggested a defect in aldosterone synthesis. Isolated aldosterone deficiency in the absence of impaired cortisol biosynthesis is associated with aldosterone synthase (CYP11B2) deficiency, which is an autosomal recessive disorder characterized by severe salt loss in early infancy. Failure to thrive and inadequate weight gain are the most important manifestations. The diagnosis of ASD can be established by measuring the appropriate mineralocorticoid precursors and mineralocorticoids, such as 11-deoxycorticosterone (DOC), corticosterone, 18-hydroxycorticosterone, and 18-hydroxy-DOC and aldosterone levels in plasma.

Plasma steroid showed normal levels of 17-OH progesterone and cortisol (0.075 and 45.1 ng/mL, respectively), thus ruling out cortisol deficiency, 21-α hydroxylase deficiency, and CAH. She finally received a diagnosis of ASD based on elevated serum corticosterone (20.1 ng/mL) and low serum aldosterone (0.035 ng/mL) levels.

The diagnosis of ASD was further confirmed by genetic testing, which revealed two pathogenic variations, c.763G > T (p. Glu255Ter) and c.554C > T (Thr185Ile), in the *CYP11B2 gene*. The segregation analysis of the parents confirmed the variations were in *trans* position. Thus, the diagnosis of aldosterone synthase type-2 deficiency was confirmed by the molecular analysis of the *CYP11B2* gene.

Typically, patients with ASD respond well to fludrocortisone therapy and may also benefit from salt supplementation, particularly in the neonatal period.[4,5] Although there are sporadic reports of pediatric cases in which fludrocortisone was no longer needed, there is no definite recommendation about when treatment can be terminated. In our case, an extensively hydrolyzed formula was administered through a feeding tube starting with 80 kcal/kg to be gradually increased daily. Despite salt supplementation, mild hyponatremia (129 to 132 mmol/L) and hyperkalemia (5.6 to 6.6 mmol/L) persisted. Once the diagnosis of ASD was made, fludrocortisone treatment was started at a dose of 0.1 mg/day. One month after the initiation of fludrocortisone treatment, salt supplementation was discontinued when serum sodium and potassium levels became normal. At follow-up visit at 1 year of age, her weight was 8.3 kg

(10th percentile) and height was 71 cm (17th percentile), which were ascertaining a catch-up growth with a favorable clinical response under mineralocorticoid therapy with fludrocortisone at a stable dose of 0.1 mg.

Case Study 16

A previously healthy 15-year-old girl was referred to our clinic by a local hospital because of persistent unconsciousness following a generalized tonic-clonic seizure. Physical examination revealed an unconscious, well-developed adolescent with normal axillary temperature, pulse rate, and blood pressure. She was neither edematous nor dehydrated. There was no cranial nerve deficit, focal neurologic sign, papilledema, or neck stiffness. The only pathologic finding was the presence of a few dental caries. Cranial computed tomography was normal.

Laboratory investigations revealed serum sodium of 118 mmol/L, potassium 3.73 mmol/L, chloride 89 mmol/L, bicarbonate 22 mmol/L, blood urea nitrogen 4.3 mg/dL, creatinine 0.36 mg/dL, glucose 98 mg/dL, calcium 9.01 mg/dL, creatinine kinase 376 U/L, C-reactive protein (CRP) 0.5 mg/L, and serum osmolality 240 mOsm/kg. Urine osmolality was 325 mOsm/kg, sodium 35 mmol/L, and creatinine 7.01 mg/dL, giving a fractional excretion of sodium (FENa$^+$) of 1.5%. Toxicological analysis of urine was negative. Evaluation of cerebrospinal fluid was normal.

Hypertonic saline infusion (6 mL/kg 3% NaCl) was started to correct hyponatremia. In addition, parenteral ceftriaxone and acyclovir treatment were initiated. Her consciousness improved rapidly along with serum sodium level, which was 129 mmol/L after 3 hours. Thereafter, hypertonic saline infusion was stopped and isotonic saline at a dose of maintenance fluid requirement was given. During follow-up, the patient was noted to be polyuric and serum sodium normalized within this period (134 mmol/L after 10 hours and 139 mmol/L after 14 hours). Along with improved serum sodium, her clinical condition also improved. Antimicrobial treatment was stopped when the culture results were reported to be sterile.

The parents stated that the patient had a toothache due to abscess formation for the last 3 days and used amoxicillin-clavulanic acid plus etodolac during this period. When the patient regained consciousness, detailed questioning revealed the cause of hyponatremia.

What is the cause of hyponatremia in this patient?

    A. Syndrome inappropriate antidiuretic hormone (SIADH)
    B. Cerebral salt wasting
    C. Reset osmostat
    D. Adrenal insufficiency

The correct answer is A
Comment: The patient reported that during the 24 hours preceding the seizure she consumed approximately 3 L of cold water and plenty of ice cubes for dental pain relief. Thus, the cause of hyponatremia was considered to be dilutional due to high water intake and also possibly due to inappropriate secretion of antidiuretic hormone (ADH), caused by persistent tooth pain in the present case.[1,2] In addition, etodolac (a non-steroidal anti-inflammatory drug [NSAID]) used for pain relief by the patient might have contributed to hyponatremia by decreasing free water excretion. NSAIDs block the synthesis of prostaglandins, which inhibit the activity of ADH on collecting ducts.[2,3]

Hypotonic hyponatremia can occur with hypovolemia, hypervolemia, or normovolemia:

    1. Hypovolemic hyponatremia is mostly due to extra renal losses like gastroenteritis. Patients have clinical symptoms of dehydration with low FENa$^+$ to conserve sodium. On the other hand, renal salt-wasting states like diuretic use, mineralocorticoid deficiency, or salt-wasting tubulopathies may cause hypovolemic hyponatremia with increased FENa$^+$.

2. Hypervolemic hyponatremia may be seen in patients with nephrotic syndrome, cirrhosis, and heart failure. These disorders are associated with low intravascular volume leading to increased ADH-related water retention, causing hyponatremia with low (< 0.5%) FENa$^+$. Hypervolemic hyponatremia and increased FENa$^+$ (> 0.5%) may develop in patients with acute or chronic kidney disease with tubular dysfunction.

3. Euvolemic (dilutional) hyponatremia is characteristic of the syndrome of inappropriate ADH secretion (SIADH). In this syndrome, abnormally increased ADH secretion causes volume expansion leading to subsequent natriuria. Higher FENa$^+$ (> 0.5%) is characteristic of SIADH. Euvolemic hyponatremia may also develop if water intake exceeds urine production leading to water intoxication.

Dilutional hyponatremia may develop iatrogenically when hypotonic intravenous fluids are used postoperatively or after trauma, both of which are associated with high circulating ADH levels. Oral fluid intake may also be associated with hyponatremia as seen in children with gastroenteritis who drink excess replacement water. Basically, any situation associated with higher water intake than the requirement determined by thirst mechanism can cause dilutional hyponatremia. Early diagnosis and treatment of dilutional hyponatremia are problematic as the symptoms of acute hyponatremia are non-specific.

This case is interesting because of the intentional consumption of a high volume of water leading to dilutional hyponatremia and acute water intoxication. Acute pulpitis is an intensely painful condition requiring prompt intervention by dental professionals for appropriate treatment. The patient utilized the analgesic effect of cold water for pain relief. However, excessive ingestion of cold water for pain control led to hyponatremic encephalopathy and seizure. On the other hand, urine osmolality was higher than plasma osmolality despite hypotonicity. Furthermore, urine sodium was increased (> 20 mmol/L) in the presence of severe hyponatremia. These findings indicate that there were also non-osmotic stimuli for ADH secretion in our patient, which include general anesthesia, stress, pain, pulmonary diseases, neurological diseases, medications including NSAIDs, and some malignant diseases. In the present case, the cause of SIADH is intense pain due to dental infection. Dental pain-related inappropriate release of ADH and ingestion of cold water to relieve pain are a well-recognized cause of hyponatremia and is thus termed dental hyponatremia.

Intrarenal prostaglandins inhibit ADH-activated adenylcyclase activity in collecting duct cells leading to attenuation of ADH-dependent transtubular water movement, and removal of the inhibitory effect of prostaglandins on ADH activity by NSAIDs can diminish free water excretion. In conditions associated with high and relatively non-suppressible levels of ADH, such as SIADH or effective volume depletion, as in patients with severe heart failure, NSAID-induced water retention can induce or worsen hyponatremia.[2] Thus, use of the NSAID might have contributed to the development of hyponatremia and associated clinical findings in our patient.

Hypertonic saline infusion was used for initial treatment since the patient had a seizure and her serum sodium was less than 125 mmol/L. Her consciousness level improved rapidly without any complication along with normalized serum sodium level. Later, physiologic saline infusion was started. The rate of correction was considerably greater than the optimal rate of recovery defined for hyponatremia (10 to 12 mmol/24 h). However, as her clinical condition was improving, we did not interrupt physiologic saline infusion until her serum sodium reached normal levels.

Case Study 17

A 12-year-old boy was referred to us with a 3-year history of recurrent fever and joint pains. Four months previously, the child had been admitted for generalized tonic–clonic convulsions, for which a computed tomography (CT) scan of the brain had been performed and reported to be normal. There was no recurrence of seizures, but the parents noticed that the child was losing weight, was very thirsty, and was passing large volumes of urine. Complaints of headache and diplopia during the preceding 10 days led to re-admission to hospital. However, the child developed progressive breathlessness and was therefore referred to us for further management.

On examination, the child was conscious, irritable, and very thirsty. The respiratory rate was 70 breaths/min, pulse was 184 beats/min, and blood pressure was 160/130 mmHg in the left upper limb, 154/130 mmHg in the right upper limb, 146/126 mmHg in the right lower limb, and 148/128 in the left lower limb. All peripheral pulses were palpable. His weight and height were 28 kg and 126 cm, respectively, both below the 5th percentile for age and sex. The skin showed no café-au-lait spots. There was no significant lymphadenopathy. On examination of the cardiovascular system, the jugular venous pressure was 7 cm above the sternal angle. The apical impulse was in the sixth left intercostal space lateral to the mid-clavicular line, and there was a gallop rhythm. Respiratory system examination revealed bilateral basal crepitations. The liver was tender and palpable 5 cm below the right costal margin. There was no abdominal bruit. The fundus showed disc edema, cotton wool exudates, focal hemorrhages, and arterio-venous nicking. Other organ systems were essentially normal.

Further tests revealed a hemoglobin of 9.8 g/dL, total white blood cell count of 11,000/mm^3 with a differential count of polymorphs of 68%, lymphocytes of 30%, and monocytes of 2%, and platelet count of 186,000/mm^3. The erythrocyte sedimentation rate was 75 mm at the end of 1 hour. Urinalysis showed microscopic hematuria and 3 + proteinuria. Serum sodium was 118 mmol/L, potassium 2.5 mmol/L. Spot urine sodium was 110 mmol/L, potassium 15 mmol/L, urinary calcium/creatinine ratio was 1.9, and urinary protein/creatinine ratio was 2.4.

Serum creatinine was 0.7 mg/dL. The Mantoux test showed no induration at 48 hours. Chest X-ray showed cardiomegaly with a cardiothoracic ratio of 0.7 and features suggestive of pulmonary edema. Abdominal ultrasonography revealed a small atrophic right kidney (6.2 × 2.3 cm) with decreased vascularity within and compensatory hypertrophy of the left kidney (11.1 × 5.2 cm). Renal Doppler showed a poor flow in the right intra-renal arteries with poor visualization of the right renal ostium. The left kidney showed hypertrophy, and the entire left renal artery was prominent with increased flow within. Two-dimensional echocardiography showed concentric hypertrophy of the left ventricle, global hypokinesia, mild aortic regurgitation, and an ejection fraction of 20%.

Plasma renin activity was 29.8 ng/mL/h (normal 0.3 to 2.9 ng/mL/h) and the serum aldosterone level was 361 pg/mL (normal 29.9 to 159 pg/mL).

On admission to the pediatric intensive care unit, the patient was started on oxygen and oral nifedipine. His blood pressure dropped to 140/110 mmHg, after which oral hydralazine was added to the treatment regimen. Intravenous fluids (normal saline) and intravenous potassium supplements were also started, but only after enalapril therapy had been initiated on treatment day 4 did the systolic blood pressure stabilize to between 130 and 120 mmHg and serum sodium and potassium levels return to normal.

A computed tomography (CT) aortogram of the thoracic and abdominal aorta revealed 50% to 60% stenosis of the proximal right subclavian artery at its origin from the brachiocephalic trunk, with post-stenotic dilatation, complete obstruction of the superior mesenteric artery at its origin and proximal part, and opacification of the distal superior mesenteric artery. The right renal artery was narrow in caliber, with faint opacification and the right kidney had decreased nephrographic density. A 99m-technicium diethylene triamine pentaacetic acid (DTPA) scan revealed poor cortical uptake and a reduced glomerular filtration rate (8.5 mL/min) in the right kidney. A right nephrectomy was done on day 27 of hospitalization. Postoperatively the blood pressure and electrolytes normalized rapidly.

A histopathological study of the nephrectomized kidney showed diffuse tubular atrophy, collapse and sclerosis of the glomeruli, and hypertensive changes in the blood vessels.

A diagnosis of Takayasu arteritis was made based on European League Against Rheumatism/ Pediatric Rheumatology European Society (EULAR/PReS) endorsed consensus criteria (angiographic abnormalities and hypertension). The child was started on immunosuppressive therapy with oral prednisolone (1 mg/kg/day) and weekly oral methotrexate (0.3 mg/kg). At discharge (15 days post-operative) the child was normotensive and off all anti-hypertensives, and serum electrolytes were normal.

What is the MOST likely cause of hypertension in this patient?

A. Hyponatremic hypertensive syndrome (HHS)
B. Pheochromocytoma
C. Renin-secreting tumor
D. Liddle syndrome

The correct diagnosis is A
Comment: Our patient had unilateral renal artery stenosis secondary to Takayasu arteritis with hyponatremia, hypokalemia, polydipsia, polyuria, weight loss, and high renin and aldosterone levels, all features compatible with a diagnosis of hyponatremic hypertensive syndrome (HHS).[1-3] Arterial hypertension, salt wasting, and hypokalemic alkalosis due to unilateral renal artery ischemia characterize this syndrome. The pathogenesis of hypertension is secondary to severe renal ischemia leading to increased secretion of renin, resulting in high circulating levels of angiotensin II (AII).[1-3] AII in turn causes arterial hypertension and induces pressure diuresis and natriuresis through the normal kidney and is responsible for polyuria and hyponatremia. AII also stimulates the secretion of aldosterone, an effect which is also aggravated by sodium depletion. Hyperaldosteronism and AII act directly on the kidney to cause renal potassium loss and hypokalemia. Hypokalemia may further stimulate renin secretion. The stimulation of thirst and release of anti-diuretic hormone (ADH) in response to the dual stimuli of AII and volume depletion would further aggravate hyponatremia. This pathophysiological mechanism presumes the presence of a normal contralateral kidney for the onset of HHS.[1-3]

The majority of patients reported with this condition have been adults, with only a few case reports of children. In most adult patients with HHS the underlying renal pathology has been atherosclerosis. In children, HHS has been described with renal ischemia due to fibromuscular dysplasia, Wilms tumor, neurofibromatosis type 1, and renal damage secondary to bladder dysfunction.

Our patient had transient hypercalciuria and nephrotic-range proteinuria, which resolved after control of blood pressure. Proteinuria has been attributed to glomerular hyperfiltration in the non-stenotic kidney due to hyperreninemia and arterial hypertension. Disorders of calcium metabolism in patients with hypertension, including a higher calcium excretion rate, have also been reported.

The correction of hyponatremic dehydration and a safe decrease of blood pressure are essential in the emergency phase of HHS. Therapy based on ACEIs and/or ARBs is the most efficient antihypertensive therapy for those with ischemic reno-parenchymal disorder. Revascularization by percutaneous transluminal angioplasty is recommended for children with renal artery stenosis and should be considered when renal function in the affected kidney can be preserved. Nephrectomy is required if an affected kidney contributes less than 10% of the global renal function, if percutaneous trans-luminal angioplasty fails, if the operative risk is too high, or in the case of extensive tumorous lesions.[1-3]

In our patient, right nephrectomy was the only option since renal function in that kidney was poor, underlying the importance of blood pressure measurements and the early detection of hypertension at any age, especially in children presenting with unexplained polyuria and polydipsia.

Case Study 18

A 15-year-old female was diagnosed with non–Hodgkin lymphoma. She was initiated on pembrolizumab therapy and achieved partial remission. Four months later, she was found to have orthostatic hypotension, with blood pressure of 90/50 mmHg sitting.

Admission laboratory findings showed serum sodium 123 mmol/L, potassium 4.2 mmol/L, chloride 110 mmol/L, bicarbonate 16 mmol/L, and serum creatinine level was 0.7 mg/dL, corresponding to estimated glomerular filtration rate greater than 60 mL/min/1.73 m². Serum osmolality was 260 mOsm/kg, and urine osmolality was 475 mOsm/kg. Urine sodium excretion was 45 mmol/L. A trial of normal saline solution led to improvement in blood pressure but did not improve hyponatremia.

Endocrine laboratory findings were corticotrophin (ACTH) 9 pg/mL, free cortisol (morning) 22 µg/dL, Prolactin 26.9 ng/mL, follicle-stimulating hormone (FSH) 3.9 IU/mL, luteinizing hormone (LH) 7.3 IU/L, thyroid-stimulating hormone (TSH) 1.38 mIU/L, free thyroxin 0.8 ng/dL, Aldosterone 4.7 ng/dL, and plasma renin direct 3.7 pg/mL.

What is the MOST likely cause of hyponatremia in this patient?

A. Gordon syndrome
B. Hyponatremia resulting from primary adrenal insufficiency
C. Pembrolizumab-induced ACTH deficiency leading to hyponatremia.
D. Hypothyroidism

The correct answer is C
Comment: The hyponatremia observed in patients with cancer usually results from nonosmotic release of vasopressin with consequent hypoosmolar hyponatremia.[1-5] Nausea, pain, and baroreceptor release of vasopressin (also known as antidiuretic hormone [ADH]) are common causes of excess ADH release, while ectopic production of ADH from tumors such as small cell lung cancer is relatively rare. Paraproteinemias, hyperlipidemia, and lipoprotein X are causes of pseudohyponatremia that are excluded here because of the documented hypoosmolality. Hypoosmolar hyponatremia may result from impaired free-water excretion associated with reduced effective arteriolar blood volume, as seen in this patient with relative hypotension. Other common causes of hyponatremia should also be considered, such as use of thiazide diuretics or other medications. A number of chemotherapeutic agents, including vincristine, vinblastine, cyclophosphamide, cisplatin, and novel targeted therapies, have been associated with enhanced ADH release, but the patient did not receive any of these agents. Finally, adrenal insufficiency consequent to adrenalitis or hypophysitis resulting from cytotoxic T lymphocyte antigen 4 (CTLA-4) and programmed cell death protein 1 (PD-1) inhibitor therapies may be observed.[6]

Case Study 19

What diagnostic tests should be performed in this patient to confirm the diagnosis? (Select all that apply)

A. Plasma renin activity
B. Serum aldosterone level
C. Free thyroxin and thyroid-stimulating hormone levels
D. Plasma adrenocorticotropic (ACTH) level

The correct answers are A, B, C, and D
Comment: An early-morning plasma cortisol test done 48 hours later in the hospital was very low, particularly in the setting of hypotension. Corticotropin (ACTH), free thyroxin, and

thyroid-stimulating hormone levels were all low, suggesting a central cause. Follicle-stimulating hormone and luteinizing hormone levels were not affected. Brain magnetic resonance imaging focused on the pituitary gland and adrenal computed tomographic scans were unremarkable. In light of these findings, the presumptive diagnosis was hyponatremia resulting from central adrenal insufficiency due to impaired ACTH synthesis.[1] The patient's hypothyroidism was thought to be at most a minor contributing factor. The patient was treated with hydrocortisone, fludrocortisone, and levothyroxine, with improvement in serum sodium concentration to 133 mmol/L over 5 days. One year later, the cancer was in remission in the context of continuing pembrolizumab treatment and the patient remained on treatment with replacement hydrocortisone and levothyroxine. The hypoosmolar hyponatremia in this patient could have been due in part to baroreceptor-mediated antidiuretic hormone (ADH) release given her hypotension, but the low aldosterone level and plasma renin activity suggest that this was not a predominant factor. Furthermore, isotonic saline solution infusion decreased the serum sodium concentration further, implying that a primary ADH effect was preventing water excretion. The prompt improvement in urinary dilution and correction of hyponatremia after hydrocortisone administration was thought to be due to its suppression of ADH release. Cortisol not only suppresses ACTH secretion but also inhibits secretion of corticotrophin-releasing hormone (CRH). CRH stimulates ADH release; thus, glucocorticoid deficiency is associated with excess CRH and ADH release, which is reversed by administration of cortisol. Cortisol deficiency may also more directly increase ADH release.

Adverse kidney effects associated with immune checkpoint inhibitors are well described, as is hyponatremia related to both PD-1 and CTLA-4 inhibitor use.[2-5] Both these agents can promote endocrine immune-related adverse events, as observed in our patient, which vary in severity and can involve damage to pituitary, adrenal, thyroid, and pancreatic beta cells. This case is unusual in that PD-1 inhibitors have not been associated with hyponatremia and less commonly induce hypophysitis than the anti–CTLA-4 class of drugs. Of the various PD-1 inhibitors, nivolumab has been most frequently reported to have endocrine adverse effects and has been linked to hypophysitis and adrenal insufficiency in 1% and 2% of patients, respectively. The potential causes of hyponatremia in patients receiving immune checkpoint inhibitors include hypovolemia, adrenal insufficiency, hypophysitis, isolated ACTH deficiency, and thyroid disorders.[2-6] The level of adrenal insufficiency can be calibrated with appropriate dosing of glucocorticoids. Because of a substantial mineralocorticoid effect, hydrocortisone may not require supplemental fludrocortisone. PD-1 inhibitors can generally be continued as part of antitumor therapy with concurrent appropriate hormone replacement, which may need to be continued even after cancer treatment has been completed. Knowledge of endocrine-related causes of hyponatremia is important for the physicians managing patients who are receiving checkpoint inhibitors.

References

Case Study 1

1. El Bitar S, Weerasinghe C, El-Charabaty E, et al. Renal tubular acidosis an adverse effect of PD-1 inhibitor immunotherapy. *Case Rep Oncol Med.* 2018. https://doi.org/10.1155/2018/8408015.
2. Herrmann SM, Alexander MP, Romero MF, et al. Renal tubular acidosis and immune checkpoint inhibitor therapy: an immune-related adverse event of PD-1 inhibitor—a report of 3 cases. *Kidney Med.* 2020;2:657–662.
3. Charmetant X, Teuma C, Lake J, et al. A new expression of immune checkpoint inhibitors' renal toxicity: when distal tubular acidosis precedes creatinine elevation. *Clin Kidney J.* 2019;13:42–45.
4. Atiq SO, Gokhale T, Atiq Z, et al. A case of pembrolizumab induced distal renal tubular acidosis. *J Onco-Nephrol.* 2021;5:23–26.
5. Barroso-Sousa R, Barry WT, Garrido-Castro AC, et al. Incidence of endocrine dysfunction following the use of different immune checkpoint inhibitor regimens: a systematic review and meta-analysis. *JAMA Oncol.* 2018;4:173–182.

6. Desikan SP, Varghese R, Kamoga R, et al. Acute hyponatremia from immune checkpoint inhibitor therapy for non-small cell lung cancer. *Postgrad Med J.* 2020;96:570–571.
7. Seethapathy H, Rusibamayila N, Chute DF, et al. Hyponatremia and other electrolyte abnormalities in patients receiving immune checkpoint inhibitors. *Nephrol Dial Transplant.* 2020. https://doi.org/10.1093/ndt/gfaa2721.

Case Study 2

1. Ellison DH, Berl T. The syndrome of inappropriate antidiuresis. *N Eng J Med.* 2007;356(20):2064–2072.
2. Hanna FW, Scanlon MF. Hyponatraemia, hypothyroidism, and role of arginine-vasopressin. *Lancet.* 1997;350(9080):755–756.
3. Skowsky WR, Kikuchi TA. The role of vasopressin in the impaired water excretion of myxedema. *Am J Med.* 1978;64(4):613–621.
4. Bartter FC, Schwartz WB. The syndrome of inappropriate secretion of antidiuretic hormone. *Am J Med.* 1967;42(5):790–806.
5. Berl T. Impact of solute intake on urine flow and water excretion. *J Am Soc Nephrol.* 2008;19(6):1076–1078.
6. Upadhyay A, Jaber BL, Madias NE. Incidence and prevalence of hyponatremia. *Am J Med.* 2006;119(7 suppl 1):S30–S35.
7. Arlt W, Allolio B. Adrenal insufficiency. *Lancet.* 2003;61(9372):1881–1893.
8. Spital A. Hyponatremia in adrenal insufficiency: review of pathogenetic mechanisms. *South Med J.* 1982;75(5):581–585.
9. DuBose Jr TD. Hyperkalemic hyperchloremic metabolic acidosis: pathophysiologic insights. *Kidney Int.* 1997;51(2):591–602.
10. Rodríguez Soriano J. Renal tubular acidosis: the clinical entity. *J Am Soc Nephrol.* 2002;13(8):2160–2170.
11. Kuwahara S, Arima H, Banno R, et al. Regulation of vasopressin gene expression by cAMP and glucocorticoids in parvocellular neurons of the paraventricular nucleus in rat hypothalamicorganotypic cultures. *J Neurosci.* 2003;23(32):10231–10237.
12. Fox B. Venous infarction of the adrenal gland. *J Pathol.* 1976;119(2):65–89.
13. Espinosa G, Cervera R, Font J, et al. Adrenal involvement in the antiphospholipid syndrome. *Lupus.* 2003;12(7):569–572.
14. Salvatori R. Adrenal insufficiency. *JAMA.* 2005;294(19):2481–2488.

Case Study 3

1. Rose BD, Post TW. *Clinical Physiology of Acid–Base and Electrolyte Disorders.* 5th ed. New York, NY: McGraw-Hill, Inc.; 2001. [chap 18, 551–571].
2. Assadi F. *Clinical Decisions in Pediatric Nephrology: A Problem-Solving Approach to Clinical Cases.* New York: Springer; 2008. [chap 2, 69–98].

Case Study 4

1. Rose BD, Post TW. *Clinical Physiology of Acid–Base and Electrolyte Disorders.* 5th ed. New York, NY: McGraw-Hill, Inc.; 2001. [chap 18, 551–571].
2. Assadi F. *Clinical Decisions in Pediatric Nephrology: A Problem-Solving Approach to Clinical Cases.* New York: Springer; 2008. [chap 2, 69–98].

Case Study 5

1. Ellison DH, Berl T. The syndrome of inappropriate antidiuresis. *N Eng J Med.* 2007;356(20):2064–2072.
2. Bartter FC, Schwartz WB. The syndrome of inappropriate secretion of antidiuretic hormone. *Am J Med.* 1967;42(5):790–806.
3. Martinez-Valles MA, Palafox-Cazarez A, Paredes-Avina JA. Severe hypokalemia, metabolic alkalosis and hypertension in a 54 year old male with ectopic ACTH syndrome: a case report. *Cases J.* 2009;2:6174.

Case Study 6

1. Adroque HJ, Madias NE. Hyponatremia. *New Engl. J Med.* 2000;342:1581–1589.
2. Adroque HJ, Madias NE. Aiding fluid prescription for the dysnatremia. *Intensive Care Med.* 2000;23:309–316.
3. Sterns RH, Nigwekar SU, Hix JK. The treatment of hyponatremia. *Semin Nephrol.* 2009;29:282–299.

Case Study 7

1. Adroque HJ, Madias NE. Hyponatremia. *New Engl. J Med.* 2000;342:1581–1589.
2. Adroque HJ, Madias NE. Aiding fluid prescription for the dysnatremia. *Intensive Care Med.* 2000;23:309–316.
3. Sterns RH, Nigwekar SU, Hix JK. The treatment of hyponatremia. *Semin Nephrol.* 2009;29:282–299.

Case Study 8

1. Adroque HJ, Madias NE. Hyponatremia. *New Engl. J Med.* 2000;342:1581–1589.
2. Adroque HJ, Madias NE. Aiding fluid prescription for the dysnatremia. *Intensive Care Med.* 2000;23:309–316.

Case Study 9

1. Adroque HJ, Madias NE. Aiding fluid prescription for the dysnatremia. *Intensive Care Med.* 2000;23:309–316.
2. Adroque HJ, Madias NE. Hyponatremia. *New Engl. J Med.* 2000;342:1581–1589.
3. Sterns RH, Nigwekar SU, Hix JK. The treatment of hyponatremia. *Semin Nephrol.* 2009;29:282–299.

Case Study 10

1. Assadi F. Hyponatremia: a problem-solving approach to clinical cases. *J Nephrol.* 2012;25(4):473–480. https://doi.org/10.5301/jn.5000060.
2. Ellison DH, Berl T. The syndrome of inappropriate antidiuresis. *N Engl J Med.* 2007;356(20). 2064–2072.8.
3. Assadi FK, John EG. Hypouricemia in neonates with syndrome of inappropriate secretion of antidiuretic hormone. *Pediatr Res.* 1985;19(5):424–427.
4. Moritz ML, Ayus JC. Hospital-acquired hyponatremia—why are hypotonic parenteral fluids still being used? *Nat Clin Pract Nephrol.* 2007;3(7). 374–382.29.
5. Palmer BF. Hyponatremia in the intensive care unit. *Semin Nephrol.* 2009;29(3):257–270.

Case Study 11

1. Assadi F, Mazaheri M. Differentiating syndrome of inappropriate ADH, reset osmostat, cerebral/renal salt wasting using fractional urate excretion. *J Pediatr Endocrinol Metab.* 2020;34(1):137–140. https://doi.org/10.1515/jpem-2020-0379.
2. Assadi FK, Agrawal R, Jocher C, et al. Hyponatremia secondary to reset osmostat. *J Pediatr.* 1986;108(2):262–264. https://doi.org/10.1016/s0022-3476(86)81000-9.
3. Assadi F. Hyponatremia: a problem-solving approach to clinical cases. *J Nephrol.* 2012;25(4):473–480. https://doi.org/10.5301/jn.5000060.
4. Moritz ML, Ayus JC. Hospital-acquired hyponatremia—why are hypotonic parenteral fluids still being used? *Nat Clin Pract Nephrol.* 2007;3(7). 374–382.29.
5. Palmer BF. Hyponatremia in the intensive care unit. *Semin Nephrol.* 2009;29(3):257–270.

Case Study 12

1. Assadi F, Mazaheri M. Differentiating syndrome of inappropriate ADH, reset osmostat, cerebral/renal salt wasting using fractional urate excretion. *J Pediatr Endocrinol Metab.* 2020;34(1):137–140. https://doi.org/10.1515/jpem-2020-0379.
2. Assadi FK, Agrawal R, Jocher C, et al. Hyponatremia secondary to reset osmostat. *J Pediatr.* 1986;108(2):262–264. https://doi.org/10.1016/s0022-3476(86)81000-9.
3. Assadi F, Mazaheri M. Differentiating syndrome of inappropriate ADH, reset osmostat, cerebral/renal salt wasting using fractional urate excretion. *J Pediatr Endocrinol Metab.* 2020;34(1):137–140. https://doi.org/10.1515/jpem-2020-0379.

Case Study 13

1. Assadi FK. Clinical quiz. *Hyponatremia Pediatr Nephrol.* 1993;7(4):503–505. https://doi.org/10.1007/BF00857585. Erratum in: *Pediatr Nephrol.* 1994;8(2):256.

2. Assadi FK, Agrawal R, Jocher C, et al. Hyponatremia secondary to reset osmostat. *J Pediatr.* 1986;108(2):262–264. https://doi.org/10.1016/s0022-3476(86)81000-9.
3. Assadi F, Mazaheri M. Differentiating syndrome of inappropriate ADH, reset osmostat, cerebral/renal salt wasting using fractional urate excretion. *J Pediatr Endocrinol Metab.* 12;34(1):137-140. https://doi.org/10.1515/jpem-2020-0379.

Case Study 14

1. Assadi FK, Agrawal R, Jocher C, et al. Hyponatremia secondary to reset osmostat. *J Pediatr.* 1986;108(2):262–264. https://doi.org/10.1016/s0022-3476(86)81000-9. Feb.
2. Assadi F, Mazaheri M. Differentiating syndrome of inappropriate ADH, reset osmostat, cerebral/renal salt wasting using fractional urate excretion. *J Pediatr Endocrinol Metab.* 12;34(1):137–140. https://doi.org/10.1515/jpem-2020-0379.
3. Assadi F, John EG. Hypouricemia in neonates with syndrome ofinappropriate secretion of antidiuretic hormone. *Pediatr Res.* 1985;19:424–427.
4. Assadi F. Hyponatremia: a problem-solving approach to clinical cases. *J Neprol.* 2012;25:473–480.

Case Study 15

1. Patti G, Guzzeti C, Di Iorgi N, et al. Central adrenal insufficiency in children and adolescents. *Best Pract Res Clin Endocrinol Metab.* 2018;32:425–444. https://doi.org/10.1016/j.beem.2018.03.012.
2. El-Maouche D, Arlt W, Merke DP. Congenital adrenal hyperplasia. *Lancet.* 2017;390:2194–2210. https://doi.org/10.1016/S0140-6736(17)31431-9.
3. Jessen CL, Christensen JH, Birkebaek NH, et al. Homozygosity for a mutation in the *CYP11B2* gene in an infant with congenital corticosterone methyl oxidase deficiency type II. *Acta Paediatr.* 2012;101:e519–e525. https://doi.org/10.1111/j.1651-2227.2012.02823.x.
4. White PC. Aldosterone synthase deficiency and related disorders. *Mol Cell Endocrinol.* 2004;217:81–87. https://doi.org/10.1016/j.mce.2003.10.013.
5. Mutlu GY, Taşdemir M, Kızılkan NU, et al. A rare cause of chronic hyponatremia in an infant: answers. *Pediatr Nephrol.* 2020;35:243–245. https://doi.org/10.1007/s00467-019-04337-0.

Case Study 16

1. Zieg J. Pathophysiology of hyponatremia in children. *Front Pediatr.* 2017;5:213.
2. Jones DP. Syndrome of inappropriate secretion of antidiuretic hormone and hyponatremia. *Pediatr Rev.* 2018;39:27–35.
3. Yildiz G, Bayram MT, Soylu A, et al. An adolescent patient presenting with hyponatremic seizure: answers. *Pediatr Nephrol.* 2019;34:1371–1372. https://doi.org/10.1007/s00467-019-04214-w.

Case Study 17

1. Ashida A, Matsumura H, Inoue N, et al. Two cases of hyponatremic-hypertensive syndrome in childhood with renovascular hypertension. *Eur J Pediatr.* 2006;165:336–339.
2. Peco-Antić A, Dimitrijević N, Jovanović O, et al. Hyponatremic hypertensive syndrome. *Pediatr Nephrol.* 2000;15:286–289.
3. Kovalski Y, Cleper R, Krause I, et al. Hyponatremic hypertensive syndrome in pediatric patients: is it really so rare? *Pediatr Nephrol.* 2012;27:1037–1040.

Case Study 18

1. Friedman TC, Yanovski JA, Nieman LK, et al. Inferior petrosal venous sampling in healthy subjects reveals a unilateral corticotrophin releasing hormone-induced arginine vasopressin release associated with ipsilateral adrenocorticotropin secretion. *Clin Invest.* 1996;97(9):2045–2050.
2. Wanchoo R, Karam S, Uppal NN, et al. Adverse renal effects of immune checkpoint inhibitors: a narrative review. *Am J Nephrol?* 2017;45(2):160–169.
3. Rahman O, El Halawani H, Fouad M. Risk of endocrine complications in cancer patients treated with immune checkpoint inhibitors: a metaanalysis. *Future Oncol.* 2016;12(3):413–425.

4. Byun DJ, Wolchok JD, Rosenberg LM, et al. Cancer immunotherapy-immune checkpoint blockade and associated endocrinopathies. *Nat Rev Endocrinol.* 2017;13(4):195–207.
5. Barroso-Sousa R, Barry WT, Garrido-Castro AC, et al. Incidence of endocrine dysfunction following the use of different immune checkpoint inhibitor regimens: a systematic review and meta-analysis. *JAMA Oncol.* 2018;4(2):173–182.
6. Caturegli P, Di Dalmazi G, Lombardi M, et al. Hypophysitis secondary to cytotoxic T-lymphocyte–associated protein 4 blockade: insights into pathogenesis from an autopsy series. *Am J Pathol.* 2016;186(12):3225–3235.

Case Study 19

1. Friedman TC, Yanovski JA, Nieman LK, et al. Inferior petrosal venous sampling in healthy subjects reveals a unilateral corticotrophin releasing hormone-induced arginine vasopressin release associated with ipsilateral adrenocorticotropin secretion. *Clin Invest.* 1996;97(9):2045–2050.
2. Wanchoo R, Karam S, Uppal NN, et al. Adverse renal effects of immune checkpoint inhibitors: a narrative review. *Am J Nephrol.* 2017;45(2):160–169.
3. Rahman O, El Halawani H, Fouad M. Risk of endocrine complications in cancer patients treated with immune checkpoint inhibitors: a metaanalysis. *Future Oncol.* 2016;12(3):413–425.
4. Byun DJ, Wolchok JD, Rosenberg LM, et al. Cancer immunotherapy-immune checkpoint blockade and associated endocrinopathies. *Nat Rev Endocrinol.* 2017;13(4):195–207.
5. Barroso-Sousa R, Barry WT, Garrido-Castro AC, et al. Incidence of endocrine dysfunction following the use of different immune checkpoint inhibitor regimens: a systematic review and meta-analysis. *JAMA Oncol.* 2018;4(2):173–182.
6. Caturegli P, Di Dalmazi G, Lombardi M, et al. Hypophysitis secondary to cytotoxic T-lymphocyte–associated protein 4 blockade: insights into pathogenesis from an autopsy series. *Am J Pathol.* 2016;186(12):3225–3235.

CHAPTER 2

Hypernatremia

Case Study 1

A 14-year-old **male** with a history of aplastic anemia underwent haploidentical stem cell transplantation, complicated by graft-versus-host disease, affecting his gastrointestinal tract. The posttransplantation course was complicated by bacteremia caused by Klebsiella species and subsequently fungal sinusitis, requiring sphenoidectomy and an extended course of antifungal therapy. One month later, nephrology was consulted for polyuria. The patient denied headache, confusion, changes in vision, weakness, or difficulty ambulating. His medications were limited to amlodipine, amphotericin B, budesonide, omeprazole, posaconazole, and terbinafine. He was receiving total parenteral nutrition and 3 L of lactated Ringer's solution daily before consultation.

On physical examination, vital signs were notable for temperature of 36.8°C, heart rate 87 beats/min, blood pressure 131/86 mmHg, respiration rate 14 breaths/min, and oxygen saturation 98% on room air. Weight was 80.5 kg. Cardiac examination findings were unremarkable, lungs were clear bilaterally, abdomen was soft without tenderness or organomegaly, extremities were without pitting edema, and there were no focal neurologic findings. The patient's urine output was 6.8 L daily. Laboratory data included serum sodium 155 mmol/L, potassium 3.4 mmol/L, chloride 115 mmol/L, bicarbonate 28 mmol/L, BUN 28 mg/dL, creatinine 1.4 mg/dL. Urine sodium was 42 mmol/L, potassium 10 mmol/L, and osmolality 155 mOsm/kg. Magnetic resonance imaging of the brain revealed stable mucosal thickening and enhancement within the sphenoid sinus, compatible with fungal sinusitis.

What is the diagnostic approach to polyuria?

    A. Nephrogenic diabetes insipidus
    B. Primary polydipsia
    C. Central diabetes insipidus secondary to invasive fungal sinusitis
    D. Reset hypernatremia

The correct answer is C
Comment: Polyuria, defined as 24-hour urine volume ≥ 3 L in patients consuming a typical Western diet, can be secondary to either solute or water diuresis.[1-3] The initial diagnostic step is to measure urine osmolality. Levels greater than 300 mOsm/kg are suggestive of an osmotic diuresis or renal concentrating defect (if solute excretion rate is < 1000 mOsm/day). Urine osmolality less than 250 mOsml/kg is suggestive of water diuresis, which can be further stratified by assessing plasma sodium concentration. A level less than 136 mEq/L suggests primary polydipsia, whereas water diuresis that persists at a plasma sodium level greater than 140 mEq/L is consistent with a diagnosis of diabetes insipidus.

In hospitalized patients, polyuria is typically secondary to iatrogenic administration of large amounts of crystalloid or high-protein enteral nutrition.[1] Alternatively, excessive urine output may be seen following relief of urinary tract obstruction, due to a reduction in the medullary concentration gradient and impaired sodium reabsorption. At the time of consultation, the urine osmolality of 380 mOsm/kg and daily solute excretion (urine osmolality multiplied by 24-hour urine volume) were significantly greater than 1000 mOsm/day, both consistent with solute diuresis. The most likely cause was iatrogenic, secondary to crystalloid infusion. After discontinuation of intravenous fluids, the patient's urine output improved to 2 L daily.

What treatment options would you consider in the short and long term?

   A. Free-water 4.5 L
   B. 0.45% saline 3.0 L
   C. 0.9% saline 1.5 L
   D. Ringer lactate 2.0 L

The correct answer is A

Comment: Given the free-water deficit of 4.5 L [$V \times (1 - (U_{Na+} + U_K)/P_{Na+})$], the patient was started on an infusion of dextrose 5% in water solution at a rate of 300 mL/h in addition to receiving desmopressin, as described.[1-3] Serum sodium level improved from 155 to 144 mEq/L during the subsequent 12 hours. He was successfully maintained on oral desmopressin treatment at a dosage of 0.1 μg daily.

Case Study 2

A 15-year-old male with a history of hypertension, hepatitis C virus infection previously treated with ledipasvir/sofosbuvir, and cirrhosis presented to an outside hospital with jaundice. His cirrhosis had been complicated by encephalopathy. He was found to have stigmata of advanced liver disease, including marked ascites and peripheral edema. Computed tomography showed a mass obstructing the biliary tree, and a biliary drain was placed. The patient's serum sodium level during this admission was 135 mmol/L and ranged from 135 to 137 mmol/L until placement of the biliary drain, after which sodium level decreased to 129 mmol/L at discharge. Before this, he had no history of hyponatremia. The hyponatremia was attributed to treatment with a thiazide diuretic that was discontinued. He was discharged with plans for further workup of the mass as an outpatient. One week later, the patient presented to the Emergency Department with persistent jaundice and was found to have a serum sodium concentration of 122 mmol/L. His presenting laboratory values were notable for serum creatinine level of 1.96 mg/dL, serum osmolarity of 272 mOsm/kg in the setting of azotemia (serum urea nitrogen, 66 mg/dL), and serum glucose level of 150 mg/dL. Total bilirubin level was elevated at 15.6 mg/dL and albumin level was 3.6 g/dL. He estimated his daily fluid intake at about 7 L. Heart rate was 73 beats/min, blood pressure was 113/62 mmHg, and oxygen saturation was 98% while breathing room air. Physical examination revealed dry mucous membranes, no jugular venous distension, no cardiac murmur, clear lung fields, a large pannus with right upper quadrant biliary drain, but no fluid wave, and edema (1 +) of the lower extremities. His laboratory data: serum sodium 122 mmol/L, potassium 4.2 mmol/L, chloride 87 mmol/L, glucose 150 mg/dL, osmolality 282 mOsm/kg, and uric acid 9.9 mg/dL, Random urine chemistry showed sodium 7 mmol/L, potassium 39 mmol/L, and osmolality 443 mOsm/kg. Daily fluid intake and urine output averaged 1070 mL and 4200 mL, respectively.

The patient was initially thought to have hypervolemic, hypotonic hyponatremia secondary to cirrhosis and treated with furosemide and fluid restriction. His biliary drain produced 2 to 3 L/day. Serum sodium level continued to decline, including after administration of 500 mL of lactated Ringer's solution. Hypertonic saline (3.0%) solution was administered at a rate of 115 mL/h with transient improvement in serum sodium concentration, but hyponatremia quickly recurred when this was discontinued.

What is the cause of hyponatremia in this patient and what additional diagnostic study should be obtained?

A. Hypovolemic, hypotonic hyponatremia from intravascular volume depletion secondary to excessive biliary output of high sodium content

B. Hyponatremia secondary to syndrome of inappropriate antidiuretic secretion (SIADH)

C. Hyponatremia secondary to polydipsia

D. Hyponatremia secondary to use of diuretics

The correct answer is A

Comment: The differential diagnosis of hyponatremia in this patient includes hypervolemic hyponatremia, hypovolemic hyponatremia, pseudohyponatremia secondary to lipoprotein X, and syndrome of inappropriate antidiuretic hormone (SIADH).[1] Patients with obstructive jaundice accompanied by extreme elevations of serum cholesterol levels can have elevation of lipoprotein X levels from the reflux of unesterified cholesterol and phospholipids into the circulation.[2,3] This can decrease the measured serum sodium level without affecting tonicity, which would be noted clinically by serum osmolality in the normal range. This is rare, and our patient was found to be hypotonic, with serum osmolality consistent with his serum sodium concentration. The presence of ascites and edema was indicative of a total-body excess of sodium and water and hypervolemic hyponatremia. A low urinary sodium concentration in such patients is common, reflecting decreased effective arterial blood volume despite the hypervolemic state due to systemic vasodilatation and splanchnic sequestration of fluid resulting in "third spacing" with the formation of ascites and edema. A hemodynamic impetus for antidiuretic hormone (ADH) release occurs, resulting in concentrated urine and hyponatremia. Although SIADH is a possibility, the diagnosis cannot be made in the face of signs of intravascular volume depletion as is seen in this patient, given his very low urinary sodium level. In SIADH, there is a slightly volume-expanded state; thus, this entity should not have a sodium-avid nephron as in intravascular volume depletion.[1]

The observed failure to sustain a response to hypertonic saline solution infusions suggested ongoing sodium chloride losses with substantial water intake. Sequestration of sodium in bile salts is responsible for bile's hypertonicity.[3] Other studies have shown electrolyte excretion into bile to be related to the flow and presence of cholelithiasis. It should be noted that most fluids, including gastric and duodenal secretions, are hypotonic to serum; however, biliary secretions are hypertonic, whereas pleural fluid, ascites, and edema are isotonic. (Diarrhea has variable tonicity.) In this patient, the high urinary osmolality indicated the presence of ADH while the low urinary sodium concentration indicated that the kidneys were in a sodium-avid state, making it likely that the stimulus for ADH secretion was hemodynamic in response to intravascular volume depletion. The continued sodium losses from his biliary drain compounded with persistent fluid intake resulted in persistent ADH stimulus and hyponatremia.

Case Study 3

This 3-year-old girl was seen in the outpatient clinic with a 2-week history of anorexia, fatigue, polydipsia, and excessive polyuria. The fluid intake had risen to 0.5 L/h, and a 24-hour urine collection yielded 10 L. Her blood pressure at home was 106/64 mmHg with a pulse of 72 beats/min, and she complained of muscle cramps. Physical examination showed a euvolemic patient in an otherwise normal condition. Laboratory investigation revealed serum sodium 144 mmol/L, potassium 3.1 mmol/L, chloride 109 mmol/L, bicarbonate 29 mmol/L, and creatinine 0.3 mg/dL. Plasma osmolality of 298 mOsm/kg and urine osmolality of 44 mOsm/kg. Random urine sodium was 5 mmol/L and potassium 3 mmol/L.

What is the MOST likely Diagnosis?

A. X-linked type of nephrogenic diabetes insipidus
B. Hypokalemia-related polyuria
C. Recessive type of nephrogenic diabetes insipidus
D. Solute induced polyuria

The correct diagnosis is C

Comment: Constellation of polydipsia and polyuria (10 L/day), elevated serum sodium (144 mmol/L), and dilute urine (urine osmolality 44 mOsml/kg) in a setting of normal blood pressure suggests the diagnosis of autosomal recessive hereditary, nephrogenic diabetes insipidus.[1,2]

In this patient, nephrogenic diabetes insipidus was caused by a homozygote mutation in the aquaporin-2 gene due to consanguine marriage. The patient's brother died at the age of 14 days, and her sister died at the age of 4 months. Aquaporin-2 channels are normally stored in the cytosol; under the influence of antidiuretic hormone, they move to and fuse with the luminal membrane, thereby allowing water to be reabsorbed down the favorable concentration gradient. The mutations may lead either to impaired trafficking of the water channels, which do not fuse with the luminal membrane, or to decreased channel function. The patient was taking amiloride-hydrochlorothiazide (Moduretic) twice daily, a combination of hydrochlorothiazide (50 mg) with amiloride hydrochloride (5 mg). The thiazide diuretic acts by inducing mild volume depletion with an increase of proximal sodium and water reabsorption, thereby diminishing water delivery to the antidiuretic hormone-sensitive sites in the collecting tubules and reducing the urine output.[1] This initial natriuresis can be enhanced by a combination therapy with amiloride.

Current conventional treatment regimen includes hydration, diuretics polyuria. Recent experimental studies have suggested that treatment with sildenafil, a selective phosphodiesterase inhibitor, may enhance cyclic guanosine monophosphate (cGMP) mediated apical trafficking of AQP2 and may be effective in increasing water reabsorption in patients with congenital nephrotic syndrome.[2]

Case Study 4

A 19-year-old male is brought into the hospital in a comatose state. He is found to have a skull fracture. It is noted that his weight is 70 kg, and his urine output is 175 mL/h. The following laboratory data are obtained: Serum sodium 168 mmol/L, potassium 4 mmol/L, chloride 130 mmol/L, bicarbonate 25 mmol/L, plasma osmolality 350 mOsm/kg, and urine osmolality 80 mOsm/kg.

What is the MOST likely diagnosis, what is the approximate water deficit and much free water is needed to lower the plasma sodium concentration to normal (assuming that the urine output has fallen to low levels)?

A. Nephrogenic diabetes insipidus
B. Central diabetes insipidus
C. Syndrome inappropriate ADH secretion
D. Essential hypernatremia

The correct answer is B

Comment: The diagnosis of central diabetes insipidus was confirmed by the good response to administration of 1-deamino-8-D-arginine vasopressin (dDAVP) or aqueous vasopressin, which raised the urine osmolality and lowered the urine volume. There was no need to do the water-restriction test since the plasma osmolality was already 350 mOsml/kg.

The water deficit can be estimated from:[1,2]

$$\text{Water deficit} = 0.5 \times 70 \times (168 / 140 - 1) \text{ or } 7\,\text{L}$$

This deficit should be replaced gradually over 56 hours at the rate of 125 mL/h. Another 50 mL/h should be added to replace continuing insensible losses. Thus, 175 mL/h can be given as dextrose in water. There is no history of sodium loss and therefore no requirement for saline administration.

Case Study 5

A 10-year-old girl presents to hospital after 2 days history of vomiting and diarrhea. She appears moderately dehydrated on exam. Her temperature is 39°C, weight 25 kg, blood pressure 110/62 mmHg, pulse 90 beats/min, and respiration 18 breaths/min. Her weight was 27 kg prior to her illness. The serum sodium concentration is 160 mmol/L and potassium 3.4 mmol/L.

What solution should be used and at what rate to correct this patient's hypernatremia?

A. 0.45% saline at 200 mL/h
B. 0.9% saline at 200 mL/h
C. 0.3% saline at 100 mL/h
D. 0.2% saline at 300 mL/h

The correct answer is A
Comment: This patient's hypovolemic hypernatremia is as a result of hypotonic sodium loss from gastrointestinal tract. She has lost both sodium and water. However, the amount of water loss is greater than sodium loss and that's why she is hypernatremic. Infusion of hypotonic fluids (such as 0.45% saline) is the most appropriate solution to correct volume depletion and reduce serum sodium concentration.

The effect of 1 L of 0.45% saline containing 20 mmol KCl/L on serum sodium change can be estimated using the following formula[1,2]:

$$\text{Na}^+ \text{ change} = \left(\text{infusate} \left(\text{Na}^+ \text{ mmo/L} + \text{infusate K}^+ \text{ mmo/L} \right) \right)$$
$$- \left(\text{serum Na}^+ \text{ mEq/L} \right) \div \left(\text{total body water (TBW) liters} + 1 \right)$$

According to this formula, the infusion of 1 L 0.45% saline containing 20 mEq K$^+$ will reduce the serum sodium concentration by 4 mmol/L $(77 + 20) - 160 \div (15 + 1)$. To reduce the serum sodium by 5 mmol/L over the next 12 hours, we would need to give 1.4 L $(5 \div 4.4)$. To account for ongoing losses, we might want to give additional 1 L for a total 2.4 L over 12 hours or 200 mL/h of 0.45% saline.

Case Study 6

What would be the anticipated duration of therapy until a normal serum (Na⁺) is restored?

A. 24 hours
B. 36 hours
C. 48 hours
D. 72 hours

The correct answer is B
Anticipated duration of therapy (hours) can be estimated as follows[1,2]

$$\left(24\,\text{hours}/10\,\text{mmol/L}\right)\times\left(\left(Na^+\right)\text{initial}-\left(Na^+\right)\text{goal}\right)\text{mmol/L or }2.4\times\left(160-145\right)=36\text{ hours}.$$

Case Study 7

A 16-year-old boy has received 5 ampules of sodium bicarbonate over a period of 1 hour during resuscitation after cardiac arrest. He is stuporous and under mechanical ventilation. His blood pressure is 136/88 mmHg, and peripheral edema (+++) is present. The serum sodium is 160 mmol/L, the body weight is 55 kg, and the urinary output is 20 mL/h.

What is the appropriate fluid for treating this patient's hypernatremia?

    A. 0.9% saline
    B. 5% dextrose in water
    C. 0.4% saline
    D. 3% saline

The correct answer is B
Comment: This patient's hypertonic hypernatremia is a result of sodium gain from hypertonic sodium bicarbonate infusion, and its correction requires the excess sodium to be removed. The administration of furosemide alone will not suffice because furosemide-induced diuresis is equivalent to one-half isotonic saline solution; thus, the hypernatremia will be aggravated. The administration of both furosemide and 5% dextrose in water will meet the therapeutic goal.

The effect of 1 L of 5% dextrose water on serum sodium change can be estimated using the following formula[1,2]

$$Na^+\text{ change}=\left(\text{infusate }Na^+\text{ mmol/L}\right)-\left(\text{serum }Na^+\text{ mmol/L}\right)\div\left(\text{TBW liters}+1\right)$$

According to the formula, infusion of 1 L of 5% dextrose water will reduce the serum Na^+ concentration by 4.7 mmol/L (0 − 160) ÷ 55 × 0.6 + 1) = −4.7 mmol/L.

Given the seriousness of the patient's symptoms the initial goal is to reduce the serum Na^+ concentration by 3 mmol/L over the next 3 hours, thus 0.63 L of 5% dextrose in water (3 ÷ 4.7), or 210 mL/h, is required. After patient's mental status is substantially improved, the goal of treatment should be to reduce serum sodium slowly by 5 mmol/L over the next 12 hours using the 0.45% saline until the target serum sodium concentration of 145 mEq/L is achieved.

Frequent monitoring of the serum sodium concentration, initially every 2 to 3 hours, is necessary in order to make further adjustments in the amount of fluid administered.

Case Study 8

A 3-year-old girl with a past medical history of nephrogenic diabetes insipidus (DI) presents to the hospital after 3 days of worsening abdominal pain and fever. Her weight on admission is 12 kg; heart rate is 78, blood pressure 104/68 mmHg, serum sodium 165 mmol/L, potassium 3.0 mmol/L, and serum creatinine 0.4 mg/dL. Her average daily urine output is 1.5 L.

What is the appropriate fluid for treating this patient's hypernatremia and would be the anticipated duration of therapy until a normal serum (Na⁺) is restored?

A. 48 hours
B. 36 hours
C. 24 hours
D. 12 hours

The correct answer is A

Comment: In this case, hypernatremia is due to pure water loss from DI. The best fluid to treat hypernatremia in a patient with DI is electrolyte-free solution. The effect of 1 L of 5% dextrose water on serum Na⁺ change can be estimated using the following formula[1–3]

$$Na^+ \text{ change} = \left(\text{infusate Na}^+ \text{ mmol/L}\right) - \left(\text{serum Na}^+ \text{ mmol/L}\right) \div \left(\text{TBW liters} + 1\right)$$

According to this formula, the infusion of 1 L of 5% dextrose water will reduce the serum sodium concentration by 20 mmol/L $(0 - 165) \div (7.2 + 1) = -20$ mEq/L. Since the goal is to reduce the serum sodium by 5 mmol/L over the next 12 hours, 0.25 L of the solution is required $(5 \div 20)$. To account for ongoing losses due to diabetes insipidus, we might add another 1.5 L for a total of 1.75 L over 12 hours or 146 mL/h. The anticipated duration of therapy (hours) can be estimated as follows:

$$\left(24 \text{ hours/10 mmol/L}\right) \times \left(\left(Na^+\right) \text{initial} - \left(Na+\right)\text{goal}\right)\text{mmol/L or } 2.4 \times \left(165 - 145\right) = 48 \text{ hours}$$

Sildenafil should be considered to prevent future fluid-electrolyte occurrence.

Case Study 9

A 4-year-old boy was brought to the Emergency Department 2 hours after drowning in seawater. His weight is 15 kg, blood pressure 110/65 mmHg, and he is on mechanical ventilator. The serum sodium is 180 mmol/L and potassium 3.0 mmol/L. He has passed 70 mL of urine since admission in the Emergency Department.

Can you estimate the ingested amount of water and Na⁺ in this child?

What is the most appropriate fluid therapy?

A. 2000 mL
B. 1800 mL
C. 1600 mL
D. 1400 mL

The correct answer is B

Comment: This patient's total body Na+ and water are both increased because of drowning and swallowing salty water (salt intoxication). The sodium excess is greater than water gain and that is why patient is hypernatremic. The concentration of salt in seawater is about 30 g/L. Each gram of salt contains 17 mmol sodium, thus each liter of seawater contains about 510 mmol sodium.

The difference between the $TBNa^+$ before and after drowning determines the amount of ingested salt as follows:

$$\left(TBNa^+ \text{ before drowning}\right) - \left(TBNa^+ \text{ after drowning}\right).$$

$TBNa^+$ before drowning = 140 mmol/L × 9 L = 1260 mmol. $TBNa^+$ after drowning = 180 mmol/L × 12 L = 2160 mmol/L. The amount of ingested salt is 900 mmol and because each liter of seawater contains 510 mmol sodium, the child should have swallowed about 1.8 L (900/510) seawater. Treatment should be initiated to remove the excess sodium and water (sodium more than water) with a loop diuretic such as Lasix. However, use of loop diuretic alone produces hypotonic urine (containing ∼70 to 80 mEq/sodium/L) compared to patient's plasma osmolality, and this may further aggravate hypernatremia. Thus, 5% dextrose water containing 20 to 30 mmol KCl/L should concurrently be administered along with loop diuretic. The 5% DW solution should contain no sodium. Addition of Na^+ would not only prolong the duration of repair but also lengthen the hospital stay.

The effect of 1 L of 5% dextrose water on serum sodium change can be estimated using the following formula:[1,2]

$$Na^+ \text{ change} = \left(\text{infusate}\left(Na^+ \text{ mmol/L} + K^+ \text{ mmol/L}\right)\right) - \left(\text{serum } Na^+ \text{ mmol/L}\right) \div \left(\text{TBW liters} + 1\right)$$

According to this formula, the infusion of 1 L of 5% dextrose water will reduce the serum sodium concentration by 15 mmol/L (0 − 180 + 30) ÷ (15 × 0.6 + 1) = −15 mmol/L. Given the seriousness of the patient's symptoms (acute severe and symptomatic hypernatremia), the initial goal is to reduce the serum sodium concentration by 1 mEq/L/h for the next 3 hours until symptoms resolve, thus 200 mL of 5% dextrose (3 ÷ 15) or 67 mL/h is required. In such patients, rapid correction improves the prognosis without increasing the risk of cerebral edema. Frequent monitoring of the serum sodium concentration, initially every 2 to 3 hours, is necessary in order to make further adjustments in the amount of fluid administered. Once patient's mental status is substantially improved, the goal of treatment is to reduce serum sodium slowly by 5 mmol/L over the next 12 hours using the 0.45% saline until the target serum Na^+ concentration of 145 mmol/L is achieved.

Case Study 10

A six-year-old girl was admitted to the hospital because of severe hypertonic dehydration. The patient was born at 40 weeks of gestation with a birth weight of 4.0 kg. Growth and development were normal until age 5 months, when she fell and suffered a severe head injury. A computed tomography (CT) scan of the head revealed diffuse intracerebral hemorrhage. The child underwent right frontal craniotomy with drainage of blood. Postoperatively, she experienced seizure requiring phenobarbital and carbamazepine for control. The child remained relatively well until the age of 2.5 years, when she experienced her first hypernatremic dehydration following an upper respiratory infection. At that time, serum sodium concentration was 181 mmol/L, creatinine 1.0 mg/dL, and urine specific gravity 1.019. Despite severe hypernatremia, she showed no interest in drinking water. Intravenous fluid therapy corrected the hypernatremia. Serum sodium concentration fell to 148 mmol/L and creatinine to 0.3 mg/dL. CT of the brain revealed left subdural effusion, enlarged third and lateral ventricles, and left cerebral atrophy. She was discharged with recommendations for a high fluid intake. At 6 years of age, 2 days before admission, she developed a low-grade fever, had decreased appetite, and experienced frequent episodes of vomiting resulting in a 3.0 kg weight loss.

On admission the patient was alert and had clinical evidence of severe dehydration. The blood pressure was 98/60 mmHg, pulse 152/min, respiration 26 breaths/min, and temperature 37°C.

Her weight was 17.0 kg (10th percentile), length 109 cm (5th percentile). Neurological deficits included right hemiparesis, wide-based gait, and mild spasticity of the left arm.

Initial serum electrolytes concentrations (mmol/L) were sodium 187, potassium 5.6, chloride 148, and bicarbonate 14. BUN was 117, serum cotinine 3.0 mg/dL, hemoglobin 14.5 g/dL, glucose 163 mg/dL, albumin 3.2 g/dL, calcium 9.3 mg/dL, and phosphorous 2.7 mg/dL. Serum and urine osmolality were 421 and 854 mOsm/kg, respectively. Urine pH was 5.0 with trace protein and no blood. Liver function study was normal. Nuclear magnetic resonance of the brain disclosed partial resolution of the subdural effusion, greatly dilated lateral and third ventricles and left cerebral atrophy with compression of the hypothalamus and pituitary stalk. Test for endocrine function was normal.

The patient was rehydrated with intravenous fluids, and within 48 hours, the serum sodium fell to 162 mmol/L and serum creatinine to 0.7 mg/dL. She did not complain of thirst throughout this entire period.

What is the underlying cause for this patient's hypernatremia?

    A. Incomplete cerebral diabetes insipidus
    B. Reset hypernatremia
    C. Selective defect in the osmoregulation of thirst
    D. Hereditary nephrogenic diabetes insipidus

The correct answer is C

Comment: This patient presented with recurrent episodes of hypertonic dehydration. She denied thirst even with serum osmolality as high as 421 mOsm/kg. The hypernatremia was associated with an ability to concentrate urine (854 mOsm/kg). Volume expansion with water corrected hypernatremia (162 to 148 mmol/L) and resulted in an increased urine flow and urine dilution (137 mOsm/kg) because of suppression of endogenous vasopressin release. With chronic forced fluid intake, the patient maintained a normal serum sodium concentration (range between 135 and 145 mmol/L). These findings are consistent with an isolated defect in the osmoregulation of thirst as the cause of the chronic hypertonic dehydration without deficiency in vasopressin secretion.[1–3]

Differentiation between disturbances in water balance due to a selective defect in the osmoregulation of thirst and those related to deficient vasopressin secretion is important because management differs according to the diagnosis.

Case Study 11

A 15-year-old boy was admitted to the hospital because of diabetic ketoacidosis. He had been well until 3 days prior to admission, when he began to complain of nausea and developed vomiting. During the next 3 days, the vomiting became increasingly severe and his parents reported the onset of polyuria, polydipsia, and marked anorexia. He was seen in his personal physician's office because of vomiting and routine laboratory studies resulted in the discovery of a blood sugar of approximately 1500 mg/dL. He was referred immediately to the hospital. Physical examination on admission disclosed a stuporous 46-kg male who was extremely dehydrated and had evident Kussmaul respirations. The odor of ketones was present on his breath. His mouth was dry. His eyes appeared sunken, the globes were soft and he had poor skin turgor. His pulse was 140/min, blood pressure 90/60 supine, but aside from his obvious increased ventilatory exchange and the physical evidence of profound dehydration, the examination was otherwise within normal limits. The initial laboratory studies at this hospital disclosed blood sugar of 1128 mg/dL. The blood urea nitrogen was 61 mg/dL and his creatinine 2.8 mg/dL. Serum sodium concentration was 158 mmol/L, potassium 3.7 mmol/L, chloride 118 mmol/L, and bicarbonate 7 mmol/L. The calculated anion gap was 33 mmol/L. His white blood cell count was 27,100, of which 82% was neutrophils, 11% lymphocytes, and 7% monocytes. His hemoglobin on arrival was 16.9 g/dL.

His hematocrit was 49%. His serum calcium was 11.1 mg/dL and phosphorus 2.0 mg/dl. The calculated total serum osmolality was 396 mOsm/kg.

What is the BEST initial fluid therapy for this patient's electrolyte disorders?

     A. Ringer's lactate solution containing 30 mmol potassium phosphate/L and 30 mmol potassium acetate at the rate of 300 mL/h plus insulin at the rate of 0.1 units/kg/h
     B. Ringer's lactate solution at the rate of 300 mL/h plus insulin at the rate of 0.1 units/kg/h
     C. 5% dextrose in water solution containing 30 mmol potassium phosphate/L and 30 mmol potassium acetate at the rate of 300 mL/h plus insulin at the rate of 0.1 units/kg/h
     D. 5% dextrose in water at the rate of 300 mL/h plus insulin at the rate of 0.1 units/kg/h

The correct answer is A

Comment: A course of therapy was planned to restore his total body fluid deficit over a 24- to 48-hour period to ensure a stable serum potassium concentration and reduce his serum osmolality to normal over a period of approximately 4 days, or at a rate of some 1.5 to 2 mOsm/h.[1,2]

The greatest threat to this patient's life (in view of the extraordinarily high osmolality of the extracellular fluids) was the risk of developing cerebral edema during treatment. To accomplish these objectives, an attempt was made to lower his blood sugar very slowly while simultaneously expanding extracellular fluid isosmotically with Ringer's lactate solution to which potassium chloride had been added to bring the tonicity of the replacement fluid to approximately that of the patient. We anticipated that during the first stage of therapy, the serum sodium would increase as the blood sugar fell, and this rise would minimize the shift of water into the central nervous system. In an effort to prevent unpredictable urinary electrolyte losses caused by perturbations in urinary electrolyte content, urine was collected and urine electrolytes measured, so urinary water and electrolytes could be replaced on a volume for volume basis. After his blood sugar reached a more physiological level and his dehydration had been largely corrected, we planned to provide sufficient water, either intravenously (IV) or orally, to gradually lower his serum sodium concentration to normal.

To accomplish these goals, three peripheral IV lines were established. Two were used to provide IV fluid therapy initially, consisting of Ringer's lactate solution to which 30 mmol potassium phosphate and 30 mmol potassium acetate were added per liter. Fluid was initially administered at the rate of 100 mL/h through each line. A Foley catheter was anchored, urine was collected, and through the third IV line, urinary water and electrolyte losses were replaced as they occurred. Urine sodium and potassium concentrations were measured every 2 hours. Initially, the urine contained approximately 30 mmol/L of sodium and 111 mmol/L of potassium. As hydration improved, the concentration of both electrolytes increased. A urine sodium concentration of 111 mmol/L at 30 hours indicated that rehydration was complete. IV insulin was provided at the rate of 0.1 units/ kg per hour. The initial body fluid deficit was estimated to be between 4 and 5 L of which 60% was assumed to be due to loss of extracellular fluid. During the first 12 hours of therapy, he received 2400 mL Ringer's lactate solution and 144 mmol potassium. His urine output was replaced with fluids of similar electrolyte composition. During this 12-hour period, his blood sugar fell to 516 mg/dL or by 31 mOsml/kg. An increase in serum sodium to 171 mEq partially attenuated the drop in serum osmolality. After 12 hours of therapy, the physical findings of extracellular dehydration were less evident, his metabolic acidosis was much improved, and his anion gap was approaching normal (13 to 17 mmol). During these 12 hours, his estimated serum osmolality fell at a rate of 1.6 mOsml/h—essentially the same as a change in serum sodium of 0.8 mEq/h.

References

Case Study 1

1. Rose BD, Post TW. *Clinical Physiology of Acid-Base and Electrolyte Disorders.* 5th ed. New York, NY: McGraw-Hill; 2001:748–767.
2. Singh I, Strandhoy JW, Assimos DG. Pathophysiology of urinary tract obstruction. In: Wein AJ, Kavoussi LR, Novick AC, Partin AW, Peter CA, eds. *Campbell-Walsh Urology.* 10th ed. Philadelphia, PA: Elsevier Saunders; 2012:1107–1108.
3. Shimizu K, Kurosawa T, Sanjo T, et al. Solute-free versus electrolyte-free water clearance in the analysis of osmoregulation. *Nephron.* 2002;91(1):51–57.

Case Study 2

1. Kaptein EM, Sreeramoju D, Kaptein JM, et al. A systematic literature search and review of sodium concentrations of body fluids. *Clin Nephrol.* 2016;86(10):203–228.
2. Wheeler HO, Ramos OL, Whitlock RT. Electrolyte excretion in bile. *Circulation.* 1960;21:988–996.
3. Reinhold JG, Ferguson LK, Hunsberger A. The composition of human gallbladder bile and its relationship to cholelithiasis. *J Clin Invest.* 1937;16(3):367–382.

Case Study 3

1. Duicu C, Pitea AM, Săsăran OM, et al. Nephrogenic diabetes insipidus in children (Review). *Exp Ther Med.* 2021 Jul;22(1):746. https://doi.org/10.3892/etm.2021.10178.
2. Assadi F, Sharbaf FG. Sildenafil for the treatment of congenital nephrogenic diabetes insipidus. *Am J Nephrol.* 2015;42(1):65–69. https://doi.org/10.1159/000439065.

Case Study 4

1. Rose BD, Post TW. *Clinical Physiology of Acid-Base and Electro-lyte Disorders.* 5th ed. New York, NY: McGraw-Hill, Inc; 2001:551–571 [Chapter 18].
2. Assadi F. *Clinical Decisions in Pediatric Nephrology: A Problem Solving Approach to Clinical Cases.* New York: Springer; 2008:69–98 [Chapter 2].

Case Study 5

1. Adroque HJ, Madias NE. Hypernatremia. New Engl *J Med.* 2000;342:1493–1499.
2. Adroque HJ, Madias NE. Aiding fluid prescription for the dysnatremia. *Intensive Care Med.* 2000;23:309–316.

Case Study 6

1. Adroque HJ, Madias NE. Hypernatremia. New Engl *J Med.* 2000;342:1493–1499.
2. Adroque HJ, Madias NE. Aiding fluid prescription for the dysnatremia. *Intensive Care Med.* 2000;23:309–316.

Case Study 7

1. Adroque HJ, Madias NE. Hypernatremia. New Engl *J Med.* 2000;342:1493–1499.
2. Adroque HJ, Madias NE. Aiding fluid prescription for the dysnatremia. *Intensive Care Med.* 2000;23:309–316.

Case Study 8

1. Adroque HJ, Madias NE. Hypernatremia. New Engl *J Med.* 2000;342:1493–1499.
2. Adroque HJ, Madias NE. Aiding fluid prescription for the dysnatremia. *Intensive Care Med.* 2000;23:309–316.
3. Assadi F, Ghaneh Sharbaf F. Sildenafil for the treatment of congenital nephrogenic diabetes insipidus. *Am J Nephrol.* 2015;42:65–69.

Case Study 9

1. Assadi F. *Clinical Decisions in Pediatric Nephrology: A Problem Solving Approach to Clinical Cases.* New York: Springer; 2008:1–68 [Chapter 2].
2. Adroque HJ, Madias NE. Hypernatremia. New Engl *J Med.* 2000;342:1493–1499.

Case Study 10

1. Assadi F, Johnson B, Dawson F, et al. Recurrent hypertonic dehydration due to selective defect in the osmoregulation of thirst. *Pediatr Nephrol.* 1989;3:438–442.
2. Robertson GL. Thirst and vasopressin function in normal and disordered states of water balance. *J Lab Clin Med.* 1983;101:351–371.
3. Assadi F, Norman ME, Parks JS, et al. Hypernatremia associated with pineal tumor. *J Pediatr.* 1977;90:605–606.

Case Study 11

1. Duck SC, Wyatt DT. Factors associated with brain herniation in the treatment of diabetic ketoacidosis. *J Pediatr.* 1988;113:10.
2. Harris GH, Fiordalisi I, Finberg L. Safe management of diabetic ketoacidosis. *J Pediatr.* 1988;113:65.

CHAPTER 3

Hypokalemia

Case Study 1

A 16-year-old young man was admitted for elective surgery for a small-bowel carcinoid tumor. Nephrology was consulted for evaluation of persistent hypokalemia and metabolic alkalosis. The patient denied abdominal pain, headache, fever, vomiting, or diarrhea. He did not use over-the-counter or herbal medications. Home medications included omeprazole, 20 mg, and daily and a monthly octreotide injection. In the hospital, he was receiving omeprazole, 20 mg daily.

On physical examination, the patient's temperature was 37.3 °C, heart rate was 90 beats/min, blood pressure was 155/95 mmHg, respiration rate was 14 breaths/min, and oxygen saturation was 97% on room air. Cardiac examination findings were unremarkable. Lungs were clear bilaterally. His abdomen was soft with no visceromegaly or tenderness. There was no edema. There were no focal neurologic findings. Laboratory studies showed serum sodium 144 mmol/L, potassium 2.8 mmol/L, chloride 9 mmol/L, bicarbonate 33 mmol/L, BUN, 16 mg/dL, creatinine 0.8 mg/dL, calcium 7.9 mg/dL, albumin 3.8 mg/dL, glucose 96 mg/dL. Arterial blood gas pH was 7.52, PCO_2 38 mmHg, HCO_3^- 32 mmol/L, plasma renin 1.06 ng/mL (reference: 0.25 to 5.82), plasma aldosterone 1 ng/dL (reference: 3 to 16), plasma cortisol 41.8 mcg/dL (reference: 6 to 26), and plasma corticotropin (ACTH) 92 pg/mL (reference: 6 to 50). In a 24-hour urine collection, cortisol was 1062 (reference: 4 to 50), creatinine 1.08 g, potassium 105 mmol, and chloride 62 mmol.

What is the MOST likely cause of hypokalemia in this patient?

    A. Liddle syndrome
    B. Hyperaldoseronim
    C. Apparent mineralocorticoid excess
    D. Ectopic ACTH-dependent Cushing syndrome from carcinoid tumor

The correct answer is D

Comment: Hypokalemia is generally due to either urinary or gastrointestinal tract losses, a shift from the extracellular to intracellular fluid compartment, or in rare cases, decreased oral intake.[1,2] In this patient, renal losses were thought to be most likely, given the elevated urinary potassium concentration.

Metabolic alkalosis is often classified as chloride responsive (urine chloride ≤20 mmol/L or less) or chloride resistant (urine chloride >20 mmol/L or more). When urine chloride excretion is greater than 20 mmol/L, the metabolic alkalosis is usually saline responsive. In metabolic alkalosis, urine chloride concentration may be a more accurate indicator of intravascular volume depletion than urine sodium concentration because bicarbonaturia in early stages of development of a chloride-depletion metabolic alkalosis results in sodium and potassium excretion in urine (as accompanying cations with bicarbonate). Thus, urine sodium and potassium concentrations may be elevated in the first 24 to 72 hours of volume depletion, and then decline subsequently. Urine chloride concentration will remain low due to ongoing sodium and chloride reabsorption in the proximal tubule due to activation of the renin–angiotensin–aldosterone axis and other factors in response to volume depletion.

This patient developed chloride-resistant metabolic alkalosis (urine chloride >20 mmol/L). Given the presence of hypertension along with urine potassium excretion greater than 20 mmol/L and low levels of both serum renin and aldosterone, the differential diagnosis includes Liddle syndrome, syndrome of apparent mineralocorticoid excess, Cushing syndrome, congenital adrenal hyperplasia, and excessive licorice use.[1-3] Liddle syndrome, syndrome of apparent mineralocorticoid excess, and congenital adrenal hyperplasia were unlikely given the patient's age. Given the patient's elevated morning cortisol level, markedly increased 24-hour urine cortisol excretion, and high serum corticotropin (adrenocorticotropic hormone, ACTH) level, ACTH-dependent Cushing syndrome was diagnosed. ACTH-dependent Cushing syndrome could be due to either an ACTH-secreting pituitary tumor or an ectopic ACTH-secreting tumor. Findings from magnetic resonance imaging of the pituitary gland and computed tomography of the chest were unremarkable. Computed tomography of the abdomen revealed peritoneal nodules consistent with his history of recurrent carcinoid tumor. Ectopic ACTH-dependent Cushing syndrome, most likely from the active carcinoid tumor, was diagnosed. There are a few case reports that describe Cushing syndrome attributed to the presence of a carcinoid tumor.

Cortisol has the capacity to bind mineralocorticoid receptors in principal cells of the cortical collecting duct.[4] Normally, this is limited by conversion of cortisol to cortisone, which is unable to bind to the mineralocorticoid receptor, by the enzyme 11β-hydroxysteroid dehydrogenasetype 2. Excess production of cortisol, as seen in our patient, saturates the enzyme, allowing cortisol to persist and activate mineralocorticoid receptors. This causes translocation of epithelial sodium channel proteins into the luminal membrane, increasing basolateral adenosine triphosphatase sodium/potassium pump activity and increasing renal outer medullary potassium channel activity, leading to sodium reabsorption and hypertension, hypokalemia, and metabolic alkalosis. Ideally, treatment in such patients is complete resection of the nonpituitary ACTH-secreting tumor. Unfortunately, the peritoneal carcinoid metastases were not respectable, and our patient's metabolic alkalosis and hypertension were treated with the mineralocorticoid receptor antagonist spironolactone. After being treated with spironolactone, 50 mg, daily for 4 weeks, the patient's blood pressure had improved to 118/77 mmHg, serum potassium concentration had increased to 3.9 mmol/L, and serum bicarbonate concentration was 25 mmol/L.

Case Study 2

A 19-year-old schoolteacher with no significant medical history or medication use presented with 3 months of lower back pain, proximal muscle weakness that limited his ability to stand, urinary frequency, and nocturia. Although denying dry mouth, dry eyes, or polydipsia, he describes frequent photophobia during this period. There was no blepharo spasm, tearing, or decreased vision. On physical examination, blood pressure was 110/70 mmHg and pulse rate was 72 beats/min. He had tenderness over his ribs bilaterally and painful restriction to flexion and extension of the ankle and knee joints. Proximal muscle strength in the upper and lower limbs was 4/5, deep tendon reflexes were present as a normal ankle jerk, superficial reflexes were normal, and there was no sensory deficit. Serum laboratory studies include the following values: Serum sodium 132 mmol/L, potassium 2.8 mmol/L, chloride 98 mmol/L, bicarbonate 18 mmol/L, creatinine 1.7 mg/dL, estimated glomerular filtration rate (GFR) 50 mL/min/1.73 m^2, glucose (fasting) 96 mg/dL, albumin 4.6 g/dL, calcium 6.8 mg/dL, phosphorous 3.1 mg/dL, ceruloplasmin 23 mg/mL (reference: 13 to 36 mg/mL), arterial blood gas pH 7.27, and PCO$_2$ 47.8 mmHg. Urinalysis showed pH 6.0, specific gravity 1.030, albumin 2+, and glucose 2+. The 24-hour urine contained 1.9 g protein, 250 potassium, 450 calcium, and 1.3 g phosphate. In addition, serological tests for antinuclear antibodies and antibodies Ro and La were negative. An ultrasound of the abdomen showed kidney sizes of 9.84.5 cm (right) and 9.64.3 cm (left); there was normal echo texture and corticomedullary differentiation.

What is the MOST likely diagnosis and what treatment is indicated?

A. Proximal tubular acidosis (RTA-2)

B. Nephropathic cystinosis-intermediate type

C. Distal renal tubular acidosis (RTA-1)

D. Tubulointerstitial nephritis

The correct answer is B

Comment: The features of polyuria, metabolic acidosis, hypokalemia, hypophosphataemia, glycosuria, and proteinuria suggest Fanconi syndrome.[1] This diagnosis is confirmed by the demonstration of generalized aminoaciduria and tubular proteinuria and should be followed by identification of the underlying cause. In adults, the major causes of Fanconi syndrome are monoclonal gammopathies, amyloidosis, membranous nephropathy, focal segmental glomerulosclerosis, and tubulointerstitial nephritis.[2] The other feature in this patient was photophobia. Sjögren syndrome presents classically with distal renal tubular acidosis and photophobia, although without the other abnormalities seen in Fanconi syndrome. Tubulointerstitial nephritis with uveitis also may present with proximal tubular dysfunction and photophobia, but most commonly is a diagnosis of exclusion in adolescent girls.

Photophobia with Fanconi syndrome is suggestive of cystinosis.[3–5] In classic nephropathic cystinosis, Fanconi syndrome appears at 6 to 12 months of age and end-stage renal disease develops at 9 years. It accounts for 95% of reported patients. Forms with late onset, as occurred in this patient, account for 5% of all cases of cystinosis. The late-onset forms are of two phenotypes. Intermediate cystinosis, also called late-onset or juvenile cystinosis, has the same features as the nephropathic form, but patients may retain kidney function into their 30s. Ocular or non-nephropathic cystinosis, previously called benign or adult cystinosis, is characterized by only ocular findings, with all systemic manifestations lacking.

Measuring the cystine usually makes the diagnosis content of peripheral leukocytes or cultured fibroblasts. The diagnosis can also be made through recognition of cystine crystals in corneal stoma, imparting a polychromatic luster on slit-lamp examination, as in this patient. Rectangular or hexagonal cystine crystals may be found in a bone marrow or kidney biopsy specimen. Because cystine crystals are water soluble, these are not retained in tissue sections after routine histological preparation with aqueous solutions. The bone marrow biopsy specimen in this patient did not show cystine crystals. The kidney biopsy specimen included eight glomeruli. Glomeruli were of normal size with patent glomerular capillaries. There was neither thickening nor irregularity of the capillary wall. Mesangial cellularity was normal. Interstitium was edematous with lymphocytic infiltrate. Cystine crystals also were not identified in the kidney biopsy specimen. *CTNS*, the gene implicated in cystinosis, encodes the protein cystinos in and maps to chromosome 17p13.

Oral cysteamine therapy is recognized as the treatment of choice for patients with nephropathic cystinosis who have not undergone transplant. Cysteamine depletes lysosomal cystine by a multistep mechanism. First, it enters into the lysosomal compartment through a specific transporter and reacts with cystine to form the mixed disulfide cysteamine–cysteine; this compound in turn exits the lysosomes through an intact lysine transporter, and when in the cytoplasm, is reduced by glutathione to cysteamine and cysteine. Cysteamine has the marked odor and taste of thiols and binds to oral mucosa and dental fillings. This patient, after 9 months of treatment with cysteamine, 50 mg/kg/day, had a serum creatinine level of 1.8 mg/dL. His joint pains, rib tenderness, and proximal muscle strength have improved.

Case Study 3

A 10-year-old girl was evaluated for uncontrolled hypertension, progressive weakness, and fatigue. High blood pressure (BP) was diagnosed at the age of 8 years during a routine clinic visit. Her BP was poorly controlled, first on atenolol therapy, and then on candesartan and amlodopine therapy.

Her course also has been notable for persistent hypokalemia, with potassium values ranging from 2.8 to 3.2 mmol/L. On physical examination, the patient's BP was 150/105 mmHg and pulse rate was 88 beats/min. Grade II retinopathy was present. Serum laboratory data included the following values: sodium 138 mmol/L, potassium, 2.9 mmol/L; bicarbonate, 33 mmol/L; creatinine, 0.7 mg/dL; estimated glomerular filtration rate, 97 mL/min/1.73 m^2, and magnesium, 1.64 mmol/L. Urinalysis showed pH 6.0; specific gravity, 1019; negative glucose, ketone, and nitrite; and 2$^+$ protein; urinary sediment was unremarkable. Twenty-four-hour urinary protein excretion ranged between 518 and 1409 mg. Echocardiography showed mild concentric left ventricular hypertrophy. Twenty-four–hour urinary excretion of free cortisol and metanephrines was normal. After felodipine and doxazosin were substituted for amlodipine and candesartan, plasma renin activity (PRA) was increased at 39.94 ng/mL/h (reference range: 1.50 to 5.70 ng/mL/h) and aldosterone level in the upright position was very high at 92.9 ng/dL (reference: 3.8 to 31.3 ng/dL).

What is the MOST likely diagnosis and how do you treat it?

    A. Renin-secreting tumor
    B. High renin essential hypertension
    C. Renovascular hypertension
    D. Hyperaldosteronism

The correct answer is A

Comment: Between 12% and 20% of patients with essential hypertension have PRA greater than the upper limit of the renin-sodium profile of normotensive control patients; however, less than 30% of these patients with high-renin essential hypertension have PRA exceeding 11 ng/mL/h, independent of daily sodium excretion.[1] Therefore one would anticipate encountering no more than 3.5% to 6% of all patients with PRA greater than this value. The persistence of unusually high PRA despite treatment with a blocker rendered the hypothesis of high-renin essential hypertension less likely in this case. High PRA may also suggest renovascular or malignant hypertension.[2–5] In a recently published series of malignant hypertension, 76% of patients had PRA greater than 4.9 ng/mL/h with 25% greater than 20 ng/mL/h.[2] However, patients with malignant hypertension usually present with a dramatic clinical picture and significant target-organ damage, including kidney damage and advanced retinopathy, neither of which was observed in our patient. Finally, the hypothesis of a renin-secreting tumor of the juxtaglomerular apparatus (TJGA) should be considered despite the rarity of this disease.[3]

    The captopril test has been used as a screening test for renovascular hypertension; however, remarkable variability exists in the diagnostic PRA cutoff values. Renal Doppler ultrasonography, computed tomography (CT), and magnetic resonance renal angiography have greater diagnostic accuracy for renovascular hypertension compared with the captopril test. Renal Doppler ultrasonography and CT renal angiography were performed in our patient and excluded renovascular disease. Abdominal CT with contrast injection also was performed for suspected Tumor of the juxtaglomerular apparatus (TJGA).

    Abdominal CT identified a 2.2 cm mass at the level of the corticomedullary junction between the middle and lower third of the left kidney, with very weak contrast enhancement in the late parenchymal phase. This location and these features are consistent with TJGA. Renal CT with contrast injection has almost 100% sensitivity for the detection of TJGA. Selective renal arteriography failed to identify these tumors, which usually appear as small hypovascularare as within the renal parenchyma in approximately 60% of patients, when this procedure was performed systematically. Renal vein sampling has at best 50% to 60% sensitivity in detecting renin lateralization, possibly due to the superficial location of these tumors draining through pericapsular veins rather than the main renal veins, variable blood dilution by extra renal veins, or secretory intermittence.

    The diagnosis was TJGA, and conservative surgery with tumor enucleation was performed. Serum potassium and BP values normalized within 7 days after surgery. At the 6-month follow-up, the patient remained normotensive (24-hour mean BP, 115/76 mmHg). Serum potassium level was 4.6 mEq/L, upright PRA was 0.67 ng/mL/h, aldosterone level was 9.0 ng/dL, and 24-hour proteinuria decreased to 60 mg of protein.

Case Study 4

A 15-year-old presented to the emergency department with 4 days of progressive muscular weakness. Weakness developed first in his legs and hands, progressed to his arms and thighs, and finally involved his torso. He denied nausea, vomiting, diarrhea, tingling or numbness in his legs and arms, recent strenuous exertion, and alcohol use. His medical history included diabetes mellitus type 2, hypertension, and hyperlipidemia. He had bilateral leg swelling for 6 to 8 months, for which he was treated with furosemide. He denied chest pain, shortness of breath, orthopnea, or decrease in urinary output. Physical examination was significant for increased BP of 182/92 mmHg, symmetrical flaccid paralysis with areflexia in all extremities, and bilateral pedal edema. Laboratory investigations showed the following values: sodium, 140 mmol/L; potassium, 1.8 mmol/L; chloride, 92 mmol/L; bicarbonate, 35 mmol/L; serum urea nitrogen, 25 mg/dL; serum creatinine, 1.7 mg/dL; estimated glomerular filtration rate, 43.2 mL/min/1.73 m^2, albumin, 2.8 g/dL, calcium, 7.8 mg/dL, and creatine kinase, 2980 U/L. Urine electrolyte values were as follows: potassium, 51.9 mmol/L, and osmolality, 500 mOsm/kg. Serum osmolality was 298 mOsm/kg. Calculated transtubular potassium gradient was 17.2. Further testing showed plasma renin activity (PRA) of 0.31 ng/mL/h (reference range for nonhypertensive upright adults: 0.65 to 5.0 ng/mL/h); serum aldosterone (upright, 8:00 AM), 3 ng/dL (reference ranges: < 28 ng/dL); thyroid-stimulating hormone, 0.70 mIU/mL (reference range: 0.34 to 4.82 mIU/mL); and cortisol, 12.61 g/dL (347.9 nmol/L (reference range: 3.09 to 16.6 nmol/L).

What is the differential diagnosis of hypokalemia in this patient and what is the treatment for this condition?

A. Cushing syndrome
B. Liddle syndrome
C. Hyperaldosteronism
D. Licorice and carbenxolone ingestion

The correct answers are A, B, C, and D

Comment: This patient had hypertension, hypokalemia, and bilateral symmetrical muscle weakness associated with low aldosterone and renin levels. Decreased potassium intake is rarely the sole cause of hypokalemia because urinary excretion of potassium can be decreased efficiently to 15 mEq/day. Hypokalemia caused by transcellular shift is transient, as seen with thyrotoxic periodic paralysis or hypokalemic periodic paralysis. Hypokalemia is more commonly caused by either increased gastrointestinal loss or urinary loss. In our patient, gastrointestinal loss could be excluded because the patient denied diarrhea. To explore the cause of hypokalemia from urinary losses associated with hypertension, PRA will narrow the differential diagnosis: (1) increased PRA: secondary hyperaldosteronism (renovascular hypertension, diuretics, renin-secreting tumor, malignant hypertension, and coarctation of the aorta); and (2) low PRA: primary hyperaldosteronism, Cushing syndrome, exogenous mineralocorticoids, Liddle syndrome, and licorice and carbenxolone ingestion.[1-3]

Plasma aldosterone levels and PRA are the most helpful laboratory tests to make the diagnosis. Both plasma aldosterone concentration and PRA were less than the reference range, which excluded the possibility of primary and secondary hyperaldosteronism. The serum cortisol level was normal; however, the increased transtubular potassium gradient suggested urinary loss of potassium. Careful history taking showed that the patient was ingesting bags of licorice, which led to this mineralocorticoid excess state.[2,3]

Licorice is made from the root of Glycyrrhiza glabra. Metabolized to glycyrrhetic acid, it inhibits the enzyme 11-hydroxysteroid dehydrogenase 2 (encoded by the *HSD11B2* gene), which converts active cortisol to locally inactive cortisone at the renal tubule. The accumulated cortisol has mineralocorticoid-like activity that acts on the receptor in the distal convoluted tubules, causing sodium retention and potassium wasting, and leads to a state of hypertension and hypokalemia.

The licorice-induced mineralocorticoid effect is usually reversible upon cessation of licorice ingestion. It also responds to spironolactone therapy. Dexamethasone may be considered because it suppresses endogenous cortisol production and thus decreases cortisol-mediated mineralocorticoid activity. The time required for correction of the potassium deficit after stopping licorice ingestion varies from days to weeks because of the large volume of distribution and long biological half-life of glycyrrhetinic acid. This patient was admitted to the intensive care unit, and after 3 days of receiving continuous supplements, serum potassium level normalized and clinical symptoms improved. He was discharged on oral potassium supplement therapy and advised not to eat licorice. At 2 weeks' follow-up, blood pressure was 140/60 mmHg and chemistry test results included the following values: potassium, 4.5 mmol/L; serum creatinine, 1.0 mg/dL; and estimated glomerular filtration rate, 79.7 mL/min/1.73 m^2 off potassium supplements.

Case Study 5

A 19-year-old woman with peptic ulcer disease reports 6 days of persistent vomiting. On physical examination, the blood pressure is found to be 100/60 mmHg without postural change, the skin turgor is decreased, and the jugular neck veins are flat. The initial laboratory data are: Serum sodium 140 mmol/L, potassium 2.2 mmol/L, chloride 86 mmol/L, bicarbonate 42 mmol/L, arterial pH 7.53, and PCO$_2$ 53 mmHg.

How would you treat this patient?

    A. Isotonic saline containing 40 mmol of potassium/L as KCl
    B. 5% Dextrose in water containing 40 mmol of potassium/L as KCl
    C. Half-isotonic saline containing 40 mmol of potassium/L as KCl
    D. Half-isotonic saline containing 80 mmol of potassium/L as KCl

The correct answer is C
Comment: This patient is both volume and potassium depleted. Thus, treatment should consist of half-isotonic saline to which 40 mmol of potassium (as KCl) should be added.[1,2] Correction of volume and chloride depletion will allow the excess bicarbonate to be excreted. Thus, the anion gap between the high urine (Na$^+$+K$^+$) concentration and low urine Cl$^-$ concentration is due primarily to HCO$_3^-$.

Note that the urine chloride concentration is still low in this patient, indicating the need for further fluid and chloride replacement; the urine sodium concentration is not an accurate estimate of volume status in this setting because the excretion of bicarbonate obligates sodium loss.

Case Study 6

A 12-year-old girl complains of easy fatigability and weakness for 1 year. She has no other symptoms. The physical examination is unremarkable, including a normal blood pressure. The following laboratory tests have been repeatedly present during this time:

    Serum sodium 141 mmol/L, potassium 2.1 mmol/L, chloride 85 mmol/L, bicarbonate 45 mmol/L, urine sodium 80 mmol/L, and potassium 170 mmol/L.

What is the differential diagnosis?

A. Bartter syndrome
B. Liddle syndrome
C. Hyperaldosteronism
D. Apparent mineralocorticoid excess

The correct answer is A

Comment: The differential diagnosis of unexplained hypokalemia, urinary potassium wasting, and metabolic alkalosis includes surreptitious diuretic use or vomiting (during the phase of bicarbonate excretion in which both sodium and potassium excretion are increased) or some form of primary hyperaldosteronism.[1,2] The normal BP in this patient excludes all of the causes of the last condition other than Bartter syndrome.

The urine chloride concentration should be measured next. A value below 25 mmol/L is highly suggestive of vomiting (which was present in this case), whereas a higher value is consistent with diuretic use or Bartter syndrome. The last two conditions can usually be distinguished by a urinary assay for diuretics.

Case Study 7

A 19-year-old woman with type 1, insulin-dependent diabetes is admitted to the hospital with a soft-tissue infection of the palate. The initial laboratory data include the following:

Serum sodium 140 mmol/L, potassium 3.8 mmol/L, chloride 110 mmol/L, bicarbonate 23 mmol/L, and glucose 147 mg/dL.

The patient eats sparingly because of pain on swallowing. To minimize the risk of hypoglycemia, her insulin is withheld. Repeat blood tests are obtained 36 hours later: Serum sodium 135 mmol/L, potassium 5.0 mmol/L, chloride 105 mmol/L, bicarbonate 15 mmol/L, glucose 270 mg/dL, anion gap 15 mmol/L, ketone 4+ arterial pH 7.32, and PCO_2 30 mmHg.

Why is the anion gap only slightly elevated despite the presence of hypokalemia and ketoacidosis?

A. β-Hydroxybutyrate and acetoacetate excretion in urine
B. Laboratory error
C. Increased serum sulfates and phosphates concentration
D. Ethylene glycol ingestion

The correct answer is A

Comment: The acidemia is due to retention of H^+ ions from the ketoacids; the associated anions (β-hydroxybutyrate and acetoacetate) were presumably excreted in the urine, resulting in only a minor elevation in the anion gap. The patient should be given insulin with glucose. This will correct the ketoacidosis without the risk of hypoglycemia.[1,2]

Case Study 8

A 12-year-old girl complains of easy fatigability and weakness. She has no other complaints. The physical examination is unremarkable, including a normal blood pressure. The following laboratory data are obtained: Serum sodium 141 mmol/L, potassium 2.1 mmol/L, chloride 85 mmol/L, bicarbonate 45 mmol/L, urine sodium 80 mmol/L, potassium 170 mmol/L, and chloride 10 mmol/L.

What is the MOST likely diagnosis?

  A. Liddle syndrome
  B. Primary hyperaldosteronism
  C. Diuretic abuse
  D. Bartter syndrome

The correct diagnosis is A

Comment: The differential diagnosis of unexplained hypokalemia, urinary potassium wasting, and metabolic alkalosis includes surreptitious diuretic use or vomiting during the phase of bicarbonate excretion in which both sodium and potassium excretion are increased and some form of primary hyperaldosteronism.[1,2] The normal BP in this patient excludes all of the causes of the last condition other than Bartter syndrome. Viewing this as a diagnostic problem of metabolic alkalosis and measuring the urine chloride concentration can distinguish these disorders. A value below 25 mmol/L is highly suggestive of vomiting (which was present in this case), whereas a higher value is consistent with diuretic use or Bartter syndrome. The last two conditions can usually be distinguished by a urinary assay for diuretics.[1,2]

Case Study 9

A 19-year-old man is found to be hypertensive and hypokalemic. A resident taking a careful history discovers that the patient is extremely fond of licorice.

Which of the following genetic defects produces a similar syndrome?

  A. Mutation in the gene for the inwardly rectifying potassium channel (ROMK)
  B. Mutation in the gene for the basolateral chloride channel CLCNKB
  C. Mutation in the gene for the sodium-chloride cotransporter
  D. Mutation in the gene for 11-β-hydroxysteroid dehydrogenase
  E. A chimeric gene with portions of the 11-β-hydroxylase gene and the aldosterone synthesis gene

The correct answer is D

Comment: Aldosterone, the most important mineralocorticoid, increases sodium reabsorption and potassium secretion in the distal nephron. Excessive secretion of mineralocorticoids or abnormal sensitivity to mineralocorticoid hormones may result in hypokalemia, suppressed plasma renin activity, and hypertension.[1-3] The syndrome of apparent mineralocorticoid excess (AME) is an inherited form of hypertension in which 11-β-hydroxysteroid dehydrogenase is defective.[1] This enzyme converts cortisol to its inactive metabolite, cortisone. Because mineralocorticoid receptors themselves have similar affinities for cortisol and aldosterone, the deficiency allows these receptors to be occupied by cortisol, which normally circulates at much higher plasma levels than aldosterone. Licorice contains glycyrrhetinic acid and mimics the hereditary syndrome because it inhibits 11-β-hydroxysteroid dehydrogenase.

Case Study 10

A 17-year-old young man presents to the emergency room with profound weakness of the lower and upper extremities on waking in the morning.

He has no history of prior episodes and denies weight loss, change in bowel habits, palpitations, heat intolerance, or excessive perspirations. He is not taking medications, including laxatives or diuretics, and denies drug or alcohol use. Blood pressure is 150/100 mmHg; heart rate,

110 per minute, respiratory rate, 20 breaths/min; and body temperature, 36.9 °C. There is a symmetric flaccid paralysis with areflexia in the lower and upper extremities. The remainder of the physical examination is unremarkable. Laboratory studies show serum levels of sodium, 142 mmol/L; potassium, 1.8 mmol/L; chloride, 104 mmol/L; bicarbonate, 24 mmol/L; calcium, 10 mg/dL, phosphate, 1.2 mg/dL, magnesium, 1.6 mg/dL, glucose, 132 mg/dL, urea nitrogen, 15 mg/dL, and creatinine, 0.8 mg/ dL. Urine potassium is 1.8 mEq/L, creatinine is 146 mg/dL, and osmolality is 500 mOsm/kg of H_2O.

What is the best treatment for this patient?

    A. Potassium chloride in dextrose 5% in water, 120 mEq over 6 hours
    B. Potassium chloride in hypertonic saline solution, 120 mEq over 6 hours
    C. Potassium phosphate in normal saline, 120 mEq over 6 hours
    D. Amiloride, 10 mg, orally
    E. Propranolol, 200 mg, orally

The correct answer is E
Comment: Hypokalemic periodic paralysis may be familial with autosomal dominant inheritance, or it may be acquired in patients with thyrotoxicosis.[1] Thyroid hormone increases sodium–potassium–adenosine triphosphate (ATP)ase activity on muscle cells, and excess thyroid hormone may thus increase sensitivity to the hypokalemic action of epinephrine or insulin, mediated by sodium–potassium–ATPase.[1,2]

    Treatment of paralytic episodes with potassium may be effective; however, this therapy may lead to post treatment hyperkalemia as potassium moves back out of the cells. Propranolol has been used to prevent acute episodes of thyrotoxic periodic paralysis and it may also be effective in acute attacks, without inducing rebound hyperkalemia.[1,2]

Case Study 11

A 13-year-old young woman complains of profound weakness and polyuria. She is taking no medications and has no gastrointestinal complaints. Pertinent clinical findings include a blood pressure of 90/50 mmHg with orthostatic dizziness. Laboratory studies show plasma/serum levels of sodium, 140 mmol/L; potassium, 2.5 mmol/L; chloride, 110 mmol/L; bicarbonate, 33 mmol/L; urea nitrogen, 25 mg/dL; and creatinine, 0.7 mg/dL. A 24-hour urine contained sodium, 90 mmol/L; potassium, 60 mmol/L; chloride, 110 mmol/L; and calcium, 280 mg/L. Plasma renin activity and aldosterone levels are elevated.

These findings are most suggestive of which one of the following?

    A. Gitelman syndrome
    B. Licorice ingestion
    C. Bartter syndrome
    D. Adrenal Adenoma
    E. Liddle syndrome

The correct answer is C
Comment: This patient is an example of classical Bartter syndrome, characterized by early onset of metabolic alkalosis, renal potassium wasting, polyuria, and polydipsia without hypertension.[1,2] Symptoms may include vomiting, constipation, salt craving, and a tendency to volume depletion. Growth retardation follows if treatment is not initiated. Unlike patients with Gitelman syndrome, their calcium excretion is elevated.

Adrenal adenoma, licorice ingestion, and Liddle syndrome are all causes of hypokalemic metabolic alkalosis, but these disorders are associated with hypertension.

Case Study 12

A 16-year-old young woman has been referred for evaluation of hypokalemia. She has no significant past medical history and does not smoke or drink alcohol, and she denies the use of any medications. Family history is negative, but she is not sure if her parents or siblings have been diagnosed with hypertension. She avoids bread, pasta, and desserts. She denies the use of licorice, but she does eat grapefruit. Her most recent clinic visit had been 3 years earlier, at which time there were no abnormal physical or laboratory findings. Recently, the patient has begun to note occasional fatigue and muscle weakness during exercise. She also experiences occasional abdominal pain for which she saw her physician.

The physical examination is generally unremarkable, without edema, but with mild lower extremity muscle weakness. Her body mass index is $25.1\,kg/m^2$; blood pressure, 152/92 mmHg with little postural change; pulse rate, 84 beats/min; respiration rate, 12 breaths/min; and body temperature, 37 °C. Laboratory studies show blood levels of sodium, 142 mmol/L; potassium, 2.9 mmol/L; carbon dioxide, 29 mmol/L; chloride, 106 mmol/L; urea nitrogen, 12 mg/dL; and creatinine, 0.8 mg/dL. Urinalysis shows a specific gravity of 1.030, otherwise negative with unremarkable sediment.

What further studies would you like to obtain at this time?

    A. Spot urine for potassium-creatinine ratio
    B. 24-hour urine for potassium and creatinine
    C. Serum aldosterone level
    D. Serum cortisol level
    E. Spot urine for anion gap

The correct answer is A
Comment: The first step is the evaluation of urinary potassium excretion. A urinary potassium–creatinine ratio value exceeding 1.5 is evidence of inappropriate urinary potassium excretion in the face of hypokalemia and helps to rule out diarrhea or laxative abuse as the cause.[1,2]

Case Study 13

The random urinary potassium-creatinine ratio value is 2.1 in the above case.

Which of the following have we ruled out as a likely cause of the hypokalemia with this measurement?

    A. Excess gastrointestinal losses
    B. Excess urinary losses
    C. Lower gastrointestinal tract potassium loss
    D. Surreptitious diuretic abuse

The correct answer is C
Comment: The urinary potassium excretion is inappropriate for someone with hypokalemia. This indicates that the likely cause is not lower gastrointestinal loss of potassium. Upper gastrointestinal loss could still be a proximate cause as the predominant mechanism for hypokalemia in that situation is renal due to secondary hyperaldosteronism and bicarbonate in the tubular fluid acting as a non-reabsorbable anion. The actual potassium loss from gastric losses is not very much, as potassium concentration is only 5 to 10 mEq/L in gastric fluid.[1,2]

Case Study 14

Which of the following conditions remain in the differential diagnosis of this patient? (Select all that apply)

A. Bartter syndrome
B. Gitelman syndrome
C. Diuretic abuse
D. Primary hyperaldosteronism
E. Secondary hyperaldosteronism
F. Apparent mineralocorticoid excess (AME)
G. Liddle syndrome

The correct answers are D, E, F, and G

Comment: The presence of hypertension and mild metabolic alkalosis indicates that all causes of primary and secondary hyperaldosteronism, as well as Liddle syndrome and the various forms of AME, have to be considered. Blood pressure would not be typically elevated with Bartter or Gitelman syndrome, but the abuse of diuretics in hypertensive patients should still be considered.[1,2]

Case Study 15

Which of the following studies would you like to order at this time? (Select all that apply)

A. Serum cortisol concentration
B. Diuretic screen concentration
C. Plasma aldosterone concentration
D. Plasma renin activity
E. Plasma magnesium concentration

The correct answers are C and D

Comment: Since we are considering the causes of hypokalemia associated with metabolic alkalosis and hypertension, measurements of plasma aldosterone concentration and plasma renin activity are necessary to differentiate the various conditions.[1,2]

Hypomagnesemia is not a cause of hypertension, nor is diuretic abuse. Diuretic abuse in a hypertensive patient might be a possibility, but it would be worthwhile to first document an elevated level of both renin and aldosterone. A plasma cortisol measurement may be of value later, but it should not be the initial test in trying to make this differentiation.

Case Study 16

Serum aldosterone level is 2.2 ng/dL (reference: 4 to 31 ng/dL) and plasma renin activity is less than 0.1 ng/mL/h (reference: 0.5 to 4 ng/mL/h).

Which of the following conditions remain under diagnostic consideration? (Select all that apply)

A. Primary hyperaldosteronism
B. Liddle syndrome
C. Renovascular hypertension
D. Diuretic abuse
E. Syndrome of apparent mineralocorticoid excess (AME)

F. Cushing syndrome
G. Deoxycorticosterone-acetate secreting tumor
H. Renin-secreting tumor

The correct answers are B and E
Comment: The data are clearly consistent with suppressed levels of aldosterone and renin. The differential diagnosis therefore now consists of conditions associated with no aldosterone-mediated mineralocorticoid excess.

Diuretic abuse and primary or secondary hyperaldosteronism are no longer considerations as all would have elevated levels of aldosterone.

Diuretic abuse and secondary hyperaldosteronism, renovascular hypertension, and renin-secreting tumor would also be associated with elevated plasma renin activity.[1,2]

Case Study 17

At this point, it might be valuable to review the patient's history.

Which of the following aspects of the patient's history might have significance to her laboratory data? (Select all that apply)

A. Social history
B. Dietary history
C. Family history
D. Current medications
E. History of present illness

The correct answers are B and C
Comment: Two aspects of the dietary history are very important. She denies ingesting licorice, but apparently ingests large amounts of grapefruit. Acquired AME is seen with ingestion of licorice and grapefruit. Dietary flavinoids present in licorice and in grapefruit inhibit the enzyme 11-β-hydroxysteroid dehydrogenase, allowing cortisol to occupy the mineralocorticoid receptor.[1,2]

Case Study 18

A decision is made to treat the patient. She is started on spironolactone, 100 mg/day. Then, she returns 10 days later. Her blood pressure is 160/90 mmHg and her serum sodium is 140 mmol/L; potassium, 3.1 mmol/L; chloride, 107 mmol/L; and bicarbonate, 30 mmol/L. She is then switched to amiloride and returns 2 weeks later. At this point, blood pressure is 127/78 mmHg.

What is the likely diagnosis?

A. Grapefruit-induced hypokalemia
B. Congenital syndrome of apparent mineralocorticoid excess (AME)
C. Liddle syndrome
D. Gitelman syndrome
E. Bartter syndrome

The correct answer is C
Comment: The differential response to amiloride is indicative of Liddle syndrome.[1,2] The mechanism of AME caused by either a genetic defect or an acquired abnormality in 11-β hydroxysteroid dehydrogenase (due to licorice or grapefruit in the latter case) is enhanced mineralocorticoid activity by virtue of occupation of the mineralocorticoid receptor by glucocorticoids. Thus, the

symptoms should respond to receptor occupant ion by spironolactone. In contrast, Liddle syndrome is due to enhanced activity of the sodium channel, which is unaffected by Spironolactone, but is blocked by amiloride.

Case Study 19

How would you confirm the diagnosis? (Select all that apply)

A. Genetic testing
B. Measurement of the ratio of cortisol to cortisone in a 24-hour urine
C. Measurement of urinary 17-hydroxysteroid
D. Measurement of plasma aldosterone level
E. Measurement of plasma renin level

The correct answers are A and B
Comment: Genetic testing can confirm the defect in Liddle syndrome.[1,2] At that point, family members should be evaluated, so that any of them with hypertension can receive appropriate treatment. Diagnosis of AME syndrome is usually done by demonstration of an excess of free urinary cortisol over free urinary cortisone in a 24-hour urine collection, although genetic testing can identify the congenital defect.

Case Study 20

A 15-year-old male presented with 3 weeks of dyspnea and cough with blood-tinged mucous. Computed tomography of the chest revealed a large mediastinal mass, and bronchoscopy with biopsy confirmed small cell lung carcinoma. There were no adrenal or brain metastases. On admission, laboratory values included potassium of 2.5 mmol/L and serum bicarbonate of 40 mmol/L. He was treated with normal saline solution infusion and potassium supple-mentation and was then discharged. The patient was readmitted with agitation, confusion, and hypoxia. On examination, he was hypertensive with systolic blood pressure of 160 to 170 mmHg. Potassium level was 2.0 mmol/L, serum bicarbonate level was 55 mmol/L, and sodium level was 149 mmol/L, and he had normal kidney function. Early-morning cortisol level was elevated at 47 mg/dL, and 24-hour urinary cortisol level was 7859 (reference: 4 to 50) mg/dL. Both low- and high-dose dexa-methasone suppression tests failed to suppress his cortisol level. Other laboratory tests showed an aldosterone level 1.0 ng/dL and low plasma renin activity. Arterial blood gas revealed pH of 7.65, PCO_2 of 64.3 mmHg, and PO_2 of 56 mmHg. Urinalysis showed specific gravity of 1.008 and urine osmolality of 266 mOsm/kg. He had polyuria during admission with urine output of 6.3 L/day. Hypokalemia persisted despite appropriate potassium supplementation.

What is the cause of this patient's polyuria and what is the appropriate treatment for this patient?

A. Primary aldosteronism
B. Renin-secreting tumor
C. Nephrogenic diabetes insipidus due to ectopic adrenocorticotropic hormone (ACTH) syndrome
D. Apparent mineralocorticoid excess (AME)

The correct answer is C
Comment: Hypokalemia can arise from a transcellular shift or increased renal and gastrointestinal losses. This patient's metabolic abnormalities persisted despite avoidance of diuretics, lack of

gastrointestinal losses, and appropriate potassium supplementation. The triad of hypertension, severe hypokalemia, and metabolic alkalosis can be seen in various conditions that can be differentiated based on the patient's renin-angiotensin-aldosterone system profile. Suppressed plasma renin activity (PRA), increased plasma aldosterone concentration (PAC), and PAC: PRA ratio ≥ 20 is characteristic of primary hyperaldosteronism.[1] Elevation of both PRA and PAC levels suggests secondary hyperaldosteronism (i.e., renovascular hypertension, diuretic use, or a renin-secreting tumor). Alternatively, suppression of both PRA and PAC levels should prompt investigation for alternative causes of severe hypokalemia and metabolic alkalosis, such as congenital adrenal hyperplasia, Liddle syndrome, or states of apparent mineralocorticoid excess.

This patient had suppressed PRA and PAC levels, which in the clinical context of lung cancer led to the diagnosis of ectopic adrenocorticotropic hormone (ACTH) syndrome.[2,3]

Under normal conditions, excess cortisol is converted to its inactive metabolite cortisone by the kidney by the enzyme 11-β-hydroxysteroid dehydrogenase. Excessive amounts of active cortisol can overwhelm the capacity of this enzyme, resulting in cross-reactivity with renal mineralocorticoid receptors. This can lead to an acquired form of apparent mineralocorticoid excess with severe hypokalemia and metabolic alkalosis. Suppression of plasma renin and aldosterone release occurs by negative feedback inhibition. Additionally, ectopic ACTH causes increased secretion of the mineralocorticoid-like hormones, such as 11 deoxycorticosterone and corticosterone, which can potentially lead to a greater degree of hypokalemia and metabolic alkalosis compared to adrenal-limited Cushing syndrome.

The differential diagnosis of polyuria includes central or nephrogenic diabetes insipidus and psychogenic polydipsia.[4,5] An osmotic load, water load, or a mix of both can drive polyuria. Osmotic diuresis is characterized by high urine osmolality (>300 mOsm/kg) and can be seen in hyperglycemia, high-protein enteral nutrition, and urea or mannitol administration. Pure water diuresis presents with low urine osmolality (<100 mOsm/kg) and results from increased free water excretion in the absence of antidiuretic hormone, reduced antidiuretic hormone responsiveness, or free water intoxication (psychogenic polydipsia). This patient's urine osmolality of 266 mOsm/kg is most consistent with mixed polyuria. Given his normal kidney function and solute and water intake, the cause was thought to be diabetes insipidus. His severe and prolonged hypokalemia (a known cause of renal tubular dysfunction) likely resulted in defective urine concentrating ability and partial nephrogenic diabetes insipidus. Lack of brain metastases made central diabetes insipidus less likely. Of note, he had only mild hypernatremia, likely due to an intact thirst mechanism and the ability to maintain free water intake.

Complete removal of an ACTH-secreting tumor is the optimal treatment of ectopic ACTH syndrome. Because this patient had a nonresectable tumor, the hypercortisolism was treated medically with an adrenal enzyme inhibitor (ketoconazole, 200 mg, three times daily). This led to near normalization of serum cortisol levels. Additionally, given concern for hypokalemia-induced nephrogenic diabetes insipidus, he was treated with a potassium-sparing diuretic (amiloride, 5 mg/day) with subsequent improvement in all electrolyte level derangements. His urine output also improved to 1.0 L/day.

Case Study 21

A 15-year-old Caucasian girl presented to the emergency department with a 2-day history of generalized body weakness, abdominal pain, and an inability to move her extremities. She reported poor appetite, fatigue, dizziness, generalized joint pains, back pain, nausea, and two episodes of vomiting. She denied having a history of diarrhea, dysuria, blood in the urine, changes in urine output, and frequent or urgent urination. She also denied having a history of recent upper respiratory symptoms, headaches, chest pain, difficulty breathing, leg or joint swelling. There was no history of seizures, rash, syncope, speech difficulty, lightheadedness, or numbness. She denied recent intense exercise, starvation, high-carbohydrate and/or low-potassium diet, and ingestion of an illicit drugs or alcohol.

Her past medical history was significant for a history of medullary sponge kidneys (MSK) and renal tubular acidosis (RTA) diagnosed 2 years ago when being worked up for generalized muscle weakness. She reported having had three previous episodes of similar presentations over the past 2 years and was told that she had low serum potassium levels. All three episodes necessitated a hospital admission lasting for about a day and the episode resolved with intravenous potassium supplements and hydration. The patient's mother was unsure of what the serum potassium levels had been between those episodes. She had been placed on daily potassium and bicarbonate supplements for the past 1-year but had not been taking it for the past 2 months. She was born at full term with a birth weight of 7.33 kg. Her growth and development were appropriate with no history of failure to thrive or repeated hospitalizations for dehydration episodes. There was no history of deafness, polyuria, or bone loss. There was no history suggestive of autoimmune disorders. She was sexually active with one male partner and had no history of sexually transmitted disease. Her family history was insignificant for consanguinity, similar problems, low serum potassium or any other renal diseases.

On physical examination, her vitals were as follows: blood pressure (BP) 114/56 mmHg manually in the right upper extremity with an adequate sized cuff (95th percentile BP: 126/82 mmHg), pulse 100 beats/min, respiratory rate 16 breath/min, temperature 36.6 °C, weight 58.9 kg (70th centile), height 157 cm (20th centile), body mass index 24 kg/m² (82nd centile), and SPO_2 99% on room air. She was alert and oriented. She was otherwise well, developed and well nourished. Extraocular movements were normal. There was no periorbital edema. There was no moon facies. There was no cervical adenopathy. She did have mild neck tenderness with restricted neck movements. Speech was not slurred. Heart sounds were normal with regular rhythm and with no murmurs. Lungs were clear to auscultation with symmetric chest expansion and no use of accessory muscles. Abdomen examination showed mild generalized tenderness. Bowel sounds were normal. There was marked tenderness in both lower extremities. Deep tendon reflexes were present but diminished and the muscle strength was two in all four extremities. Tone was diminished in all four extremities, more so in the lower extremities. Pain sensation was intact. There were no cranial nerve deficits.

Laboratory investigations showed normal complete blood count and liver function test. Initial arterial blood gas showed pH 7.18, PCO_2 28 mmHg, PO_2 129 mmHg, bicarbonate 10 mmol/L and base excess -18 mmol/L. Initial serum electrolytes showed serum Na^+ 140 mmol/L, K^+ less than 1 mmol/L, Cl^- 116 mmol/L, bicarbonate 13 mmol/L, BUN 17 mg/dL, creatinine 1.19 mg/dL, calcium 8.1 mg/dL, P 1.5 mg/dL, which later increased to 4 mg/dL, magnesium 2.6 mg/dL, lactate less than 0.3 mmol/L, anion gap 11, albumin 3.6 g/dL, and serum osmolality of 290 mOsm/kg. Urine osmolality was 400 mOsm/kg, spot urine sodium 68 mmol/L, spot urine potassium 20 mmol/L, spot urine creatinine 24 mg/dL, spot urine calcium 12 mg/dL, spot urine protein 16 mg/dL, and positive urine myolobin. Transtubular potassium gradient (TTKG) was elevated at 14.5 (value >2 during hypokalemia indicates renal loss). Spot urine calcium to creatinine ratio was 0.5. Initial urinalysis showed pH of 7.5 (which remained persistently at 7 to 7.5 on repeat tests), specific gravity 1.008, no glucose, no ketones, no protein, 164 white blood cells per high power field (HPF), positive blood with 10 red blood cells per HPF, many bacteria and large leukocyte esterase and negative nitrites. Urine culture was negative. Urine toxicology was negative. Urine anion gap was + 4. Urine electrophoresis showed non-selective proteinuria. Blood culture showed no growth. Plasma renin activity was 1.5 ng/mL/h and serum aldosterone was 1.8 ng/dL. Serum 25 hydroxy vitamin D level was 28 ng/mL, intact parathyroid hormone was 52 pg/mL, and she had a normal thyroid profile. Lupus serologies were negative. Total creatine kinase level was elevated at 1392 U/L. Electrocardiography showed evidence of normal sinus rhythm, with a rate of 98 beats/min with a normal axis but generalized ST segment depression and T wave inversion with QTC 432 ms. Renal sonogram showed a right kidney of 12.4 × 4.2 × 4.3 cm and a left kidney measuring 11.7 × 4.1 × 4.3 cm. A CT scan of the abdomen and pelvis without contrast agent was performed.

She was admitted to the pediatric intensive care unit and aggressive electrolyte replacement and acidosis correction were initiated. Acidosis and electrolytes improved with replacement of potassium acetate, potassium phosphate, and bicarbonate infusions. After treatment, her venous blood gas showed pH 7.37, PCO_2 41 mmHg, PO_2 34 mmHg, bicarbonate 24 mEq/L, and a base deficit of 1.4 mEq/L. Serum bicarbonate, creatinine, and potassium on discharge were 24 mmol/L, 1.03 mg/dL, and 3.4 mmol/L, respectively. Muscle weakness and pain also resolved. Patient was discharged in a stable condition on potassium and bicarbonate supplements.

What is the MOST likely diagnosis?

A. Hypokalemic familial periodic paralysis (HFPP)
B. Primary hypoaldosteronism
C. Pseudohperadosteronism
D. Medullary sponge kidney (MSK)

The correct answer is D

Comment: Hypokalemic paralysis, as the name implies, encompasses paralysis, muscle weakness, and is seen with severe hypokalemia.[1,2] Various causes of such are mentioned above. However, the most important challenge is to differentiate between the recurrent paralyses caused by RTA, mainly the distal type, and that caused by HFPP, an entirely different condition.[3,4] The latter can be caused either by hypokalemia (most commonly) or by hyperkalemia. Hypokalemia in HFPP is not due to loss of potassium as observed in distal RTA (dRTA), but to abnormalities in its redistribution between intra- and extracellular compartments. Often, the predisposing factors are strenuous exercise, high carbohydrate diet, and other triggers. They usually have normal physical growth unlike patients with dRTA. Acidosis is not a typical feature and nephrocalcinosis is not observed. Mutations in two genes encoding subunits of skeletal muscle voltage-gated calcium or sodium channels (CACNL1A3 and SCN4A) have been identified in hypokalemic HFPP. Most of the cases are hereditary, mostly autosomal dominant (AD), but acquired cases can occur with thyrotoxicosis. Management in hypokalemic HFPP involves administration of potassium supplements and/or potassium-sparing diuretic; bicarbonate is not required, as it may worsen the paralysis by redistributing potassium intracellularly. This is in opposition with hypokalemia in dRTA where both potassium and bicarbonate supplements are required.

dRTA is characterized by an impaired capacity of the distal tubules to secrete hydrogen ions and hence ammonium secretion. Urine anion gap provides a rough estimate of urinary ammonium excretion. Besides normal serum anion gap and hyperchloremic metabolic acidosis, patients with dRTA have an abnormally high urine pH (≥ 5.5) for the degree of systemic acidemia in addition to positive urine anion gap.[4] The most common cause of dRTA in children is primary, mostly familial; it can be either autosomal dominant (AD) or recessive (AR). AD dRTA is mainly due to mutations causing defects in the kidney anion exchanger (kAE1) in the distal tubule α-intercalated cells. The AR form of dRTA is mainly due to the mutations causing defects in beta subunit of H^+ ATPase in the apical membrane of α-intercalated cells. Most of the children have some degree of growth failure. In adults, the dRTA can be associated with hypergammaglobulinemia, autoimmune conditions, e.g., systemic lupus erythematous, rheumatoid arthritis, etc., and drugs, e.g., lithium, amphotericin B, ifosfamide, etc. Other secondary causes of dRTA are hypercalciuric conditions, e.g., hyperparathyroidism, vitamin D intoxication, and sarcoidosis. Hypercalciuria is common in dRTA due to effects of chronic acidosis on both bone resorption and the renal tubular reabsorption of calcium. Hypercalciuria eventually leads to nephrocalcinosis and nephrolithiasis. Association of nephrocalcinosis with MSK has been described.

Our patient had a known diagnosis of MSK and also had typical features of bilateral diffuse medullary nephrocalcinosis. Patients with MSK can have medullary nephrocalcinosis along with renal tubular acidification defects, both proximal and dRTA have been described.[3] The latter is thought to be due to tubular disruption by cysts. MSK is a congenital disorder manifested by the formation of medullary cysts secondary to dilatation of the collecting ducts in the pericalyceal region of the renal pyramids. The gold standard test to diagnose MSK is an intravenous urography. Another diagnostic modality may be a CT scan with contrast showing persistence of the contrast enhancement in the renal collecting tubules and may be as useful as an intravenous pyelogram (IVP). MSK is usually diagnosed incidentally when being worked up for some other condition. However, growth failure can be associated with it and hence may be diagnosed in patients as early as 5 or 12 years old. In fact, most cases of dRTA described in the literature in association with MSK presented with growth failure. Severe hypokalemia in dRTA has been described in association with MSK and nephrocalcinosis. Our patient had recurrent hypokalemic paralysis secondary to dRTA but presented with normal growth. Evaluation of her growth charts prior to the diagnosis of dRTA and prior to being on potassium and bicarbonate supplements revealed normal height and weight. This may suggest an incomplete dRTA; however, we do not have an ammonium chloride test to confirm this.

dRTA is commonly associated with varying degrees of hypokalemia. However, the exact mechanism of hypokalemia is not very clear. The accepted hypothesis is that when H^+ secretion is impaired, there is simultaneous amplification of potassium secretory mechanisms involving the potassium channel, ROMK, or the epithelial sodium channels. However, some forms of dRTA can present with normal or even high serum potassium. Also, the autosomal recessive (AR) form of dRTA usually presents with more severe hypokalemia and acidosis as compared to the AD form. The primary form of dRTA can present sporadically as in our patient (most likely), as there was no similar family history or history of consanguinity. However, we could not perform mutation analysis of the kAE1or H^+ ATPase, as the patient was lost to follow-up.

Transtubular potassium gradient (TTKG) is an index of potassium secretary activity in the distal tubules. There is a positive correlation between aldosterone activity and the TTKG; a high TTKG value during hypokalemia generally reflects increased aldosterone production or increased distal tubule response to aldosterone. TTKG less than six (in adults) and less than four (in children) indicates an inappropriate renal response to hyperkalemia, whereas value greater than two during hypokalemia generally points to renal loss. Hence, the expected value of the TTKG must be interpreted as per the serum concentration of potassium. Our patient had inappropriately high TTKG in the setting of hypokalemia. The possible causes of such include hyperaldosteronism or pseudohyperaldosteronism. Her serum aldosterone level was not elevated. Additionally, the CT scan of the abdomen showed no adrenal lesions. Hypokalemia in association with hyperaldosteronism secondary to adrenal tumor has been described. Causes of pseudohyperaldosteronism including Cushing's syndrome, AME, licorice ingestion, etc., were unlikely given normal physical examination and normotension and no alkalosis.

References

Case Study 1

1 Gennari FJ. Hypokalemia. *N Engl J Med.* 1998;339(7):451–458.
2 Rose BD, Post TW. *Clinical Physiology of Acid-Base and Electrolyte Disorders.* 5th ed. New York, NY: McGraw-Hill, Inc.; 2001:551–571 [Chapter 18].
3 Lococo F, Margaritora S, Cardillo G, et al. Bronchopulmonary carcinoids causing Cushing syndrome: results from a multicentric study suggesting a more aggressive behavior. *Thorac Cardiovasc Surg.* 2016;64(2):172–181.
4 Morris DJ, Souness GW, Brem AS, et al. Interactions of mineralocorticoids and glucocorticoids in epithelial target tissues. *Kidney Int.* 2000;57(4):1370–1373.

Case Study 2

1 Van't Hoff WG. Fanconi syndrome. In: Davison AM, Cameron JS, Grunfeld JP, eds. *Oxford Textbook of Clinical Nephrology.* Oxford: Oxford University Press; 2005:961–973.

2 Vohra S, Eddy A, Levin AV, et al. Tubulointerstitial nephritis and uveitis in children and adolescents. Four new cases and a review of the literature. *Pediatr Nephrol.* 1999;13(5):426–432.
3 Servais A, Morinière V, Grünfeld J-P, et al. Late-onset nephropathic cystinosis: clinical presentation, outcome, and genotyping. *Clin J Am SocNephrol.* 2008;3(1):27–35.
4 Gahl WA, Theone JG, Schnei-der JA. Cystinosis. *N Engl J Med.* 2002;347(2):111–121.
5 Bonnardeaux A, Bichet DG. Inherited disorders of the renal tubule. In: Brenner BM, ed. *Brenner and Rectors' the Kidney.* Philadelphia: Saunders Elsevier; 2008:1390–1427.

Case Study 3

1 Brunner HR, Laragh JH, Baer L, et al. Essential hypertension: renin and aldosterone, heart attack and stroke. *N Engl J Med.* 1972;286:441–449.
2 Van den Born B-JH. Koopmans RP, van Montfrans GA: The renin-angiotensin system in malignant hypertension revisited: plasma renin activity, microangiopathic hemolysis, and renal failure in malignant hypertension. *Am J Hypertens.* 2007;20:900–906.
3 Wong L, Hsu THS, Perlroth MG, et al. Reninoma: case report and literature review. *J Hypertens.* 2008;26:368–373.
4 McVicar M, Carman C, Chandra M, et al. Hypertension secondary to renin-secreting juxtaglomerular cell tumor: case report and review of 38 cases. *Pediatr Nephrol.* 1993;7:404–412.
5 Vasbinder GB, Nelemans PJ, Kessels AG, et al. Diagnostic tests for renal artery stenosis in patients suspected of having renovascular hypertension: a meta-analysis. *Ann Intern Med.* 2001;135:401–411.

Case Study 4

1 Yasue H, Itoh T, Mizuno Y, et al. Severe hypokalemia, rhabdomyolysis, muscle paralysis, and respiratory impairment in a hypertensive patient taking herbal medicines containing licorice. *Intern Med.* 2007;46(9):575–578.
2 Armanini D, Fiore C, Mattarello MJ, et al. History of the endocrine effects of licorice. *Exp Clin Endocrinol Diabetes.* 2002;110(6):257–261.
3 Van den Bosch AE, van der Klooster JM, Zuidgeest DMH, et al. Severe hypokalaemic paralysis and rhabdomyolysis due to ingestion of liquorice. *Neth J Med.* 2005;63(4):146–148.

Case Study 5

1 Gennari FJ. Hypokalemia. *N Eng J Med.* 1998;339(7):451–458.
2 Rose BD, Post TW. *Clinical Physiology of Acid–Base and Electrolyte Disorders.* 5th ed. New York, NY: McGraw-Hill, Inc; 2001:551–571 [Chapter 18].

Case Study 6

1 Thomas D, Dubose J. Disorders of acid–base balance. In: Skorecki K, Chertow GM, Marsden PA, et al., eds. *Brenner & Rector's the Kidney.* 10th ed. Philadelphia: Elsevier; 2016:511–558.
2 Assadi F. *Clinical Decisions in Pediatric Nephrology: A Problem Solving Approach to Clinical Cases.* New York, NY: Springer; 2008:69–98 [chapter 2].

Case Study 7

1 Rose BD, Post TW. *Clinical Physiology of Acid–Base and Electrolyte Disorders.* 5th ed. New York, NY: McGraw-Hill, Inc.; 2001:551–571 [Chapter 18].
2 Assadi F. *Clinical Decisions in Pediatric Nephrology: A Problem Solving Approach to Clinical Cases.* New York, NY: Springer; 2008:69–98 [Chapter 2].

Case Study 8

1 Assadi F. *Clinical Decisions in Pediatric Nephrology: A Problem Solving Approach to Clinical Cases.* New York, NY: Springer; 2008:69–98 [Chapter 2].
2 Bonnardeaux A, Bichet DG. Inherited disorders of the renal tubule. In: Brenner BM, ed. *Brenner and Rector's the Kidney.* Philadelphia: Saunders Elsevier; 2008:1390–1427.

Case Study 9

1 White PC. 11beta-hydroxysteroid dehydrogenase and its role in the syndrome of apparent mineralocorticoid excess. *Am J Med Sci.* 2001;322:308–315.
2 Rose BD, Post TW. *Clinical Physiology of Acid–Base and Electrolyte Disorders.* 5th ed. New York, NY: McGraw-Hill; 2001:836–856.
3 Assadi F. Diagnosis of hypokalemia: a problem-solving approach to clinical cases. *Iran J Kidney Dis.* 2008;2(3):115–122.

Case Study 10

1 Lin SH, Lin YF, Halperin ML. Hypokalaemia and paralysis. *QJM.* 2001;194:133–139.
2 Assadi F. Diagnosis of hypokalemia: a problem-solving approach to clinical cases. *Iran J Kidney Dis.* 2008;2(3):115–122.

Case Study 11

1 Assadi F. Diagnosis of hypokalemia: a problem-solving approach to clinical cases. *Iran J Kidney Dis.* 2008;2(3):115–122.
2 Shaer AJ. Inherited primary renal tubular hypokalemic alkalosis: a review of Gitelman and Bartter syndromes. *Am J Med Sci.* 2002;322:316–332.

Case Study 12

1 Gennari FJ. Hypokalemia. *N Engl J Med.* 1998;339:451–458.
2 Groeneveld JHM, Sijpkens YWJ, Lin S-H, et al. An approach to the patient with severe hypokalaemia: the potassium quiz. *QJM.* 2005;98:305–316.

Case Study 13

1 Gennari FJ. Hypokalemia. *N Engl J Med.* 1998;339:451–458.
2 Groeneveld JHM, Sijpkens YWJ, Lin S-H, et al. An approach to the patient with severe hypokalaemia: the potassium quiz. *QJM.* 2005;98:305–316.

Case Study 14

1 Palmer BF, Alpern RJ. Metabolic alkalosis. *J Am Soc Nephrol.* 1977;8:1462–1469.
2 Assadi F. Diagnosis of hypokalemia: a problem-solving approach to clinical cases. *Iran J Kidney Dis.* 2008;2(3):115–122.

Case Study 15

1 Palmer BF, Alpern RJ. Metabolic alkalosis. *J Am Soc Nephrol.* 1977;8:1462–1469.
2 Assadi F. Diagnosis of hypokalemia: a problem-solving approach to clinical cases. *Iran J Kidney Dis.* 2008;2(3):115–122.

Case Study 16

1 Assadi F. Diagnosis of hypokalemia: a problem-solving approach to clinical cases. *Iran J Kidney Dis.* 2008;2(3):115–122.
2 Morineau G, Sulmont V, Salomon R, et al. Apparent mineralocorticoid excess: report of six new cases and extensive personal experience. *J Am Soc Nephrol.* 2006;17:3176–3184.

Case Study 17

1 Ishiguchi T, Mikita N, Iwata T, et al. Myoclonus and metabolic alkalosis from licorice in antacid. *Intern Med.* 2004;43:59–62.
2 Assadi F. Diagnosis of hypokalemia: a problem-solving approach to clinical cases. *Iran J Kidney Dis.* 2008;2(3):115–122.

Case Study 18

1 Assadi F. Diagnosis of hypokalemia: a problem-solving approach to clinical cases. *Iran J Kidney Dis.* 2008;2(3):115–122.
2 Botero-Velez M, Curtis JJ, Warnock DG. Brief report: Liddle's syndrome revisited—a disorder of sodium reabsorption in the distal tubule. *N Engl J Med.* 1994;33:178–181.

Case Study 19

1 Assadi F. Diagnosis of hypokalemia: a problem-solving approach to clinical cases. *Iran J Kidney Dis.* 2008;2(3):115–122.
2 Botero-Velez M, Curtis JJ, Warnock DG. Brief report: Liddle's syndrome revisited—a disorder of sodium reabsorption in the distal tubule. *N Engl J Med.* 1994;33:178–181.

Case Study 20

1 Blumenfeld JD, Sealey JE, Schlussel Y, et al. Diagnosis and treatment of primary hyperaldosteronism. *Ann Intern Med.* 1994;121(11):877–885.
2 Martinez-Valles MA, Palafox-Cazarez A, Paredes-Avina JA. Severe hypokalemia, metabolic alkalosis and hypertension in a 54 year old male with ectopic ACTH syndrome: a case report. *Cases J.* 2009;2:6174.
3 Jammalamadaka D, Shahnia S, Buller G. Refractory hypokalemia- from ectopic adrenocorticotropic hormone secreting thymic tumor. *Webmed-Central.* 2010;1(10). WMC00912.
4 Bhasin B, Velez JCQ. Evaluation of polyuria: the roles of solute loading and water diuresis. *Am J Kidney Dis.* 2016;67(3):507–511.
5 Khositseth S, Uawithya P, Somparn P, et al. Autophagic degradation of aquaporin-2 is an early event in hypokalemia-induced nephrogenic diabetes insipidus. *Sci Rep.* 2015;5:18311.

Case Study 21

1 Gamakaranage CS, Rodrigo C, Jayasinghe S, et al. Hypokalemic paralysis associated with cystic disease of the kidney: case report. *BMC Nephrol.* 2011;12:16.
2 Fontaine B, Lapie P, Plassart E, et al. Periodic paralysis and voltage-gated ion channels. *Kidney Int.* 1996;49(1):9–18.
3 Kasap B, Soylu A, Oren O, et al. Medullary sponge kidney associated with distal renal tubular acidosis in a 5-year-old girl. *Eur J Pediatr.* 2006;165:648–651.
4 Battle D, Moorthi KM, Schlueter W, et al. Distal renal tubular acidosis and the potassium enigma. *Semin Nephrol.* 2006;26(6):471–478.

CHAPTER 4

Hyperkalemia

Case Study 1

A 6-year-old boy with mild chronic renal failure is started on a low-sodium diet for hypertension. Two weeks later, he notices that he is unable to lift himself out of a chair. On physical examination, slightly decreased skin turgor and marked proximal muscle weakness are found. Blood pressure was 112/68 mmHg. The electrocardiograph (ECG) reveals peaked T waves and some widening of the P wave and QRS complex. The following blood test results are obtained: Sodium 130 mmol/L, potassium 9.8 mmol/L, chloride 98 mmol/L, bicarbonate 17 mmol/L, creatinine 2.7 mg/dL, and arterial pH 7.32.

What are the most likely factors responsible for the hyperkalemia and how would you treat the hyperkalemia?

    A. Pseudohyperkalemia
    B. Increased potassium intake
    C. Adrenal insufficiency
    D. Hyperkalemic distal renal tubular acidosis (RTA-4)

The correct answer is B
Comment: The underlying renal insufficiency, superimposed volume depletion (due to sodium wasting after the acute institution of a low-sodium diet), and metabolic acidosis may all play a contributory role.[1,2] However, many patients have these problems without life-threatening hyperkalemia. Therefore, the patient should be questioned about increased potassium intake; this patient gave a history of using large quantities of potassium chloride (KCl)-containing salt substitute.

    The patient has both severe muscle weakness and electrocardiographic changes. By definition, pseudohyperkalemia produces no symptoms or signs of potassium intoxication. Therefore, therapy should be initiated with calcium gluconate, followed by glucose, insulin, and sodium bicarbonate to temporarily drive potassium into the cells. For example, 500 mL of 10% dextrose in saline plus 10 units of regular insulin plus 45 mmol of sodium bicarbonate infused over 30 minutes will lower the plasma potassium concentration, raise the plasma sodium concentration, and produce volume expansion. Sodium polystyrene sulfonate should be given orally and repeated as necessary to remove the excess potassium. Dialysis will not be required since the patient does not have severe renal failure.

Case Study 2

A 14-year-old man with no prior medical history complains of chronic fatigue. The positive physical findings include a blood pressure of 100/60 mmHg and increased skin pigmentation. The skin turgor is relatively normal. The laboratory data are as follows: Serum sodium 130 mmol/L, potassium 6.8 mmol/L, Chloride 100 mmol/L, bicarbonate 20 mmol/L, glucose 90 mg/dL, osmolality 275 mOsm/kg, BUN 28 mg/dL, and creatinine 1.2 mg/dL, Urine sodium 50 mmol/L, potassium

34 mmol/L, osmolality 550 mOsm/kg. The electrocardiogram (EEG) shows mild peaking of the T waves in the precordial leads. An infusion of glucose and insulin in appropriate proportions results in an episode of hypoglycemia.

What is the most likely diagnosis and how would you treat this patient?

    A. Chronic kidney disease
    B. Primary adrenal insufficiency
    C. Acute renal failure
    D. Metabolic acidosis

The correct answer is B
Comment: By definition, patients with chronic hyperkalemia have a defect in renal potassium excretion, since normal subjects would rapidly excrete the excess potassium in the urine. Thus, the urine potassium concentration of 34 mmol/L is inappropriately low.

The transtubular potassium gradient (TTKG) can be calculated in this patient to assess the degree of aldosterone effect:

$$TTKG = \left[\left(Uk^+ \div \left(U_{osm} \right) \div P_{Oam} \right) \div PK^+ \right]$$

$$TTKG = [34 \div (550 \div 275) \div 6.8 \text{ or } 2.5$$

The TTKG is low in this patient, a finding that is consistent with some form of mineralocorticoid deficiency or resistance.

The findings of low blood pressure, increased skin pigmentation, a low TTKG, and hypoglycemia after the administration of glucose and insulin all point to the probable diagnosis of primary adrenal insufficiency.[1,2]

Acutely, sodium polystyrene sulfonate can be given to lower the plasma K^+ concentration. Chronically, both glucocorticoid and mineralocorticoid replacement will be required because of the persistent adrenal dysfunction.

Case Study 3

A 16-year-old female was admitted for the management of elevated blood pressure. Past medical history was uneventful except for a history of chronic kidney disease secondary to recurrent urinary tract infections diagnosed at 2 years of age. Physical examination on admission revealed a well-nourished and developed adolescent female. She weighed 55 kg and was 157 cm tall. The blood pressure was 148/92 mmHg, pulse 81 beats/min, and respiratory rate 19 breaths/min. Chest was clear to auscultation and percussion. Examination of the eyes, ears, nose, and throat was unremarkable. The remaining physical examination was also normal.

Laboratory investigation on admission showed serum sodium 138 mmol/L, potassium 4.0 mmol/L, chloride 106 mmol/L, bicarbonate 25 mmol/L, BUN 31 mg/dL, and creatinine 1.2 mg/dL. The estimated glomerular filtration rate (eGFR) was 67 mL/min/1.73 m². Urinalysis revealed a pH of 6.0, specific gravity 1.015, 2 + protein and small blood.

Treatment with enalapril (5 mg twice daily) was initiated. After 2 weeks of antihypertensive therapy the blood pressure fell to 128/81 mmHg. A repeat of serum electrolytes at this time showed serum sodium 141 mmol/L, potassium 5.9 mmol/L, chloride 110 mmol/L, total carbon dioxide 26 mmol/L, BUN 38 mg/dL, and serum creatinine concentration 1.5 mg/dL (GFR 54.3 mL/min/1.73 m²).

Which ONE of the following statements is TRUE regarding this patient condition?

A. She is likely to have bilateral renal artery stenosis and should be evaluated

B. The angiotensin converting enzyme inhibition (ACEI) should be stopped because of hyperkalemia and the worsening renal function

C. Stopping ACE inhibitor is a mistake because of long-term benefits on protection against the progression of renal disease

D. An angiotensin-converting blocker (ARB) should be substituted for ACE inhibitor because it may not affect serum creatinine values

The correct answer is B

Comment: Inhibition of renin-angiotensin system (RAS) by either ACEI or ARB slows the progression of renal disease in patients with preexisting renal insufficiency. The patient's serum creatinine returned to levels not different from baseline after the 6 weeks of ACEI therapy and remained unchanged during a 2-year follow-up, an observation that supports the notion that the initial rise in serum creatinine is not only reversible but the rate of progression of renal disease can be retarded despite prolonged use of ACEI.[1,2] Answer A should be considered in individuals when a rise in serum creatinine is 30% or greater above baseline or in patients with decreased effective circulating volume in whom rehydration has not reduced serum creatinine to baseline values within a few weeks. Answer B is incorrect because the initial rise in serum creatinine associated with ACEI use is reversible and stabilizes to baseline values within 2 to 4 weeks of therapy. Withdrawal of an ACEI should occur only when the rise in serum creatinine is greater than 30% above baseline value with the first 8 weeks of ACEI therapy. Answer D is also incorrect. The transient rise in serum creatinine levels has been reported with both ACEI and ARB. Answer E is wrong. Blood pressure reduction clearly slows renal disease progression. Furthermore, many clinical trials demonstrate additional protection against progression of renal disease when ACEI or ARB are used as an antihypertensive medication. The patient's prognosis for adverse renal outcomes would be better with controlled blood pressure than those whose blood pressure has not been adequately controlled.

Case Study 4

A 7-year-old girl with Rett syndrome (RS) was referred to the nephrology service for evaluation of persistent metabolic acidosis. She was the first child of unrelated healthy parents, born at 38 weeks' gestation, and with a birth weight of 3.0 kg (75th percentile), length 50.2 cm (75th percentile), and head circumference 39 cm (50th percentile). The neonatal period was uneventful. The family history was unremarkable. She grew normally until the age of 9 months, when she was found to have failure to thrive, developmental delay, and hypotonia. She was diagnosed with RS at 2 years of age, following an investigation for seizures complicated by gross motor dysfunction, hand wringing, decelerated head growth, loss of speech, and periodic breathing. She was treated with oxcarbazepine (Trileptal) oral suspension 900 mg daily for seizure control. On examination at 7-years of age, her weight was 18.2 kg, height was 112 cm (both below the 3rd percentile), and head circumference was 47 cm (below the 2nd percentile). Her temperature was 37.0°C, pulse 103 beats/min, respirations 22 breaths/min and blood pressure 94/69 mmHg. There was no clinical evidence of dehydration. Her craniofacial appearance was normal. The lungs were clear to auscultation bilaterally. Her heart had normal sinus rhythm without a murmur. Her abdomen was soft without masses or organomegaly. No rashes or edema were noted. Genital examination findings were normal. On neurological examination, she clearly had significant delay for age. She had limited vocalization. She was unable to sit, creep, or crawl. She exhibited stereotypical hand movements, including alternate opening and closing of the fingers, and twisting of wrists and arms were noted. Her pupils had normal reaction to light. She did not fix or follow. Her facial movements were symmetric, and she did not drool. There was no arching. Her tendon reflexes were 2 + and normal.

Initial laboratory studies revealed serum sodium 139 mmol/L, potassium 5.8 mmol/L, chloride 111 mmol/L, bicarbonate 18 mmol/L, blood urea nitrogen was 7.0 mg/dL, creatinine 0.3 mg/dL, glucose 88 mg/dL, calcium 9.2 mg/dL phosphate 5.3 mg/dL alkaline phosphatase 232 U/L, cortisol 8.8 ng/L, aldosterone 17 ng/dL, and plasma renin activity 1.9 ng/mL/h. White cell count was 4200 with 75% neutrophils. Hemoglobin was 13.1 g/dL hematocrit 40% and platelet count was 275,000. Urinalysis showed a pH of 7.0, specific gravity of 1.014, negative dipstick test result for protein, and blood with unremarkable features on microscopy. The urine culture was sterile. Urine anion gap was positive $(Na^+ + K^+) - (Cl^-)$=10 mmol/L, fractional excretion of Na^+ and K^+ were 0.6% and 4.6%, respectively. Renal ultrasound results were normal. MRI of the brain and spinal canal showed normal findings.

Alkaline therapy with sodium bicarbonate (35 mEq orally, daily for 10 days) failed to lower urine pH below 5.5 or to increase potassium excretion. Therapy with hydrochlorothiazide (HCT), 25 mg orally, daily for 7 days resulted in a fall in urine pH below 5.5, an increase in potassium excretion, and the complete resolution of acidosis. The effect of therapy was remarkable in that the child's weight and length increased by 1.3 kg and 2.0 cm, respectively, in the following 4 months, exceeding the 3rd percentile weight and height values on the growth chart.

What is the MOST likely diagnosis?

    A. Hyperkalemia distal renal tubular acidosis associated with Rett syndrome
    B. Hyperkalemia related to adrenal insufficiency
    C. Hyperkalemia related to chronic kidney disease
    D. Adrenal insufficiency

The correct answer is A
Comment: This patient had the classic phenotype of Rett, including normal early development followed by loss of purposeful use of hands, distinctive hand movements, slow head growth, apraxia, seizures, periodic apnea, and mental retardation. The finding of hyperchloremic metabolic acidosis in the presence of normal glomerular function suggests the diagnosis of renal tubular acidosis (RTA).[1,2] The finding of urinary pH above 5.5 and positive urinary anion gap during acidosis, combined with hyperkalemia, suggests the presence of hyperkalemic distal RTA.[3,4]

The cause of hyperkalemic distal RTA includes disorders that affect adrenal aldosterone synthesis, the renal response to aldosterone, and a voltage-dependent type of derangement in the distal nephron.[3-5] The normal values for cortisol, plasma renin activity (PRA) and plasma aldosterone levels in this patient exclude hypoaldosteronism as the cause of impaired urinary acidification. Furthermore, therapy with sodium bicarbonate failed to lower urine pH below 5.5 or increase potassium excretion. Administration of HCT resulted in a fall in urine pH below 5.5 and an increase in urine potassium excretion to normal, suggesting that a voltage-dependent defect, rather than aldosterone deficiency, was responsible for the altered urinary acidification observed in our patient.

Case Study 5

A 4-month-old former term female infant born to a 36-year-old healthy mother was admitted to the hospital for evaluation and management of right neck abscess and cellulitis. Outpatient treatment, including an incision and drainage done in clinic the day prior and two doses of oral antibiotics, resulted in no improvement. Past medical and surgical history was unremarkable. Family history was significant for an unspecified seizure and movement disorder in her older sister. She had appropriate growth for her age, with weight, length, and head circumference all measuring around the 20th percentile. Vitals were unremarkable on presentation, and she remained normotensive during her stay at the hospital. Exam was within normal limits, aside from erythema and induration consistent with her abscess.

Initial blood chemistry panel showed an alarmingly high potassium level of 8.4 mmol/L with slight hemolysis (normal for age is 4.1 to 5.3) with repeat of 7.3 without hemolysis. She had a low bicarbonate level of 10 mmol/L (normal for age is 19 to 24), high chloride level of 116 mmol/L (normal for age is 97 to 108), and elevated creatinine of 0.56 mg/dL (normal for age is 0.2 to 0.4). Anion gap was normal at 10 mmol/L. No electrocardiogram changes were noted. She was promptly transferred to the pediatric intensive care unit for care of her abscess and these incidental findings of hyperkalemia and non-gap metabolic acidosis. Intravenous calcium gluconate, sodium acetate, and Kayexalate (sodium polystyrene sulfonate) were given for hyperkalemia. The following morning, her potassium normalized to 5.8 mEq/L and then further to 4.7 mmol/L. Her bicarbonate level improved to 20 mmol/L, and her serum creatinine improved to 0.19 mg/dL. Renal ultrasound revealed no abnormalities.

After transfer to the general pediatrics floor, she again developed hyperkalemia of 7.5 mmol/L and non-gap metabolic acidosis. A subsequent dose of Kayexalate was given. Additional lab work revealed urine potassium of 15 mmol/L, urine sodium of 90 mmol/L, and urine chloride of 65 mmol/L, resulting in a positive urine anion gap of 40 mmol/L. She had a normal serum aldosterone level of 22 ng/L (normal for age is 6 to 89) but low renin activity of 0.2 ng/mL/h (normal for age is 2 to 37). Her hyperkalemia and metabolic acidosis were treated with fludrocortisone, high dose sodium citrate/citric acid, and kayexalate. During the hospital admission, the patient's abscess significantly improved after repeat incision and drainage and intravenous antibiotics. The family was discharged home with oral antibiotics, fludrocortisone, sodium citrate/citric acid, and Kayexalate with close nephrology follow-up.

What is the MOST likely diagnosis and how would you treat it?

A. Renal tubular acidosis type 4 (RTA-4)
B. Primary adrenal insufficiency
C. Pseudohypoaldostronism (PHA)
D. Interstitial nephritis

The correct answer is C
Comment: This patient had severe recurrent hyperkalemia, hyperchloremic metabolic acidosis, and positive urine anion gap in a setting of low plasma renin and aldosterone levels. RTA-4 was suspected.[1] Differential diagnosis of RTH-4 in children includes sequelae to critical illness, such as obstructive nephropathy, interstitial nephritis, diabetic nephropathy, primary adrenal insufficiency, or medications such as NSAIDs or ACE inhibitors.[1-3] Our patient had no history of failure to thrive or significant medical history, so likelihood of RTA-4 secondary to chronic conditions or medications was unlikely.

To elucidate whether she may have possible PHA, a genetic analysis was performed and revealed a de novo heterozygous c.1376A greater than T (p. K459M) likely pathogenic variant in the Cullin 3 (*CUL3*) gene consistent with type PHP (PHA-II).[2] This explained the low renin, hyperchloremia, severe hyperkalemia, and metabolic acidosis.

PHA-I and PHA-II are exceedingly rare genetic disorders that are caused by aldosterone resistance or reduced aldosterone production, respectively. When PHA-I occurs, patients often present with sodium wasting, hypovolemia, metabolic acidosis, and hyperkalemia in the neonatal period. PHA-II presents with hyperkalemia and hypertension in variable ages of patients, though most cases have been reported in adolescence or young adulthood. Severe hypertension tends to develop later in life in the majority of cases.

The mainstay of treatment for PHA type II is thiazide diuretic, which quickly corrects metabolic abnormalities and hypertension within 1 week. In general, dosing is titrated to normalization of blood pressure. Prognosis is good on thiazide treatment. Most patients do not have long-term sequelae as long as vitals are closely monitored over time.[2]

This patient was treated with fludrocortisone, sodium citrate/citric acid, and Kayexalate after hospital discharge. She maintained relatively stable electrolytes on this regimen, but medication dosage adjustments were frequently needed. She was promptly started on hydrochlorothiazide after genetic results confirmed PHA type II. Her other medications were weaned rapidly. To date, her blood pressure measurements have remained within normal range for age, and she is meeting all growth milestones.

Case Study 6

An 8-day-old male baby presented to our emergency unit with lethargy and poor feeding and reduced urine output since 3 days. He was a second born child of a third-degree consanguineous marriage, born at term with a birth weight of 1.8 kg with no history of significant perinatal events. However, a history of sibling death following a similar illness at day 15 of life was reported.

On examination, the child was dehydrated, the skin was mottled, and peripheral pulses were weak. The child was in shock and had a convulsion while in the emergency department. He received saline boluses and supportive management was instituted, while his investigations were awaited. He had severe respiratory distress due to pneumonia for which he required mechanical ventilation and inotropes were started for shock. Intravenous antibiotics were started in view of positive screen for sepsis. His serum potassium was 11.9 mmol/L at admission and serum sodium was 119 mmol/L. Blood urea was 78.42 mg/dL and serum creatinine was 1.41 mg/dL initially, which was subsequently documented normal (23 mg/dL, 0.4 mg/dL respectively). In view of severe hyperkalemia, he was started on peritoneal dialysis (PD) along with supportive management with sodium bicarbonate, salbutamol nebulization and potassium binding resins through nasogastric tube.

The infant improved after supportive management for sepsis and was off inotropes after 48 hours of admission. His potassium improved after 12 hours of PD (K^+ = 3.7 mEq/L), after which PD was stopped. Forty-eight hours later, the child was weaned off the ventilator, but he again developed hyperkalemia (serum potassium of 9.6 mmol/L) and hyponatremia (serum sodium of 114 mmol/L) and PD had to be instituted again. The child developed a skin rash (miliaria rubra) the following day which improved a week later and during his prolonged course of stay in the hospital he developed pneumonia, which again required him to be ventilated for 7 days. During his hospital stay, the child required a total of eight PD sessions, each time owing to uncontrollable hyperkalemia.

Additional laboratory studies revealed serum cortisol 15.94 µg/dL (reference: 2 to 11 µg/dL); 17–OH progesterone 8.13 ng/dL (reference: 3 to 90 ng/dL); aldosterone 171.1 ng/dL (reference: 2.52 to 39.2 ng/dL); and renin 6.11 ng/mL (reference: 0.15 to 2.33 ng/mL).

What is the cause of hyperkalemia in this neonate?

    A. Sepsis-induced acute kidney injury
    B. Congenital adrenal hyperplasia
    C. Type 4 renal tubular acidosis (RTA-4)
    D. Hereditary pseudohypoaldosteronism type-I (PHA-I)

The correct answer is D

Comment: The first differential considered was late onset sepsis with acute kidney injury (AKI) and electrolyte abnormalities. Since this newborn had hyperkalemia with hyponatremia, out of proportion to his AKI and sepsis, congenital adrenal hyperplasia (CAH-salt wasting type) was also considered. CAH due to 21-hydroxylase deficiency leads to decreased cortisol and aldosterone, which may present clinically like aldosterone resistance. In girls, virilization may be seen while in boys only increased pigmentation may be noted, which was absent in this child. Other inborn errors of metabolism and pseudo-hypoaldosteronism (PHA) (primary or secondary) were also considered as rare differentials.[1-3] Secondary/transient type 1 PHA occurs in the setting of obstructive urinary tract malformation or a urinary tract infection and usually gets corrected after adequate fluid resuscitation and management of infections, while other types of PHA are genetically mediated disorders of tubular transport of potassium and sodium. Type 4 renal tubular acidosis (RTA) and was also considered in view of deranged renal functions and hyperkalemia, but it occurs in setting of obstructive uropathy or diabetic nephropathy, which were absent in the child.[1-3]

Sepsis induced AKI as a primary cause for his illness was ruled out as the child continued to have severe hyperkalemia despite improvement in sepsis and initial resuscitation. CAH was ruled out as serum cortisol level was elevated and 17–OH progesterone was suppressed. Serum ammonia, lactate, and blood sugar were normal, which ruled against inborn errors of metabolism.

RTA type 4 and secondary or transient PHA was also ruled out as renal dysfunction improved after correcting the initial shock and fluid bolus, and ultrasound of kidneys and urinary tract did not reveal any obstructive pathology.

Serum aldosterone and renin activity were normal. When both elevated, favoring a diagnosis of PHA, likely of genetic etiology as secondary and transient forms were ruled out.

Among the various types of PHA that are described, the PHA type 1 may be (a) systemic/multiple site form or (b) renal limited. The former occurs due to defects in epithelial sodium channel (ENaC) or defective mineralocorticoid receptor at multiple sites. Since the ENaC is expressed in all epithelial tissues, it is associated with widespread systemic manifestations such as pulmonary infections. One may find a high sweat or salivary sodium level, which provides a clue to multisystem involvement. This helps to differentiate it from the renal limited form, which occurs due to defects in receptors for mineralocorticoid on tubular epithelial cells.[1,2]

Since our patient had skin as well as respiratory system infections, the possibility of type 1 autosomal recessive variant of PHA was considered, which could be confirmed further by performing a genetic analysis.

PHA occurs due to renal tubular unresponsiveness to the action of aldosterone. Aldosterone acts on the aldosterone receptor and then through nuclear transcription pathways and increases the activity of basolateral Na^+/K^+ adenosine triphosphate (ATP)ase, luminal expression of epithelial sodium channel (ENaC) and the activity of luminal renal outer medullary potassium (ROMK) channels. A defective mineralocorticoid receptor function or a failure of ENaC would lead to sodium wasting and failure of potassium excretion.

Multiple site type 1 PHA (ar-PHA1) is inherited as an autosomal recessive trait due to mutations in *SCNN1A* located in 12p13.31, *SCNN1B*, and *SCNN1G*, both situated in the locus 16p12.2. Each of these three genes is responsible for making one of the subunits of the ENaC protein complex. When homologous mutations are introduced into alpha, beta, or gamma subunits of ENaC, they all bring about a change in sodium channel gating, causing a reduction in sodium channel opening probability.

Renal form (ad-PHA1) shows autosomal dominant inheritance and is due to heterozygous mutation of *NR3C2* located at 4q31.1, which is responsible for making the mineralocorticoid receptor protein. Various mutations have been described worldwide in coding regions of ENaC subunit genes. Most of these cases are attributed to mutations in the alpha subunit gene (*SCNN1A*). In the present case, a known homozygous mutation in the *SCNN1B* gene was identified, which is relatively uncommon, as well as a new variant.

In the acute phase of illness, the child may require adequate fluid resuscitation, supportive measures for hyperkalemia and even transient dialysis for management of refractory hyperkalemia. For AD-PHA, only sodium supplementation may be required that generally becomes unnecessary by 3 years of age, which may be due to maturation of renal salt conserving ability. In children with AR-PHA, management entails lifelong salt supplementation and intensive monitoring for management of systemic features like respiratory complications. The requirement of sodium may sometimes be very high, reaching up to 15 to 20 g a day. A diet low in potassium or measures to reduce potassium content of foods should be instituted for every child. The use of potassium binding resins, like sodium polystyrene, helps to excrete large amounts of potassium. In refractory cases, indomethacin may be used to reduce loss of sodium in urine, as it helps inhibit prostaglandin synthesis. Though fludrocortisone is effective in congenital adrenal hyperplasia, the same is not true for PHA as the defective ENaC channel causes resistance to both aldosterone and fludrocortisone.

Case Study 7

A 13-year-old girl was admitted with a history of periorbital edema for 10 days and intermittent fever and arthralgia of 6 months duration. She had been diagnosed with urinary tract infection several times before her admission based on the presence of leukocytes in her urine. There was no history of drug intake, facial rash, or joint pains. Her weight and height were within normal ranges. Vital signs, including blood pressure (BP), were normal. Physical examination was remarkable for periorbital edema. There were no signs of oral ulcer, rash, lymphadenopathy, or joint swelling.

The laboratory results on admission were as follows: hemoglobin, 10.7 g/dL, total white blood cell count 4500/mm^3, lymphocyte count 1000/mm^3, platelet count 127,000/mm^3, erythrocyte sedimentation rate 102 mm/h, sodium 130 mmol/L, potassium 6.7 mmol/L, chloride 111 mmol/L, bicarbonate, 16.8 mEq/L, blood urea nitrogen 25 mg/dL, creatinine 1.42 mg/dL, total protein 6 g/dL, albumin, 2.6 g/dL. Venous pH was 7.31, pCO$_2$ 34.5 mmHg, base excess −8 mEq/L. The anion gap was calculated to be 13. Urinalysis revealed a pH of 5.5, protein of 250 mg/dL, and 10 to 15 red blood cells. The 24-hour urinary protein excretion was 113 mg/m^2/h, and creatinine clearance was positive. The antinuclear antibody (ANA) titer was 1:320, and the antinative DNA antibody titer was negative. Serum complement levels were low; with a C3 of 0.18 (normal 0.8 to 2) g/L and a C4 of 0.06 (normal 0.15 to 0.5) g/L. Anti-cardiolipin immunoglobulin G (IgG) and IgM were 92 (normal 0 to 10) and 300 (normal 0 to 18) g/L, respectively.

She was diagnosed with systemic lupus erythematous (SLE) according to the American College of Rheumatology criteria, based on Coombs test-positive anemia, thrombocytopenia, nephrotic syndrome, positive ANA, and positive anticardiolipin antibody. Renal biopsy revealed severe diffuse proliferative glomerulonephritis (Renal Pathology Society/International Society of Nephrology World Health Organization class IV). There was also severe interstitial mononuclear cell infiltration and widespread tubulitis. While she was being investigated for hyperkalemia and metabolic acidosis, intravenous methylprednisolone therapy (1 g daily) was given for 3 days, along with sodium bicarbonate and calcium polystyrene sulfonate. This was followed by treatment with prednisone and oral cyclophosphamide 2 mg/kg for 3 months. Her condition improved remarkably, and her renal function and proteinuria remained normal at the 1-month follow-up clinic visit. Admission laboratory values were sodium 130 mEq/L, potassium 6.7 mEq/L, chloride 111 mEq/L, creatinine 1.4 mg/dL, blood pH 7.31, bicarbonate 16.8 mEq/L, urine pH 5.5, urine sodium 88 mEq/L, urine potassium 43 mEq/L, urine osmolality 360 mOsm/kg, and plasma osmolality 280 mOsm/kg.

What is the MOST likely diagnosis?

A. Primary hypoaldosteronism
B. Hyperkalemic renal tubular acidosis (RTA-4)
C. Congenital adrenal hyperplasia
D. Addison disease

The correct answer is B

Comment: Our patient initially presented with lupus nephritis and hyperkalemia, with a normal anion gap and hyperchloremic metabolic acidosis. A wide range of conditions has to be taken into account in the differential diagnosis for hyperkalemia. Based on our patient's laboratory findings, acute renal failure, drugs, blood transfusion and hemolysis were ruled out. Persistent hyperkalemia and normal anion gap metabolic acidosis led us to suspect the presence of type 4 RTA.[1,2] This is included in the general classification of RTA as its cardinal feature is hyperkalemia with a mild (normal anion gap) metabolic acidosis and normal measured urinary acidification.

Unlike distal RTA, in which proton secretion is defective, causing high urine pH, the main defect in type 4 RTA is transport abnormality of the distal tubule, which is secondary to aldosterone deficiency, resistance, or inhibition. The primary effect of aldosterone on the collecting duct is to stimulate sodium reabsorption and potassium secretion in principle cells, which results in an increase in the negative electrical potential of the lumen, promoting proton secretion. Aldosterone also directly affects the alpha intercalated cells to promote proton secretion by upregulating the expression of the proton ATPase as well as carbonic anhydrase. Thus, patients who are aldosterone deficient or resistant to aldosterone have increased sodium excretion. Our patient also had mildly increased of sodium excretion.

The preferred method to estimate potassium excretion by the distal tubule is the TTKG. Our patient's TTKG was 5 in the presence of hyperkalemia (normal >10), which indicates a defect in potassium secretion. A low TTKG is associated with aldosterone deficiency or resistance. The renin activity was 2.3 (5 to 27.8) pg/mL and the aldosterone level was 10 (reference: 13 to 34 pg/L) in the presence of high plasma levels of potassium. She appeared to have two distinct disorders, namely, renin–aldosterone deficiency or hyperkalemic distal RTA. Her urine pH was 5.5 when the blood pH was 7.3, and the HCO_3^- was 16.8 mEq/L, which are suggestive of hyporeninemic hypoaldosteronism (type 4 RTA).

Type 4 RTA is the most common form of renal tubular acidosis and occurs in various disorders. The most common causes of hyporeninemic hypoaldosteronism include diabetic nephropathy, tubulointerstitial disease and, in particular, interstitial nephritis associated with non-steroidal anti-inflammatory drugs (NSAIDs). Other causes in which hypoaldosteronism is present but not matched by hyporeninism include adrenal destruction (whether surgical, malignant, or hemorrhagic), Addison disease, angiotensin converting enzyme inhibitor therapy or angiotensin receptor blockade, and the inhibition of aldosterone synthesis by heparin. Our patient was investigated for the other causes of hyperkalemic RTA (diabetes, monoclonal gammopathies, NSAIDs), which were all ruled out.

Since our patient had a low renin level, other causes, which are characterized by hypoaldosteronism, such as primary hypoaldosteronism, congenital adrenal hyperplasia, and Addison disease, were ruled out. Within 3 days our patient showed a dramatic response to steroid treatment, with a normal potassium level. After treatment of lupus nephritis with prednisolone, plasma renin activity and plasma aldosterone concentration were elevated.

Case Study 8

A male infant presented with recurrent episodes of hyperkalemia and acidosis since birth. He was born by normal vaginal delivery at term weighing 2.7 kg (9th percentile) with a head circumference of 33 cm (9th percentile) to a mother with a known history of alcohol abuse. There were no perinatal problems. Mother's antenatal ultrasound scan at 20 weeks' gestation did not identify any fetal abnormalities.

At 1 month of age, the boy was admitted to the local hospital with a week's history of "funny spells," where he had extensor posturing of his trunk and limbs and cried out. These lasted for 2 to 3 minutes at a time. There was no apparent relationship to feeding or passing bowel motions. On examination, the child was noted to be thriving, with a weight of 3.29 kg (2nd percentile), a head circumference of 36 cm (9th percentile), and a length of 52 cm (9th percentile). Blood pressure was 78/52 mmHg. Clinical examination was unremarkable. He was not dehydrated on clinical assessment. The external genitalia appeared normal.

Initial blood investigations (performed by venipuncture) showed serum potassium 7 mmol/L, sodium 135 mmol/L, chloride 112 mmol/L, bicarbonate 19 mmol/L, urea 2.1 mmol/L, and creatinine 0.3 mg/dL. The complete blood count showed normal hemoglobin, white blood cell and platelet values. Liver function tests were within normal limits. Calcium, phosphate, and magnesium were within the normal range. Serum ammonia, lactate and creatinine kinase were normal. Capillary blood gas showed a mild metabolic acidosis with a base deficit of 5.2 mmol/L.

A working diagnosis of sepsis was originally considered, and he was treated with antibiotics intravenously. A complete septic screen was negative. Cerebrospinal fluid (CSF) lactate, plasma, and CSF amino acids; random cortisol; thyroid function tests; and 17-hydroxyprogesterone were all within the normal range. Serum aldosterone was entirely normal for age at 454 pmol/L (reference: 300 to 1500 pmol/L). Plasma renin activity was low at less than 0.2 mmol/L/h (reference: 1.1 to 2.7 nmol/L/h). Urinary potassium was 10 mmol/L; urine osmolality 151 mOsm/kg and plasma osmolality 290 mOsm/kg Urinary screen for drugs and toxins was negative. An ultrasound scan of the renal tract demonstrated two normal kidneys with no evidence of hydronephrosis or hydroureter.

The child had a trial of sodium bicarbonate, fludrocortisone, and calcium at 2 months of age. However, these were not sufficient to correct the hyperkalemia, which at this stage was associated with poor weight gain (3.7 kg). He was then commenced on low-potassium-containing milk. This corrected the hyperkalemia. He was discharged home with serum potassium 3.8 mmol/L, sodium 139 mmol/L, chloride 100 mmol/L, urea 12 mg/dL, and creatinine 0.3 mg/dL.

What is the MOST likely cause of hyperkalemia in this infant?

　　A. Gordon syndrome
　　B. Acute renal failure
　　C. Congenital adrenal hyperplasia
　　D. Tubulointrestitial disease

The correct answer is A
Comment: The child has presented in infancy with hyperkalemia associated with a hyperchloremic metabolic acidosis and a normal anion gap of 11 (normal 10 to 14). His estimated glomerular filtration rate (eGFR) is normal. Hyperkalemia in the presence of eGFR greater than 15 mL/min/1.73 m² is generally due to aldosterone deficiency or aldosterone resistance in the distal nephron.

A variety of conditions can be associated with aldosterone deficiency or aldosterone resistance in the distal nephron including pseudohypoaldosteronism type 1 and type 2, systemic lupus erythematous, amyloidosis, obstructive uropathy, sickle cell nephropathy and drugs such as potassium sparing diuretics and pentamidine.[1,2]

Our patient had a reduced transtubular potassium gradient (TTKG) [Urine K⁺ × Plasma osm]/Urine osm × Plasma K⁺] of 2.7 in the presence of hyperkalemia (normal range in infants 4.9 to 15.5), suggesting aldosterone deficiency or end organ resistance. The differential diagnosis would thus include congenital adrenal hyperplasia or hypoplasia, hypoaldosteronism or insensitivity to aldosterone.[1,2]

In view of the early presentation and the fact the infant was not on any medication and in the presence of a normal serum aldosterone makes end-organ resistance to this mineralocorticoid the most likely cause.

Type I PHA reflects the apparent lack of aldosterone effect on sodium reabsorption and potassium secretion and thus features hypotension and hyperkalemia. These children have renal salt wasting and often have hyponatremia. Plasma renin levels are elevated, as are plasma levels of aldosterone. The latter finding, as well as the lack of response to mineralocorticoid replacement therapy, differentiates them from infants with selective aldosterone deficiency that otherwise have a similar constellation of clinical findings. There are autosomal dominant and autosomal recessive forms of this disease, caused by mutations of the mineralocorticoid receptor and epithelial Na^+ channel (ENaC), respectively. Therapy with salt supplementation is effective in treating both the salt depletion and the hyperkalemia. As in other instances of mineralocorticoid deficiency, volume contraction with decreased distal delivery of salt and water appears necessary for overt hyperkalemia to develop. Spontaneous recovery usually occurs by the age of 2 years, although episodic hyperkalemia may still occur during episodes of acute illness.

PHA type II (Gordon's syndrome or familial hypertension with hyperkalemia) exhibits an autosomal dominant mode of transmission and is usually seen in late childhood or adulthood. These patients also have hyperkalemia and hyperchloremic metabolic acidosis, but do not exhibit renal salt wasting, have low plasma renin levels and are usually hypertensive.[2] Aldosterone levels are normal or high and most of these patients have a normal eGFR. This syndrome is also characterized by short stature, intellectual impairment, dental abnormalities, and muscle weakness. Recent positional cloning has linked mutations of *WNK1* (on chromosome 12p) and *WNK4* (on chromosome 17q21) to type II PHA. With-no-lysine [K] (WNK) kinases are a new family of large serine–threonine protein kinases with an atypical placement of the catalytic lysine. Wild type WNK1 and WNK4 inhibit the thiazide-sensitive sodium chloride co-transporter in the distal tubule. Mutations of these proteins are associated with gain of function and increased co-transporter activity, excessive chloride and sodium reabsorption and volume expansion. Hyperkalemia, another hallmark of this syndrome, might be a function of diminished sodium delivery to the cortical collecting tubule. Sodium reabsorption provides the driving force for potassium excretion, which is mediated by the renal outer medullary potassium channel (ROMK). Alternatively, the same mutations in *WNK4* that result in gain of function of the Na–Cl co-transporter (NCC) might inhibit ROMK activity, resulting in hyperkalemia. Treatment consists of either a low salt diet or thiazide diuretics, aimed at decreasing chloride intake and blocking Na^+–Cl^- co-transporter activity (NCC), respectively.

The presence of hyperkalemia in association with hyperchloremic metabolic acidosis, a low serum renin, a normal serum aldosterone and an adequate GFR in this child makes PHA type II the most likely diagnosis. In this syndrome, hypertension tends to develop in the third decade, so its absence in our patient does not exclude the diagnosis. As the condition is inherited in an autosomal dominant pattern, we proceeded to screen the child's father, who was 28 years old and asymptomatic. He was hypertensive with a blood pressure reading of 160/90 mmHg. His serum potassium was elevated at 6.4 mmol/L. His renal function and acid base status was normal. The father and the infant were commenced on chlorothiazide, which led to normalization of the serum potassium (and blood pressure in the father) and eliminated the need for dietary restriction of potassium. Initial genetic screening for *WNK1* and *WNK4* gene mutations in our patient was negative. However, further mutation studies are ongoing.

Case Study 9

A 5-month-old male infant was referred to our medical center with a possible diagnosis of Bartter syndrome. The patient had been admitted, 2 days before referral, to a local hospital with gastroenteritis and abdominal distension. Repeated investigations there had shown hypokalemia (K^+ 2.0

to 2.6 mEq/L), (Cl⁻ 92 to 95 mEq/L) metabolic alkalosis (pH 7.5 to 7.58, HCO_3^- 38 to 42 mEq/L, and base excess + 8 to + 14 mEq/L). The patient had been treated with IV fluids and potassium replacement. Results from other investigations were: urea 10.0 mg d/L, creatinine 0.3 mg/dL, Hb 10.1 g/dL WBC 9700/mL, and platelets 3.12 × 10⁶ mL; abdomen ultrasound revealed normal-sized kidneys and no abnormality.

The patient had been born at term with a birth weight of 2.8 kg and had an uneventful perinatal period. The patient thrived well on breast feeds and formula milk feeds until approximately 7 weeks of age. The patient then started to suffer from repeated episodes of watery diarrhea and was diagnosed as milk protein/lactose intolerant and switched to soya-based formula. The patient was thriving well on this formula until 15 days before this illness when his parents switched to ordinary formula milk feeds. Development was normal for his age.

Examination revealed an active, 5.5-kg male (growth 25th centile), length 61.5 cm (25th centile), and head circumference 40 cm (25th centile) with stable hemodynamics, mild dehydration, abdominal distension, and reduced bowel sounds. Investigations revealed K⁺ 2.0 mEq/L with pH 7.59, PCO_2 52 mmHg, PO_2 73 mmHg, HCO_3^- 48 mEq/L, BE + 28 mEq/L, Na⁺ 129 mEq/L, Cl⁻ 95 mEq/L Hb 9.2 g/dL, WBC 6400/mL platelets 2.1 × 10⁶/mL, urea 16.0 mg/dL, creatinine 0.3 mg/dL. Plain X-ray abdomen was suggestive of adynamic ileus. Simultaneous urine electrolytes were K⁺ 3 mEq/L and Na⁺ 40 mEq/L. A provisional diagnosis of pseudo-Bartter syndrome was made, and the patient was started on intravenous hydration and potassium supplementation K⁺ 30 mEq (deficit) plus maintenance, over 24 hours. Sixteen hours after starting the treatment potassium was 3.8 mEq/L with blood pH 7.36, HCO_3^- 32 mEq/L, and BE + 2 mEq/L, diarrhea and abdominal distension improved, and the patient was started on soya-based formula.

On the third day after admission the patient became irritable and was sweating more than his usual. He was otherwise sucking well, had infrequent loose motions, passed urine freely, and was afebrile. Repeat investigations revealed Hb 9.0 g/dL, WBC 5700/mL, platelets 2.56 × 10⁶/mL, K⁺ 9.3 mEq/L, Na⁺ 129 mEq/L, urea 18 mg/dL, creatinine 0.4 mg/dL, and normal blood gas (pH 7.34, PCO_2 40 mmHg, PO_2 86 mmHg, HCO_3^- 23 mEq/L, BE 1.5 mEq/L), blood sugar 102 mg/dL. Repeat sample ruled out any hemolysis. Electrocardiogram (ECG) showed tall-tented T waves with broad QRS complex (0.12 second) and increased QT_c (0.5). The patient was given one bolus of calcium gluconate (2 mmol/kg) intravenously over 15 minutes, which resulted in normalization of ECG. The patient was started on treatment for hyperkalemia with continuous intravenous calcium infusion (1 mEq/k/h), intravenous hydration (120 mL/kg/day) and salbutamol nebulization (1 mg per dose every 2 hours).

Other investigations revealed urea 18 mg/ dL, creatinine 0.3 mg/dL, CPK 790 IU/L (normal reference range: 25 to 175 IU/L), SGOT 81 IU/L, SGPT 71 IU/L; calcium 8.2 mg/dL, bilirubin 0.3 mg/dL pH 7.38, PCO_2 36 mmHg, PO_2 123 mmHg, HCO_3^- 21 mEq/L, and BE 1.5 mEq/L.

What is the MOST likely cause of hyperkalemia in this infant?

    A. Rhabdomyolysis
    B. Sepsis
    C. Adrenal insufficiency
    D. Inborn error of metabolism

The correct answer is A
Comment: In our patient rhabdomyolysis was the cause of hyperkalemia.[1,2] Evidence that rhabdomyolysis was present were extremely high CPK levels and results from urine examination suggestive of myoglobinuria. There was no evidence of renal failure.

The patient was managed for hyperkalemia.[3] Potassium levels gradually decreased to normal by the end of 24-hour treatment, maximum being 10.4 and 3.8 mEq/L at the end of 24-hour. The total potassium intake in the 24-hour preceding hyperkalemia was 4 mEq/kg/day. CPK decreased to 490 IU/L after 24-hour. The urine was positive for hemoglobin and there were no red blood cells (RBCs) in the urine, indicating likely presence of myoglobin in the given clinical setting. A week later, the patient on follow-up was normal, abdominal distension had decreased and serum potassium, CPK, and renal function tests were normal.

Rhabdomyolysis is defined as an acute increase in serum creatinine phosphokinase to more than five times the normal with/without associated acute renal failure and hyperkalemia. Various causes of rhabdomyolysis have been identified and may be subdivided into traumatic, exercise-induced, toxicological, environmental, metabolic, infectious, immunological, and inherited causes.[1,2,4] The occurrence of rhabdomyolysis in hypokalemia is found to be independent of the etiology and degree of hypokalemia. It has been reported that sub-clinical rhabdomyolysis is a common complication of hypokalemia, which is detected only as elevated muscle enzymes and, as a result, hypokalemia as a cause of rhabdomyolysis goes unnoticed because of the counteracting response of rhabdomyolysis on serum potassium concentration.

Clinical presentation of rhabdomyolysis varies between patients. Muscle pain and myoglobin-uria are not always found on presentation. The usual laboratory features of rhabdomyolysis are acute renal failure with or without hyperkalemia, hyperkalemia without renal failure, and myo-globinuria. Other uncommon features are hyperphosphatemia, hypocalcemia, hyperuricemia, and disseminated intravascular coagulopathy (DIC).

Case Study 10

A 2-month-old female infant was admitted with 2 days history of poor feeding and lethargy. She was born to a 28-year-old primary gravid at 38 weeks gestation via normal vaginal delivery with a birth weight of 2.9 kg. The neonatal period was uneventful.

On admission to the hospital, her weight was 3.7 kg, blood pressure 92/55 mmHg, pulse 139 beats/min, and temperature 90.1°C. Examinations of lung, heart, and abdomen were normal. Laboratory data: white blood cell counts $17 \times 10^3/\mu L$ with a shift to the left, platelets $107 \times 10^3/\mu L$, hematocrit 33.2%, serum sodium 129 mmol/L, chloride 111 mmol/L, potassium 9.2 mmol/L, bicarbonate 9.1 mmol/L (anion gap 8.9 mmol/L), creatinine 0.8 mg/dL, BUN 32 mg/dL, calcium 8.1 mg/dL phosphate 4.4 mg/dL, and urate 6.1 mg/dL. Estimated glomerular filtration rate (eGFR) using the original Schwartz equation was $32.1 \, mL/min/1.73 \, m^2$. Repeated measurements of serum potassium confirmed the initial value. Urinalysis revealed pH 6.5, specific gravity 1.009, without proteinuria or hematuria. Urine culture was positive for *Escherichia coli*. Arterial blood gas determinations on room air showed pH 7.24, PCO_2 18 mmHg, bicarbonate 11.4 mmol/L, base excess −8.2. A renal ultrasound showed bilateral obstructive hydronephrosis. The diagnosis of ureteropelvic junction obstruction (UPJO) was suspected and confirmed by diuretic ^{99}mTc diethylenetriamine pentaacetic acid (DTPA) renography. Serum renin activity was 18.8 ng/mL/h (normal range 0.1 to 3.1), aldosterone 198 ng/dL (normal range 3 to 16) and cortisol 36.1 ug/dL (normal range 2.3 to 11.9). The admission electrocardiogram (EEG) showed normal sinus rhythm, normal PR, QRS, and T waves morphology.

After therapy with intravenous 0.9% saline, antibiotic, sodium bicarbonate, glucose and insulin, nebulized salbutamol (β_2 agonist), and sodium-potassium ion exchange resins and insertion of nephrostomy tubes, the serum potassium concentrations returned to normal; her BUN and serum creatinine concentrations also returned to normal values of 12 mg/dL, and 0.4 mg/dL, respectively. A repeat EEG when the serum potassium concentration was 4.4 mEq/L, was unchanged compared to that taken on admission.

Which of the following statements is correct? (Select all that apply)

A. Pseudo hyperkalemia without ECG manifestations
B. True hyperkalemia without ECG manifestations
C. Both of the above
D. None of the above

The correct answer is B

Comment: The finding of normal ECG in our patient with severe hyperkalemia suggests the ECG findings may not be a reliable indicator in patients with chronic kidney disease or a useful observation to monitor therapy aimed to lower the serum K$^+$ concentration.[1-5]

The etiology of hyperkalemia in our patients was the impaired K$^+$ excretion as a result of acute or chronic kidney disease. Hyperkalemia is usually not seen until the glomerular filtration rate falls below 30 mL/min/1.73 m^2. One possible explanation for the absence of typical ECG changes may be the slow rises in serum K$^+$ concentrations and the presence of chronic kidney disease in five of our patients. It is known that patients with CKD tolerate higher levels of serum K$^+$ concentration than patients without chronic kidney disease. It is not known if the present observation can be applied to patients with other hyperkalemic syndromes

The **rate** of increase in serum K$^+$ can also potentiate the cardiotoxic effect of hyperkalemia and influence the development of ECG abnormalities.

Hyperkalemia is defined as a serum K$^+$ level greater than 5.5 mmol/L. Clinical symptoms including cardiac arrhythmias, muscle weakness and paralysis usually develops at levels higher than 7.0 mmol/L, but the rate of change is more important than the level of K$^+$ concentration.

Mild to moderate hyperkalemia (serum K$^+$ concentrations between 6 and 7 mmol/L) is associated with the appearance of tall, peaked T waves, known as tenting T wave. As potassium levels rise further, the PR interval increases, and p wave amplitude decreases followed by widening QRS complex and disappearance of p waves.

Calcium gluconate is the first line of therapy in patients with evidence of cardiac toxicity. Insulin and glucose will lower serum K concentration by allowing the K$^+$ back into the cells. A common practice is 10 units of regular insulin given with 50 mL of 50% dextrose solution. Beta-2adrenergic agents such as albuterol will also shift K$^+$ intracellular. Sodium bicarbonate is given in patients with metabolic acidosis. Loop diuretics may be helpful in non-oliguric and volume overload patients by enhancing the urinary K$^+$ excretion.[6,7] Gastrointestinal cation exchangers such as patiromer or sodium polystyrene sulfonate may be administered in patients with renal insufficiency. Hemodialysis should be considered in patients with severe renal injury (GFR $\leq$ 30 mL/min/1.73 m^2).[6,7]

Case Study 11

A 2.5-month-old girl was admitted to our emergency department with a 1-day history of fever and vomiting. She was born at the 35th week of gestation by cesarean section and admitted to the neonatal intensive care unit. Her past medical history was significant for urinary tract infection in the neonatal period and congenital anomalies of the kidney and urinary tract (CAKUT), which was completely identified at 4 weeks of age. She had antenatal hydronephrosis and was diagnosed with right multicystic dysplastic kidney and severe left ureterovesical junction (UVJ) obstruction with imaging tests including 99m Tc-mercaptoacetyltriglycine (MAG3) scintigraphy and voiding cystourethrography (VCUG). When she was 3 weeks old, a double J catheter was inserted due to severe left UVJ obstruction. VCUG did not demonstrate any vesicoureteral reflux (VUR). She was on prophylactic antibiotics. Her weight was 4210 g (3rd to 10th percentile), height 56 cm (10th percentile), head circumference 37 cm (3rd to 10th percentile), and blood pressure 110/70 mmHg (95th percentile 98/65 mmHg). She had signs of mild–moderate dehydration with dry mucosal membranes and normal female external genitalia on physical examination. While there was no abnormality in the previous biochemical parameters of the patient, the results of the laboratory examination at the time of admission were blood urea nitrogen (BUN), 25 mg/dL (5 to 20 mg/dL); serum creatinine, 0.34 mg/dL (0.3 to 1 mg/dL); sodium, 111 mmol/L (135 to 145 mmol/L); potassium, 7.4 mmol/L (3.5 to 5 mmol/L); chloride, 98 mmol/L (98 to 115 mmol/L); glucose, 88 mg/dL (50 to 90 mg/dL); hemoglobin, 13 g/dL; leukocytes, 16,870/mm^3 (7000 to 15,000/

mm^3); and platelets, 656,000/mm^3 (150,000 to 450,000/mm^3). Hormonal analysis showed elevated plasma renin greater than 500 pg/mL (reference: 2.77 to 61.8 pg/mL) and serum aldosterone greater than 1500 pg/mL (reference: 50 to 900 pg/mL). Random adrenocorticotrophic hormone (ACTH) was 30.8 pg/mL (reference: 8.6 to 46.3 pg/mL) and cortisol was 7.2 µg/dL (reference: 1 to 24 µg/dL). Venous blood gas analysis was pH 7.20, pCO_2 38 mmHg, bicarbonate 11 mmol/L, and base excess −13 mmol/L. Her urine analysis results were pH 5, density 1025, leukocyte esterase (3 +) positive, nitrite positive, and leukocyturia with bacteriuria in microscopic examination. She was hospitalized with a diagnosis of acute pyelonephritis.

What is your diagnostic approach to hyperkalemia and hyponatremia?

A. Liddle syndrome
B. Congenital adrenal hyperplasia
C. Pseudohypoaldosteronism (PHA)
D. Primary aldosteronism

The correct answer is C

Comment: Diagnosis of pseudohypoaldosteronism (PHA) was confirmed with hyponatremia, hyperkalemia, metabolic acidosis, and elevated levels of renin (>500 pg/mL) and aldosterone (>1500 pg/mL).[1-5] After pyelonephritis treatment, biochemical parameters were completely normal, and renin and aldosterone levels decreased to normal limits. Based on clinical and laboratory results, she was diagnosed with secondary (transient) PHA type 1. Congenital adrenal hyperplasia (CAH) and other aldosterone synthesis defects were excluded by clinical course as well as female genitalia with normal pigmentation, and the hormonal profile of the patient.[1-5]

This patient was treated with appropriate antibiotic therapy for urinary tract infection (UTI), and appropriate fluid and electrolyte therapy for hyponatremia and hyperkalemia.[6] After initiation of UTI treatment, serum sodium, potassium, bicarbonate, renin, and aldosterone levels normalized within a few days, which confirmed the diagnosis of secondary PHA1. Infants with secondary PHA1 require long-term follow-up of serum electrolytes after surgical treatment of obstruction.

Pseudohypoaldosteronism is a rare heterogeneous syndrome of mineralocorticoid resistance that is characterized by systemic or renal tubular unresponsiveness to aldosterone. Two different forms of PHA have been described, type 1 (PHA1) and type 2 (PHA2). PHA1 has been sub classified into primary and secondary (transient) PHA1. Primary PHA1 is caused by mutations in the epithelial sodium channel (ENaC) genes or mineralocorticoid receptor (MR) gene. The secondary (transient) form of PHA1 is associated with urinary tract malformations and/or infections during infancy. Therefore, a urinary ultrasound examination should be performed in infants with salt loss and hyperkalemia. Other causes of secondary PHA1 are systemic lupus erythematous, acute renal allograft rejection, chronic allograft nephropathy, and sickle cell nephropathy. The common presenting symptoms in children with PHA are poor feeding, failure to thrive, polyuria, dehydration, and vomiting. Clinical features of PHA are hyperkalemia, metabolic acidosis, and elevated plasma aldosterone levels. Our patient presented with vomiting and dehydration. Severe hyponatremia, hyperkalemia, and metabolic acidosis were detected.

References

Case Study 1

1. Assadi F. *Clinical Decisions in Pediatric Nephrology: A Problem Solving Approach to Clinical Cases.* New York: Springer; 2008:1–68 [Chapter 2].
2. Rose BD, Post TW. *Clinical Physiology of Acid–Base and Electrolyte Disorders.* 5th ed. New York, NY: McGraw-Hill, Inc.; 2001:551–571 [Chapter 18].

Case Study 2

1. Assadi F. *Clinical Decisions in Pediatric Nephrology: A Problem Solving Approach to Clinical Cases.* New York: Springer; 2008:1–68 [Chapter 2].
2. Rose BD, Post TW. *Clinical Physiology of Acid–Base and Electrolyte Disorders.* 5th ed. New York, NY: McGraw-Hill, Inc.; 2001:551–571 [Chapter 18].

Case Study 3

1. Assadi F. Rising serum potassium and creatinine concentrations after prescribing renin-angiotensin-aldosterone system blockade: how much should we worry? *World J Pediatr.* 2021 Oct;17(5):552–554. https://doi.org/10.1007/s12519-021-00455-8. Epub September 2, 2021.
2. Barkis GL, Weir MR. Angiotensin-converting enzyme inhibitor-associated elevations in serum creatinine: is this a cause for concern? *Arch Intern Med.* 2000;160:685–693.

Case Study 4

1. Assadi F, Crowe C, Roohi O. Hyperkalemic distal renal tubular acidosis associated with Rett syndrome. *Pediatr Nephrol.* 2006;21(4):588–590. https://doi.org/10.1007/s00467-006-0029-2. Epub March 2, 2006.
2. Hagberg B, Hanefeld F, Percy A, Skjeldal O. An update on clinically applicable diagnostic criteria in Rett syndrome. *Eur J Paediatr Neurol.* 2002;6:293–297.
3. Batlle DC, Hizon M, Cohen E, Gutterman C, Gupta R. The use of the urinary anion gap in the diagnosis of hyperchloremic metabolic acidosis. *N Engl J Med.* 1988;318:594–599.
4. Battle DC, Aruda JAL, Kurtzman NA. Hyperkalemicdistal tubular acidosis associated with obstructive uropathy. *N Engl J Med.* 1981;304:373–380.
5. Assadi FK, Ziai M. Impaired renal acidification in infants with fetal alcohol syndrome. *Pediatr Res.* 1985;19:850–853.

Case Study 5

1. Riepe FG. Clinical and molecular features of type 1 pseudohypoaldosteronism. *Horm Res.* 2009;72:1–9. https://doi.org/10.1159/000224334.
2. Yu G, Hashim F, Macmurdo Hanna C. Persistent hyperkalemia in an otherwise healthy 4-month-old female: answers. *Pediatr Nephrol.* 2020;35:2099–2100. https://doi.org/10.1007/s00467-020-04575-7.
3. Geller DS, Zhang J, Zennaro MC, et al. Mechanisms of type I and type II pseudohypoaldosteronism. *J Am Soc Nephrol.* 2010;21:1842–1845.

Case Study 6

1. Furgeson SB, Linas S. Mechanisms of type I and type II pseudohypoaldosteronism. *J Am Soc Nephrol.* 2010;21:1842–1845.
2. Nobel YR, Lodish MB, Raygada M, et al. Pseudohypoaldosteronism type 1 due to novel variants of SCNN1B gene. *Endocrinol Diabetes Metab Case Rep.* 2016;2016, 150104.
3. Mittal A, Khera D, Vyas V, et al. Dangerous hyperkalemia in a newborn: answers. *Pediatr Nephrol.* 2019;34:813–815. https://doi.org/10.1007/s00467-018-4102-4.

Case Study 7

1. Karet FE. Mechanisms in hyperkalemic renal tubular acidosis. *J Am Soc Nephrol.* 2009;20:251–254.
2. Marks SD, Shah V, Pilkington C, et al. Renal tubular dysfunction in children with systemic lupus erythematosus. *Pediatr Nephrol.* 2005;20:141–148.

Case Study 8

1. Proctor G, Linas S. Type 2 pseudohypoaldosteronism: new insights into renal potassium, sodium, and chloride handling. *Am J Kidney Dis.* 2006;48:674–693.
2. Garovic VD, Hilliard AA, Turner ST. Monogenic forms of low-renin hypertension: Gordon's syndrome. *Nat Clin Pract Nephrol.* 2006;2:624–630.

Case Study 9

1. Lane R, Phillips M. Rhabdomyolysis. *BMH.* 2003;327:115–116.
2. Rosenberry C, Stone F, Kalbfleisch K. Rhabdomyolysis-induced severe hyperkalemia. *West J Emerg Med.* 2009;10(4):302.
3. Weisberg LS, Dellinger RP. Management of severe hyperkalemia. *Crit Care Med.* 2008;36:3246–3251.
4. Park SE, Kim DY, Park ES. Hyperkalemia in a patient with rhabdomyolysis and compartment syndrome—a case report. *Korean J Anesthesiol.* 2010;59(suppl):S37–S40. https://doi.org/10.4097/kjae.2010.59.S.S37.

Case Study 10

1. Assadi F, Mazaheri M, Malakan-Rad E. Electrocardiography is unreliable to detect potential lethal hyperkalemia in patients with non-dialysis chronic kidney disease. *Pediatr Cardiol.* 2022;43(5):1064–1070. https://doi.org/10.1007/s00246-02826-y.
2. Assadi F. Clinical disorders associated with altered potassium metabolism. In: Elzouki AY, Harif HA, Nazer H, Stepleton FB, Oh W, Whitley RJ, eds. *Textbook of Clinical Pediatrics.* 2nd ed. Vol 4. New York: Springer; 2011:2663–2670.
3. Szerlip HM, Weiss J, Singer I. Profound hyperkalemia without electrocardiographic manifestations. *Am J Kidney Dis.* 1986;7:461–465.
4. Martinez-Vea A, Bardaji A, Garcia C, Oliver JA. Severe hyperkalemia with minimal electrocardiographic manifestations of electrocardiography. *J Electrocardiol.* 1999;32:45–49.
5. Sharna S, Gupta H, Ghosh M, Padmanabhan A. Severe hyperkalemia with normal electrocardiogram. *Indian J Crit Care Med.* 2007;11:215–217.
6. Lemonie L, Le Bastard Q, Montassier E. An evidenced-based narrative review of the emergency department management of acute hyperkalemia. *J Emerg Med.* 2021;60:599–606.
7. Lopes MB, Rocha PN, Pecoits-Filho R. Updates on medical management of hyperkalemia. *Curr Opin Nephrol Hypertens.* 2019;28:417–423.

Case Study 11

1. Torun-Bay ram M, Soylu A, Kasap-Demir B, et al. Secondary pseudohypoaldosteronism caused by urinary tract infection associated with urinary tract anomalies: case reports. *Turk J Pediatr.* 2012;54:67–70.
2. Abraham MB, Larkins N, Choong CS, et al. Transient pseudohypoaldosteronism in infancy secondary to urinary tract infection. *J Paediatr Child Health.* 2017;53:458–463.
3. Riepe FG. Pseudohypoaldosteronism. *Endocr Dev.* 2013;24:86–95.
4. Casas-Alba D, Vila Cots J, Monfort Carretero L, et al. Pseudohypoaldosteronism types I and II: little more than a name in common. *J Pediatr Endocrinol Metab.* 2017;30:597–601.
5. Krishnappa V, Ross JH, Kenagy DN, et al. Secondary or transient Pseudohypoaldosteronism associated with urinary tract anomaly and urinary infection: a case report. *Urol Case Rep.* 2016;8:61–62.
6. Atmis B, Turan İ, Melek E, Bayazit AK. An infant with hyponatremia, hyperkalemia, and metabolic acidosis associated with urinary tract infection: answers. *Pediatr Nephrol.* 2019;34:1739–1741. https://doi.org/10.1007/s00467-019-04254-2.

CHAPTER 5

Metabolic Alkalosis

Case Study 1

A 15-year-old male patient with cirrhosis and ascites secondary to Wilson disease is admitted to the hospital with acute gastrointestinal bleeding due to ruptured esophageal varices. He is taken to surgery, where a portacaval shunt is performed. He is given a total of 19 units of blood before and during the surgery. Although the ascites was removed during the surgery, it begins to reaccumulate postoperatively. His laboratory tests were normal preoperatively, but the following values are obtained 12 hours after surgery: Arterial pH 7.53, PCO_2 50 mmHg, and bicarbonate 40 mmol/L.

What is responsible for the development of metabolic alkalosis and how would you correct the alkalosis?

A. Citrate load from multiple blood transfusion
B. Hepatic insufficiency
C. Hyperventilation

The correct answer is A
Comment: The acute metabolic alkalosis is due to the citrate load from the multiple blood transfusions. Acetazolamide is the preferred therapy, both to remove the excess fluid and to cause a preferential HCO_3^- diuresis. Saline loading is not indicated since it will result in a marked increase in ascites formation.[1]

Case Study 2

A13-year-old girl presented with 2 days of progressive dyspnea, weight gain, and peripheral edema. She was treated with azithromycin for a cough 2 weeks prior, with resolution of symptoms. Her history was significant for chronic kidney disease (CKD) secondary to hypertension and prior use of non-steroidal anti-inflammatory drugs. She also had a history of chronic hyperkalemia (treated with sodium polystyrene therapy), osteoporosis, and gastroesophageal reflux disease. She denied use of herbal or over-the-counter medications, change in diet, or nausea or vomiting. Blood pressure was 150/79 mmHg, heart rate 76 beats/min, respiratory rate 24 breaths/min, and oxygen saturation 92% breathing room air. On examination, she had jugular venous distension, bibasilar inspiratory rales, tenderness of the right chest wall, and pitting edema (3+) in the legs bilaterally. The radiograph of the chest showed new small bilateral pleural effusions and mildly displaced fractures of the right 8th, 9th, and 10th ribs attributed to severe coughing. Laboratory testing revealed serum sodium 138 mmol/L, potassium 2.0 mmol/L, chloride 82 mmol/L, bicarbonate 46 mmol/L, calcium 8.3 mg/dL, magnesium 1.5 mg/dL, albumin 3.0 g/dL, creatinine 0.9 mg/dL, and estimated glomerular filtration rate 36 mL/min/1.73 m^2. Urine chloride was 95 mmol/L, pH 7.0, and urine protein-creatinine ratio 400 mg/g.

Arterial blood gas showed pH of 7.55, PCO_2 of 52 mmHg, PO_2 of 70 mmHg, and bicarbonate level of 45 mmol/L.

What is the cause of the metabolic alkalosis in this patient?

    A. Apparent mineralocorticoid access

    B. Hyperaldosteronism

    C. High-dose sodium polystyrene use with concomitant calcium carbonate and magnesium hydroxide

    D. Pseudohyperaldosteronism

The correct answer is C

Comment: The patient's blood tests indicate a simple metabolic alkalosis characterized by three clinical features: an increase in plasma pH (> 7.40), an increase in plasma bicarbonate concentration, and an increase in PCO_2 due to adaptive hypoventilation. Although the differential diagnosis of metabolic alkalosis is broad, simple blood and urine tests combined with a detailed history can often lead to a diagnosis.[1] Urine pH is an important and often overlooked initial step in this process. The patient's elevated urine pH indicates alkali loading, resolving metabolic alkalosis, or very recent vomiting prior to establishing a new steady state. With an alkaline urine pH, additional testing often is unnecessary because all other causes of metabolic alkalosis are associated with aciduria. It should be noted that although urine chloride is usually advocated as the initial diagnostic test in the case of alkali loading, urine pH could reveal the diagnosis prior to testing urinary chloride. Caution also should be used when interpreting urine chloride results after administration of diuretics because this would mask the presence of a chloride-dependent alkalosis. In our patient, urine chloride levels were found to be elevated on admission.

Further examination of the patient's history revealed that she was unsure of the dose of sodium polystyrene she took after the medication's formulation was changed from liquid to powder 1 month prior to admission. The patient's family believed that she might have been taking higher doses than prescribed. Coadministration of sodium polystyrene and antacids (calcium carbonate and magnesium oxide, in this case) has been reported to cause metabolic alkalosis in patients with end-stage renal disease and advanced stages of CKD.[2-5]

In the absence of sodium polystyrene, antacids containing calcium and magnesium first react with hydrogen chloride secreted in the stomach to form calcium chloride and magnesium chloride, respectively. These moieties enter the duodenum, where they react with the secreted sodium bicarbonate to subsequently form carbonates of the cations. Because there is equal secretion and consumption of hydrogen chloride and sodium bicarbonate, there is no change in the net acid-base balance.

When calcium-, magnesium-, or even aluminum-containing antacids are administered concomitantly with sodium polystyrene, there is a similar equal secretion of hydrogen chloride and sodium bicarbonate. However, the sodium bicarbonate secreted in the duodenum is not consumed; rather, it is reabsorbed, resulting in a salt and alkali load. Alkali loading in the presence of reduced kidney function leads to metabolic alkalosis despite alkaline urine pH.

It is not known yet whether the newer agents for management of hyperkalemia (patiromer and sodium zirconium cyclosilicate) may have a similar complication.[6,7] Patiromer reportedly has nonspecific cation binding similar to sodium polystyrene, whereas sodium zirconium cyclosilicate selectively binds potassium. Based on this consideration, we would hypothesize that a similar effect could be seen with patiromer use.

Hypokalemia can contribute to maintenance of the metabolic alkalosis through several mechanisms including increased ammoniagenesis and increased hydrogen secretion at the intercalated epithelial cell in the collecting duct.

In this case, we attributed hypokalemia to cellular shift along with enhanced gastrointestinal and kidney losses. It is difficult to know whether hypokalemia was contributing to maintenance of the metabolic alkalosis via increased tubular hydrogen secretion in the setting of alkaline urine.

In previous case reports, it has been shown that stopping coadministration of sodium polystyrene and oral antacids results in improvement in metabolic alkalosis.

This should be adequate unless serum pH requires rapid correction for symptoms related to electrolyte abnormalities or alkalemia. This can be achieved by administration of acetazolamide (with close monitoring of serum potassium level) or rarely with dilute hydrochloric acid.

In our patient, both metabolic alkalosis and hypokalemia improved after withdrawing sodium polystyrene and administering supplemental potassium and acetazolamide. The alkalosis and hypokalemia did not recur with appropriate sodium polystyrene dosing (changed back to liquid formulation) and spacing of calcium carbonate and magnesium oxide administration.

Case Study 3

A 15-year-old male has a history of hypertension, which is treated with a diuretic. The following arterial blood values are obtained on room air:

Arterial pH 7.8, PCO_2 51 mmHg, bicarbonate 36 mmol/L, PO_2 73 mmHg,

What is the MOST likely acid-base disturbance?

A. Metabolic alkalosis
B. Metabolic acidosis
C. Respiratory acidosis
D. Mixed metabolic alkalosis and respiratory acidosis

The correct answer is B
Comment: Metabolic alkalosis, with the elevated PCO_2 reflecting the appropriate respiratory compensation.[1,2]

Case Study 4

A 19-year-old woman with adequately controlled diabetes mellitus and previously normal renal function presents with fever, dysuria, nausea, recurrent vomiting, flank pain, and polyuria that have become progressively more severe over 4 days. The physical examination reveals a temperature of 39.6°C, reduced skin turgor, estimated jugular venous pressure below 5 cmH_2O, postural hypotension, and marked tenderness over the right costovertebral angle. The urine shows pyuria and bacteriuria, and a diagnosis of acute pyelonephritis is made. Other laboratory data reveal the following: Serum sodium 135 mmol/L, potassium 2.6 mmol/L, chloride 87 mmol/L, bicarbonate 30 mmol/L, BUN 32 mg/dL, creatinine 4 mg/dL, ketones 4+, arterial pH 7.36, PCO_2 37 mmHg, glucose 570 mg/dL.

The electrocardiogram shows prominent U waves in the precordial leads and occasional multifocal premature ventricular beats.

What is the acid-base disturbance on admission and what would be your initial therapeutic regimen?

A. Metabolic alkalosis
B. Laxative abuse
C. Mixed metabolic acidosis and metabolic alkalosis
D. Aldosteronism

The correct answer is C
Comment: The patient has both diabetic ketoacidosis and a superimposed metabolic alkalosis due to vomiting.[1,2] Notice that the anion gap is 28 mmol/L (16 mmol/L above normal), which should

be associated with a reduction in the plasma bicarbonate concentration to about 10 mmol/L. The substantially high value in this case is indicative of the underlying metabolic alkalosis. Dehydration undoubtedly is responsible for much of the decline in renal function. In addition, acetoacetate is measured as creatinine in the standard assay, resulting in a further apparent elevation in the plasma creatinine concentration.

The major electrolyte problems in this patient are hypokalemia and volume depletion. The hyperglycemia and metabolic acidosis are relatively mild; immediate correction of these disturbances with insulin is not necessary and may be deleterious by driving potassium into the cells, possibly inducing arrhythmias. Thus, the initial therapy should consist of isotonic or half-isotonic saline to which 40 mmol/L of KCl is added. This regimen will correct the hypokalemia and volume depletion and will slowly ameliorate the hyperglycemia, both by dilution and by improving renal function, thereby enhancing glucose excretion. The patient should also be started on antimicrobial therapy for presumed acute pyelonephritis. This infection was probably responsible for the loss of diabetic control.

Case Study 5

A 13-year-old girl was admitted to the hospital complaining of persistent vomiting of 10 days' duration. Her past history was otherwise unremarkable. Physical examination showed a thin white girl who appeared somewhat confused. Blood pressure was 100/80 mmHg, pulse 110 beats/min, and respiratory rate was 10 breaths/min. The remainder of the physical examination was unremarkable except for moderate mid-epigastric tenderness. Blood electrolytes were sodium 130 mmol/L, potassium 2.2 mmol/L, chloride 50 mmol/L, and bicarbonate 60 mmol/L. The creatinine was 4 mg/dL, blood urea nitrogen 80 mg/dL, and glucose 85 mg/dL. The urine sodium concentration was 62 mEq/L.

What is the MOST likely cause of this patient's renal failure and electrolyte disorders?

    A. Interstitial nephritis
    B. Glomerular disease
    C. Obstructive nephropathy
    D. Pre-renal azotemia

The correct diagnosis is D
Comment: The differential diagnosis of this patient's electrolyte disorders rests between renal failure of undetermined cause, which results in uremia and vomiting, and vomiting which results in severe volume depletion and prerenal azotemia. The finding of high urine sodium might point to the former diagnosis.[1,2] The urine sodium as a means of distinguishing between renal failure due to parenchymal disease and renal failure due to under perfusion is not useful in patients who have metabolic alkalosis secondary to vomiting. The rise in bicarbonate concentration seen in this disorder results in spillage of some bicarbonate into the urine. This bicarbonaturia obligates the excretion of cations, some of which will be sodium.[3] The critical test in this patient is to measure the urine chloride concentration.[4] In this patient, this was 1 mEq/L. Thus, the kidney retained the capacity to reabsorb all the filtered chloride. This finding, plus the patient's severe hypokalemic metabolic alkalosis, suggests vomiting is the primary disorder. The BUN, which is typically elevated out of proportion to the rise in creatinine in patients with prerenal azotemia, will not rise in this fashion in patients who vomit, owing to the lack of nitrogen intake. The infusion of large amounts of sodium chloride and potassium chloride not only corrected the hypokalemic metabolic alkalosis in this patient, but also resulted in the restoration of renal function to normal within 13 days.

Case Study 6

A 10-year-old boy admitted to the pediatric nephrology outpatient clinic with the complaints of fatigue lasting more than 2 months, and abdominal pain. He never had polyuria or polydipsia and did not complain about muscle cramps or contractions. He had never experienced dehydration attacks, and his growth was normal. The patient's mother and grandmother were hypertensive, and the patient's mother had chronic kidney disease with an estimated glomerular filtration rate (eGFR) of 25 mL/min/1.73 m².

Physical examination revealed high blood pressure (190/130 mmHg). The weight and height percentiles were both between 25th and 50th percentile. The patient had diffuse and vague tenderness on abdomen. The patient had hypokalemia (serum potassium 2.1 mmol/L) and hypochloremia (serum chloride 78 mmol/L) accompanying metabolic alkalosis with a blood pH of 7.5, and a serum bicarbonate level of 32 mmol/L. Serum creatinine and serum sodium were normal, 0.7 mg/dL and 138 mmol/L, respectively. The patient was hospitalized for hypertensive urgency and further evaluation. Fractional excretion of sodium was 0.01%, and fractional excretion of potassium was 30%. Tubular phosphorus reabsorption was 92%. Renin activity was 1.22 ng/mL/h; aldosterone level was reported as less than 3.7 ng/dL, both of which were at the lowest ranges of their references. Serum cortisol urine catecholamines were within normal ranges.

What is the MOST likely diagnosis and how do you treat it?

A. Congenital adrenal hyperplasia
B. Pheochromocytoma
C. Liddle syndrome
D. Glucocorticoid remediable aldosteronism

The correct answer is C
Comment: This patient presented with hypertension associated with hypokalemic metabolic alkalosis, and low plasma renin and aldosterone levels. Our patient also had medullary nephrocalcinosis.

The differential diagnosis of severe hypertension and hypokalemia and metabolic alkalosis includes glucocorticoid remediable aldosteronism, the syndrome of apparent mineralocorticoid excess, congenital adrenal hyperplasia (11 beta hydroxylase and 17 alpha hydroxylase deficiencies), pseudohypoaldosteronism type 2 (Gordon syndrome), and Liddle syndrome.[1–4] The combination of hypertension with hypokalemia and metabolic alkalosis is also seen with hyperaldosteronism. Genetic testing confirms the correct diagnosis.

Liddle syndrome is inherited in an autosomal dominant fashion and characterized by early onset hypertension with low plasma renin and aldosterone levels together with hypokalemic metabolic alkalosis. The renal epithelial sodium channel (ENaC) consists of alpha, beta, and gamma subunits.[1,2,4] Mutations in the sodium channel in the distal collecting tubules cause an increase in sodium reabsorption, leading to intravascular volume expansion resulting as hypertension. Together with sodium reabsorption, potassium and hydrogen ion wasting occurs mimicking hyperaldosteronism.

When we evaluate the genetic heterogeneity of the disease, there are three different genes involved: *SCNN1A*, *SCNN1B*, and *SCNN1G*. LS-1 is caused by heterozygous mutation in the *SCNN1B* gene, encoding the beta subunit of ENaC. LS-2 is caused by mutation in the *SCNN1G* gene encoding the ENaC gamma subunit. More than 20 pathogenic variants in the β and γ subunits of the ENaC have been identified. A newly discovered type, LS-3, is caused by mutation in the *SCNN1A* gene encoding the ENaC alpha subunit.[1,2,4]

In our patient, we could only screen for genetic mutation in the *SCNN1B* gene, and we were not able to demonstrate any mutation. However, it is known that in addition to the *SCNN1B* gene, the *SCNN1G* and *SCNN1A* genes are involved. When there is a high clinical suspicion of LS, and in the presence of hypertensive family members such as in our patient, to confirm the genetic diagnosis, other genes such as *SCNN1G* and *SCNN1A* should also be screened.

Liddle syndrome should be suspected in hypertensive young patients when there is a history of a family member with early-onset hypertension and accompanying hypokalemia.[3] There may also be mild or atypical cases with vague features. Liddle syndrome should always be kept in mind for the diagnosis of early-onset (typically between late childhood and adolescence) hypertension even when there is no positive family history since certain cases without hypertensive family members were previously reported.

The suppression of renin and aldosterone is the hallmark of the disease. Due to the continuous reabsorption of sodium from ENaC, potassium is lost via the Na^+/K^+-ATPase pump. Enhanced sodium reabsorption results in negative ion charge in the lumen of the renal tubules, leading to a rise in the excretion of hydrogen ion from the ROMK (renal outer medullary potassium) channel and hydrogen-ATPase pump on alpha-intercalated cells leading to mild metabolic alkalosis. Increased sodium levels and associated volume expansion result in suppression of renin. Suppression of aldosterone is relatively less when compared with renin, yielding an elevated aldosterone/renin ratio, which may also be used as a screening test.

Treatment mainly involves a low-salt diet and the use of a direct ENaC inhibitor and potassium-sparing diuretics such as amiloride or triamterene to control blood pressure. Our patient's hypertension could be controlled after triamterene administration. Mutated ENaC channels are not regulated by mineralocorticoids; for this reason, spironolactone is not beneficial. In the management of hypertension, a low-sodium diet is advised which is also useful in the regulation of the mutated ENaC.

Case Study 7

A 12-year-old girl, born to second-degree consanguineous parents, was brought to the pediatric emergency with complaints of weakness and inability to use all four limbs for 1 day. She was apparently asymptomatic until the previous day, after which she developed weakness and was unable to use all four limbs from the time she woke up in the morning the following day. She had symmetrical weakness of both proximal and distal muscles of the limbs and the trunk. There was no history of dysphagia or nasal regurgitation of feeds, nor did she have deviation of angle of mouth. She did not have any sensory disturbance, or bladder/bowel dysfunction. There was no history of fever, rash, any recent vaccination, intramuscular injection, dog/snake bite, trauma, or intake of any drug in the recent past. Further inquiry revealed that she had polyuria and nocturia since childhood, which had not been quantified. She also had constipation over the last 2 weeks. There was no history of fractures, polydipsia, vomiting, tetany, seizures, dental caries, night blindness, photophobia, dry skin, neck flop, or muscle weakness in the past. Her scholastic performance had been good.

Her anthropometric evaluation revealed that she was severely wasted (weight 22 kg, −4.5 Z-score) and stunted (height 130 cm, −2.6 Z-score) with severe thinness (BMI 13, −4.1 Z-score). At admission, she was hemodynamically stable with a heart rate of 81 beats/min, respiratory rate of 19 breaths/min, blood pressure of 105/70 mmHg, and oxygen saturation of 98%. There was no pallor, icterus, lymphadenopathy, edema, rash, or signs of dehydration. Oral examination revealed yellowish-brown pigmentation of all surfaces of her teeth and delayed eruption of permanent teeth. The ophthalmological examination was negative for corneal crystals and Kayser-Fleischer rings. The pure-tone audiometry was normal. There was no bony deformity or any other features of rickets. On examination, she was alert, conscious, and oriented. The neurological examination revealed generalized hypotonia (with neck flop) and areflexia in all four limbs, power of 1/5 in all four limbs, normal muscle bulk, and no cranial nerve/sensory deficit. The rest of the systemic examination was unremarkable.

Initial investigations showed hypokalemia, hypophosphatemia, metabolic acidosis, normal anion gap (12 mmol/L), normal BUN, serum creatinine, and calcium levels. Her random blood glucose was normal (128 mg/dL). The electrocardiogram showed T-wave inversion and prominent U-waves. She was confirmed to have polyuria after admission (urine output 5.5 mL/kg/h). The 24-hour urine analysis revealed hypercalciuria, phosphaturia (maximum tubular reabsorption [TmP]/glomerular filtration rate [GFR] 1.5 mg/dL), and aminoaciduria. Urine Benedict's test was negative and the urine calcium:creatinine ratio was elevated. The thyroid function tests were normal. Radiographic imaging of kidneys did not reveal any evidence of nephrocalcinosis. There was also no radiographic evidence of rickets.

Further probing revealed that the index child had a 9-year-old sister, who also had polyuria and nocturia for 2 years. She had bony deformities in the form of genu varum. There was no history of fractures, polydipsia, tetany, neck flop, or weakness of muscles. She also had yellowish-brown pigmented teeth since infancy. The parents were advised to bring her for evaluation and her blood investigations also revealed a normal anion gap metabolic acidosis and hypokalemia. Her radiographic images confirmed the presence of rickets and ultrasonography of kidneys revealed nephrocalcinosis. However, she did not have phosphaturia, glycosuria, or aminoaciduria. The fractional excretion of bicarbonate was 3.3%.

What is the MOST likely diagnosis and how would manage this patient?

 A. Wilson disease
 B. Cystinosis
 C. Lowe syndrome
 D. Amelogenesis imperfecta

The correct diagnosis is D

Comment: The child had normal anion gap metabolic acidosis (NAGMA) with hypokalemia. This is mainly caused by an increased bicarbonate loss from either the kidney or gut or impaired acidification in the kidney. She did not have any history of diarrhea, making the bicarbonate loss from the gut unlikely. The constellation of symptoms—polyuria since childhood, hypokalemia, and NAGMA—in the presence of normal estimated glomerular filtration rate favored the diagnosis of renal tubular acidosis (RTA).[1-3] Considering the fractional excretion of bicarbonate (4.1%), alkaline urine pH, and increased urinary calcium:creatinine ratio in our patient, a diagnosis of distal RTA (dRTA) was more likely. The major etiologies for dRTA include hereditary tubulopathies (due to mutations in *SLC4A1*, *ATP6V0A4*, and *ATP6V1B1*) or acquired disorders such as drugs or Sjögren syndrome. However, the child had some features of proximal tubular dysfunction in the form of phosphaturia and aminoaciduria. Hence, the major etiologies of proximal tubular dysfunction—namely Wilson disease, cystinosis, and Lowe syndrome—were ruled out with appropriate investigations and clinical tests. Our patient additionally had yellowish-brown discoloration of her teeth. This abnormality in the background of dRTA aroused the suspicion of amelogenesis imperfecta (AI).[4] Clinical exome sequencing unveiled a pathogenic homozygous nonsense variation in exon 2 of the *WDR72* gene (chr15: g.54025259G > A; Depth: 58x) that resulted in a stop codon and premature truncation of the protein at codon 30 (p. Arg30Ter; ENST00000396328.1), confirming the diagnosis of AI (hypomaturation type).

WDR72 mutation has recently been implicated in the causation of dRTA. The index case, although having dRTA, showed some features of proximal RTA in the form of aminoaciduria and phosphaturia. The exact pathogenesis in the occurrence of additional proximal tubular dysfunction in some cases of dRTA is not clear. The common hypotheses proposed are that defective vacuolar-ATPase (V-ATPase) and hypokalemic nephropathy resulted in defective acidification of the endosome, which is in turn responsible for proximal tubular dysfunction. However, the proximal tubular cells of the kidney do not express β1 subunit of V-ATPase, and therefore, in patients harboring *ATP6V1B1* mutation, proximal RTA cannot be attributed to a defective V-ATPase. Hypokalemia, in the long run, causes a tubulointerstitial injury that can lead to dysfunction of proximal tubules. Emery et al. demonstrated increased excretion of β2 microglobulin in 45% of hypokalemic patients, which was corrected after potassium supplementation. Hypokalemic nephropathy is outlined by tubular cell atrophy and destruction and vacuolization of proximal tubular cells. This leads to intrarenal hypoxia due to microvascular injury, which in turn is responsible for tubulointerstitial damage. CLC-5 chloride channel and V-ATPase activity are essential for orderly acidification of the sorting endosomes. V-H⁺ ATPase is contained on both the apical membranes of proximal and distal renal tubular cells. V-H⁺ ATPase dysfunction leads to a more severe intracellular acidosis in proximal tubular cells in the presence of preexisting acidosis, which results in endosomal dysfunction that culminates in proximal tubular dysfunction. Acidosis also hinders CLC-5 function as an aftermath of a decrease in driving force for exchange caused by the pH gradient. This may contribute to proximal renal tubular dysfunction in dRTA patients prior to initiating treatment.

The management of this patient can be summarized into two aspects: management of the complications and management of the underlying disease. Our index child presented with hypokalemic paralysis, which is a life-threatening complication. Therefore, she was immediately started on potassium correction at 40 mmol/L in the maintenance intravenous fluids under strict cardiac monitoring, until potassium normalized and then switched to oral potassium supplements. Her limbs restored normal power after potassium correction. Management of the underlying disease involves correction of acidosis and hypokalemia. Correction of acidosis restores normal growth rate and reduces calcium losses associated with bone buffering of some of the retained acid, thereby diminishing the risk of osteopenia. Alkali therapy also reverses hypercalciuria and reduces the rate of nephrolithiasis and nephrocalcinosis. Additionally, it reduces urinary potassium losses, correcting the associated hypokalemia. A part of potassium depletion is also due to a reduction in proximal sodium reabsorption induced by metabolic acidosis. The goal of alkali therapy must be to achieve a normal serum bicarbonate level (22 to 24 mmol/L). Our patient required potassium citrate (4 mmol/kg/day) to neutralize the acidosis and hypokalemia. The child also had hypophosphatemia due to phosphaturia and required treatment with neutral phosphate supplementation at 50 mg/kg/day initially. On follow-up at 2 months, the serum bicarbonate was 22.5 mmol/L, serum potassium was 3.7 mEq/L, and serum phosphorus was 3.5 mmol/L. She gradually outgrew the neutral phosphate supplementation on follow-up. She was advised to follow up in dentistry to plan regarding crowns or tooth implants for the teeth discoloration.

Case Study 8

A 10-year-old Caucasian female presented to an emergency department for evaluation for acute bilateral upper and lower limb weakness and inability to walk. The patient was in her usual state of health until the morning of presentation when she woke up and slid off the bed while trying to stand up. She described feeling a heavy sensation in her lower limbs and an inability to lift them or bear any weight on them. She denied any pain or paresthesia; there was no shortness of breath or loss of bowel or bladder continence. She had difficulty holding herself up and had to be carried around by her father. Due to the acuity of the paralysis, patient was brought to the emergency department by her parents. The patient and her parents denied any recent upper respiratory infection symptoms, fever, skin rash, insect bites, drug ingestion, dark urine, trauma, or any recent travel. The parents reported that along with the paresis, patient had slow speech and difficulty finding correct words, but denied any facial drooping, confusion, altered mental status, or previous history of muscle weakness. In fact, the patient went swimming 2 days prior to presentation. Immunizations were up to date.

Past medical history was significant for a seizure disorder with onset at age five *83*
been treated and was under control on lamotrigine. Last seizure episode was 6 month
this presentation. The parents also reported a history of recurrent urticarial rash with 6
proximately 11 months prior to this presentation. She was referred to an allergist who o.
lab work that demonstrated serum sodium 138 mmol/L, potassium of 4.1 mmol/L, chlor.
mmol/L, bicarbonate 30 mmol/L, ANA that was positive at 1280, speckled pattern, neg
thyroid antibodies, and a chronic urticaria index of greater than 50. Patient was initially managu
with systemic steroids that led to a 9 kg weight gain. Treatment was later changed to omalizumab
injections that brought it under control without needing to continue systemic steroids.

Vital signs upon arrival on admission included a temperature of 36.4, heart rate of 122 beats/
min, respiratory 22 breaths/min, blood pressure of 120/min, blood pressure of 120/67 mmHg,
oxygen saturation of 100% on room air, weight of 52.2 kg (97th percentile for age), height of 157.5
cm (98th percentile for age), and BMI of 21.04 kg/m². Physical exam was remarkable for an alert,
coherent, and oriented female with no respiratory distress and intact cranial nerves but decreased
motor strength of 3/5 of both upper and lower extremities against gravity and weak hand grip.
Deep tendon reflexes were 2/4 bilateral biceps, brachioradialis, patellae, and ankles. Sense of light
touch was preserved throughout. Normal muscle tone and bulk × 4 extremities. Initial evaluation
was remarkable for a critically low serum potassium level of 2.0 mmol/L, bicarbonate of 15
mmol/L, normal anion gap of 7.0 mmol/L, normal BUN, creatinine, calcium. Serum phosphorus
was initially low at 2.3 mg/dL. Urinalysis was unremarkable except for dilute urine with specific
gravity of 1.004, pH of 7.0. Venous blood gas confirmed primary metabolic acidosis. Erythrocyte
sedimentation rate was elevated at 62, urine drug screen was negative except for amphetamine
(patient was on ADHD medication), lactic acid level was normal, and Lyme antibodies were
negative. Initial ECG was remarkable for first-degree AV block with a prolonged PR interval of
220 ms. A head computed tomography (CT) was unremarkable for any acute intracranial process.
The patient was admitted to the pediatric intensive care unit for close monitoring and telemetry.
Over the course of 48 hours, the patient's hypokalemia and metabolic acidosis were corrected,
initially by intravenous supplementation, then orally with potassium citrate. There was concurrent
normalization of electrocardiogram changes and improvement of muscle weakness.

What is the MOST likely diagnosis?

A. Primary hyperaldosteronism
B. Sjogren syndrome
C. Familial hypokalemic periodic paralysis (FHPP)
D. Fanconi syndrome

The correct answer is B
Comment: Hypokalemia can be caused by an intracellular shift of potassium, a decrease in potassium
intake, or an increase in potassium loss (GI or renal). The patient did not take medications that
can cause intracellular shift, such as beta-adrenergic agonist, antipsychotic medications, insulin,
and catecholamines. There was no family history to suggest familial hypokalemic periodic
paralysis (FHPP), which causes transient hypokalemia and muscle weakness and is inherited in
an autosomal dominant trait, and in addition, metabolic acidosis is not characteristic of FHPP.
The patient was on a normal diet, which makes decreased potassium intake unlikely. There was no
history of vomiting or diarrhea, which makes gastrointestinal loss unlikely. Urine tests confirmed
renal K⁺ loss. The majority of renal K⁺ wasting conditions such as diuretic use, Bartter syndrome,
Gitelman syndrome, Liddle syndrome, or primary hyperaldosteronism are accompanied by
metabolic alkalosis not metabolic acidosis.

Workup for the etiology of hypokalemia and non-anion gap metabolic acidosis was initiated.
Calculation of transtubular potassium gradient (TTKG = 8) and fractional excretion of potassium

%) indicated renal potassium wasting. Renal tubular acidosis (RTA) was suspected due to inappropriately high urine pH relative to the metabolic acidosis. The low serum K^+ level ruled it type 4 RTA. Bicarbonate wasting from the proximal tubule (type 2 RTA) as part of Fanconi syndrome was entertained, especially since the initial serum phosphorus level was low; however, there was no glucosuria or evidence of renal phosphate wasting (urine phosphorus < 10), and subsequent serum PO_4 levels were normal. Type 1 distal RTA was confirmed due to positive urine anion gap, presence of hypercalciuria with urine calcium creatinine ratio of 0.47, and a kidney ultrasound that demonstrated a non-obstructing 6-mm lower pole calculus in the left kidney.

RTA in pediatrics is generally caused by a genetic abnormality or congenital urinary tract anomalies. We suspected that this was an acquired RTA due to the absence of short stature, which is typically seen in longstanding untreated metabolic acidosis, and we had lab evidence that she had normal serum K^+ and total CO_2 levels 8 and 10 months prior to presentation.

Further investigation revealed that 8 months prior to the presentation, because of the elevated erythrocyte sedimentation rate (ESR) and ANA titer, the allergist treating the patient for recurrent urticaria had referred her to a pediatric rheumatologist at another medical facility. A more extensive evaluation for autoimmune disease was initiated which included a repeat CBC that was unremarkable, urinalysis that demonstrated a specific gravity of 1.028, pH of 6.0, negative for blood or protein, repeat ESR of 22 (patient was on prednisone 10 mg BID), elevated ANA titer of 1280, negative anti-dsDNA, normal C3 and C4 complements, normal C1Q binding assay, SM antibody IgG negative, normal TSH, negative thyroperoxidase antibody, negative thyroglobulin antibody, RNP IgG negative, SM antibody IgG negative, SCL 70 IgG negative, and SSA IgG positive. The patient was diagnosed with primary Sjogren syndrome.[1,2] Due to improvement of ESR, albeit the patient was on prednisone at that time, and absence of sicca symptoms, the rheumatologist elected not to treat the patient, with notation that hydroxychloroquine would be considered if the patient becomes symptomatic. With this new information, we repeated SS-A/Ro IgG which came back elevated at greater than 8.0; SS-B/La IgG also came back elevated at 2.1. Repeat ANA was again positive at 1:1280, anti-dsDNA was negative, and C3 and C4 complements were normal. Additional tests were conducted to support the diagnosis of Sjogren syndrome, and this included a positive rheumatoid factor, hyperimmunoglobulinemia (elevated IgG and IgA levels). Despite the absence of symptoms of dry mouth and dry eyes, we performed a Schirmer test to assess for adequate tear production, and this was positive with only 3 and 5 mm of tear production (normal should be ≥ 10 mm) in the patient's right and left eyes, respectively.

Case Study 9

A 3-year-old male patient was admitted to the otolaryngology department for cochlear implantation plan with the diagnosis of bilateral sensorineural deafness. During the preoperative evaluation, severe hypokalemia (serum potassium, 2.4 mmol/L) was observed and referred to the pediatric nephrology department. There was not any history of diarrhea, vomiting, or polyuria. He was born at 33 weeks of gestational age with a history of polyhydramnios from healthy non-consanguineous parents. His birth weight was 2.1 kg. He was the third child with two healthy siblings.

On admission, the patient's weight was 10 kg and length was 86 cm, all of which were below the 3rd percentile for the age. He did not have facial dysmorphism. He was normotensive.

In biochemical investigation, serum creatinine was 0.46 mg/dL and urea was 16 mg/dL. Serum electrolytes showed hyponatremia (serum sodium, 130 mmol/L), severe hypokalemia (serum potassium, 2.4 mmol/L), and hypochloremia (serum chloride, 87 mmol/L). Serum calcium was 9.5 mg/dL, serum phosphate was 5.1 mg/dL, and serum magnesium was 2.4 mg/dL, all of which were in normal ranges. The patient had metabolic alkalosis (blood gas pH, 7.55; HCO_3^-, 28.4 mmol/L) together with high plasma renin activity (983 pg/mL; reference range: 3.18 to 32.61 pg/mL) and elevated aldosterone level (2891 pg/mL; reference range: 12 to 340 pg/mL).

Ultrasonographic evaluation did not reveal any pathology such as nephrocalcinosis. Oral sodium supplements and potassium chloride treatment were administered. Subsequently, the electrolyte levels became normal (sodium and potassium levels after supplementation were 140 mmol/L and 3.7 mmol/L, respectively). The patient underwent surgery for cochlear implantation.

What is the MOST likely diagnosis?

A. Bartter syndrome type 4 with sensorineural defenses
B. Liddle syndrome
C. Congenital adrenal hyperplasia
D. Apparent mineralocorticoid excess (AME)

The correct answer is A
Comment: Sensorineural hearing loss is seen in Pendred syndrome, Jervell and Lange-Nielsen syndrome, Waardenburg syndrome, Usher syndrome, CHARGE syndrome (Coloboma, Heart Anomaly, Choanal Atresia, Retardation, Genital, and Ear anomalies), and Alport syndrome, and in other rare syndromes like CINCA (Chronic Infantile Neurologic Cutaneous and Articular) syndrome, Bartter syndrome type 4, and Donnai-Barrow syndrome.[1-5] Diagnosing these rare syndromes might be difficult in a patient group who has mild symptoms. The patient presented in the case was not symptomatic and hypokalemia was detected in routine laboratory workup before surgery.

In this child, the sensorineural hearing loss was associated with polyuria, renal salt wasting, hypokalemic metabolic alkalosis, and normotensive hyperreninemic hyperaldosteronism, which point to the diagnosis of Bartter syndrome type 4.

There are several reports about *SLC12A1*, *KCNJ1*, *BSND*, *CLCNKA*, *CLCNKB*, and *CASR* mutations that cause Bartter syndrome *BSND* and *CLCNKA* and *CLCNKB* mutations cause BS with sensorineural hearing loss (BS type 4a and 4b, respectively). *BSND* gene is located at chromosome 1p31 locus, and it codes barttin protein, which is a subunit for CLC-Ka and ClC-Kb chloride channels. Barttin is expressed at tubular segments beginning from thick ascending limb to cortical collecting tubules. At inner ear, barttin is also expressed at potassium-secreting epithelial cells, and this is the reason *BSND*-mutated patients have sensorineural hearing loss. There are several "disease-causing mutations" in *BSND* gene, affecting function of ClC-K channels. Some of these are R8L, R8W, G10S, Q32X, G47R, and G10S. Three of them (R8L, R8W, G10S) disturb the function of ClC-K channels; however, insertion of channel-to-surface membrane is not affected. On the other hand, G47R mutation causes mild renal phenotype, and in this type of mutation, bounding of mutant barttin to ClC-K channel is less effective.

In our patient, sequence analysis of all coding exons and exon-intron boundaries presented "NM_057176.2:c.139G greater than C (p. Gly47Arg)(p. G47R) (homozygote) mutation" in exon 1 of 4 of *BSND* gene, while his parents were heterozygotes. This is a known variant (rs74315289/ HGMD (Human Gene Mutation Database)-Public-CM035675) and closely related with BS type 4a but mostly presents a mild clinical phenotype. This variant was also given in OMIM (Online Mendelian Inheritance in Man) database. As clinical confirmations and segregations were documented before, this variant was classified as a "pathogenic variant" due to ACMG (American College of Medical Genetics and Genomics) criteria.

In Bartter syndrome, prompt treatment with intravenous fluids is needed. Indomethacin has limited effects in type 4 Bartter syndrome. Oral sodium and potassium supplements were sufficient to normalize his serum electrolytes.

Case Study 10

A 7-year-old girl was transferred to hospital for the evaluation of failure to thrive. She was born at term with a birth weight of 3.0 kg and without perinatal problems. At the age of 3 years and 4 months, she was examined at a hospital for poor weight gain and difficulty in running and climbing stairs. At that time, her height was 92.4 cm (5th to 10th percentile) and weight was 11.8 kg (< 3rd percentile). Neurologic development and cognitive and social language skills were found to be normal. The laboratory tests, including those for serum electrolyte levels and thyroid function, revealed no abnormality. At the age of 6 years, she was diagnosed with bilateral sensorineural hearing loss and she started wearing a hearing aid.

At the first visit to our hospital (age 7 years), her height was 104 cm (< 3rd percentile) and weight was 13.45 kg (< 3rd percentile). Her blood pressure was 99/53 mmHg. She did not eat well and had a mildly poor motor function, especially in climbing upstairs, while her intelligence was normal. Laboratory tests revealed Bartter-like electrolyte imbalance: serum sodium, potassium, chloride, and bicarbonate levels were 133, 2.7, 93, and 31.4 mEq/L, respectively, and the arterial blood pH was 7.504. Serum creatinine level was 0.34 mg/dL and creatinine clearance was 79.7 mL/min/1.73 m². The serum albumin (4.9 g/dL) level was normal. Serum calcium, phosphorus, and magnesium levels were 9.5 mg/dL, 3.9 mg/dL, and 1.1 mEq/L, respectively. Serum uric acid level was 1.4 mg/dL. Plasma renin activity was 70.64 (normal 1 to 2.5) ng/mL/h and serum aldosterone level was 125.7 (normal 3 to 16.0) ng/dL. Urinalysis revealed 1 + albumin and 1 + glucose. In the spot urine test, the protein/creatinine ratio was 1.72 mg/mg, the calcium/creatinine ratio was 0.06 mg/mg, the β2-microglobulin level was 28.0 (reference: 0 to 0.37) μg/mL, and the N-acetyl-β-glucosaminidase level was 40.3 (reference: 0 to 5.6) IU/g creatinine. The trans-tubular potassium gradient was 7. The tubular maximum phosphorus reabsorption/glomerular filtration rate was 3.46 (reference: 2.6 to 4.4) mg/dL, and uric acid excretion/glomerular filtration rate was 0.52 (reference: < 0.56) mg/dL. Plasma organic acid profile revealed lactic acid to be 3909.85 (reference: 500 to 1500) μmol/L and pyruvic acid to be 165 μmol/L (reference: 50 to 500), while the urinary organic acid profile was normal. Immediately following this, intermittent hypocalcemia (the lowest serum ionized calcium level was 0.83 mmol/L) was noted during follow-up. The serum intact parathyroid hormone level was less than 5 pg/mL (reference: 10 to 65 pg/mL), and serum 25 (OH)-vitamin D3 level was 16.0 (reference: 9.0 to 37.6) ng/mL.

What is the MOST likely diagnosis?

  A. Kearns-Sayre syndrome
  B. Bartter syndrome
  C. Cystinosis
  D. Tubulointerstitial disease

The correct diagnosis is A

Comment: The patient presented multiorgan-involving symptoms and signs sequentially: lower extremity muscle weakness at 3 years and 5 months, sensorineural hearing loss at 6 years, and Bartter-like renal tubulopathy and hypoparathyroidism at 7 years. The initial clinical diagnosis made at the age of 7 years was that of Bartter syndrome with an uncertain genotype. The presence of Gitelman syndrome-like features, i.e., normal or low urinary calcium excretion level and hypomagnesemia, suggested Bartter syndrome type III due to mutations in *CLCNKB*.[1-3] Meanwhile, sensorineural hearing loss and hyperparathyroidism are typical findings of Bartter syndrome type IV due to mutations in *BSND* and Bartter syndrome type V due to gain-of-function mutations in *CASR*, respectively. Initially, we thought that the muscle weakness was related to chronic hypokalemia and/or hypocalcemia. However, mutational studies of all five genes (*SLC12A1*, *KCNJ1*, *CLCNKB*, *BSND*, and *CASR*) implicated in Bartter syndrome revealed no pathogenic mutation.

Notably, the patient also presented other proximal tubular dysfunctions, including low-molecular-weight proteinuria and hypouricemia, which are not detected in patients with the classic forms of Bartter syndrome. Therefore, at the age of 8 years, a biopsy of the left thigh muscle was performed to enable a correct diagnosis, with the biopsy revealing findings typical of mitochondrial myopathy. Genetic analysis using a peripheral blood sample then revealed a homoplasmic 8932-bp deletion (m.6130_15061del) in the mitochondrial DNA (mtDNA). In addition, an electrocardiogram taken before the muscle biopsy revealed left axis deviation, left bundle branch block, and borderline degree of left ventricular hypertrophy and QT interval prolongation. One month after the muscle biopsy, a decrease in visual acuity with bilateral ptosis was noted in the school physical examination, and the results of an ophthalmologic examination revealed pigmentary retinopathy. With these additional cardiac and ocular findings, the diagnostic criteria for Kearns-Sayre syndrome (KSS) were fulfilled.

Case Study 11

A 2-year-old boy was admitted for the evaluation of failure to thrive. The patient was born at 36 weeks of gestation with a birth weight of 2850 g as the first living child of consanguineous apparently healthy parents. The pregnancy had been complicated by polyhydramnios. The mother reported two previous pregnancies, one resulting in early abortion, and the other in an anencephalic neonate. After birth, the patient showed prolonged jaundice, vomiting, and dehydration with hypokalemia, and the clinical diagnosis of neonatal Bartter syndrome was made. Initial treatment included intravenous fluids to correct hypovolemia and oral potassium solutions. The further clinical course was characterized by persistent diarrhea (8 to 9 stools daily) complicated by frequent episodes of dehydration and water-electrolyte-imbalances leading to repeated hospitalizations. Because of the unremitting course and progressive failure to thrive, it was decided to refer the patient to our institution for further diagnosis and therapy.

A review of previous hospital records showed that the patient had needed daily potassium supplements. Since the child strongly disliked the salty flavor of potassium chloride, an oral potassium gluconate solution had been given at a dose of 8 mmol/kg/day. Medication and feeding had remained difficult and the child had never developed normal eating patterns, resulting in a dependence on continuous oral feeding by relatives with occasional intravenous alimentation; however, application by a nasogastric tube had been refused by the parents. Celiac disease had been excluded by intestinal biopsy. Medication with omeprazole and domperidone was without effect. Altogether, the child had spent almost half of his life in hospitals.

Upon admission, at the age of 2 years, the child appeared severely malnourished and weight (8900 g), height (81.5 cm), and head circumference (45 cm) were far below appropriate percentiles for his age. Apart from abdominal distension and paleness, clinical examination revealed no further abnormalities and no congenital malformations. Blood gas analysis showed severe metabolic alkalosis (pH 7.58, bicarbonate 46 mmol/L, and base excess + 21 mmol/L). Serum electrolytes were as follows: potassium 2.0 mmol/L, sodium 131 mmol/L, and chloride 68 mmol/L. Further clinical observation after rehydration and during a period of minimal intravenous fluid replacement showed that the patient had a spontaneous total caloric intake of approximately 20% of his recommended dietary allowance and a spontaneous fluid intake of about 200 mL.

What is the MOST likely diagnosis?

  A. Congenital Bartter syndrome
  B. Congenital chloride diarrhea (CLD)
  C. Apparent mineralocorticoid excess
  D. Liddle syndrome

The correct answer is B
Comment: Chronic diarrhea and absence of polyuria and polydipsia are not typical for patients with Bartter syndrome. Congenital chloride diarrhea (CLD) is a rare autosomal recessive disease occurring mainly in people in Arabian countries, Finland, and Poland. It is characterized by unremitting watery diarrhea with high fecal losses of chloride, failure to thrive, and renal impairment in

older children and adults if the disease is left untreated.[1,2] Prenatal symptoms include polyhydramnios and dilated intestinal loops; birth is often premature, and postnatal mortality rates are high due to severe dehydration and electrolyte imbalances. The disease is caused by a defective anion exchange protein, an epithelial chloride/bicarbonate exchanger located in the brush border of the ileum and colon, resulting in defective intestinal chloride absorption and secretion of bicarbonate, with a secondary defect in sodium/hydrogen (Na^+/H^+) transport, altogether leading to intestinal losses of both sodium and water, hypochloremia, hyponatremia, and metabolic alkalosis.

Some of the clinical features may resemble Bartter syndrome, which had been suspected in this case, namely, polyhydramnios, failure to thrive, and hypochloremic metabolic alkalosis. However, all forms of Bartter syndrome are characterized by high urinary losses of Na^+, K^+, and Cl^- due to defective tubular reabsorption. Thus, a simple spot urine measurement may rule out Bartter syndrome, as in this case. Urinary concentrations of Na^+ and Cl^- were 14 mmol/L and 15 mmol/L, respectively. However, misdiagnosis of Bartter syndrome in CLD patients has been described in a number of cases. Differential diagnosis further includes cystic fibrosis, which (especially in hot climates) may result in high Cl^- losses, hypochloremic metabolic alkalosis, gastrointestinal symptoms, and failure to thrive and should be ruled out by a sweat chloride test (normal in this case).

Measuring chloride in stool is a simple clinical test to confirm the clinical diagnosis of CLD. Chloride concentrations of greater than 90 mmol/L are reportedly diagnostic for the disease. In this case, the value was 89 mmol/L (after rehydration and chloride substitution). However, genetic testing is now available in specialized laboratories to establish the definitive diagnosis.

Patients with CLD harbor mutations in both copies of the *SLC26A3* (solute carrier family 26, member 3, or DRA) gene on chromosome 7q31. Altogether, 36 different mutations distributed within exons 3 to 19 of the gene have been identified in patients with CLD. However, certain founder mutations are particularly frequent in patients in Arabian countries, Finland, and Poland, and account for the majority of CLD cases. No genotype-phenotype correlation has emerged. Direct sequencing of the *SLC26A3* gene detects point and splice-site mutations and small insertions and deletions, with an overall mutation detection rate of greater than 95%. In this case, both parents were found to harbor the heterozygous mutation c.559G > T (p. G187X), resulting in a homozygous mutation of the patient at this locus. This mutation results either in severe protein truncation or in nonsense-mediated RNA decay, with no protein produced at all.

Case Study 12

A 13-year-old boy was admitted to our hospital with recurrent headaches that had been localized to the occipital region for the past year. His medical history was unremarkable, with no known history of kidney disease. The family history was also unremarkable, and consanguinity was not present between his parents. His weight and height were within normal ranges; casual blood pressure was measured as 150/100 mmHg. The systemic examination revealed no abnormal results. Ambulatory blood pressure monitoring (ABPM) obtained mean 24-hour, daytime, and nighttime systolic and diastolic blood pressures of 140/99, 148/106, and 135/95 mmHg, respectively; the daytime and nighttime systolic and diastolic blood pressure load were 100%, and abnormal dipping (8%) was present. The laboratory findings were: hemoglobin, 14.8 g/dL; white blood cells, 8400/mm³; platelets, 479,000/mm³; BUN 17 mg/dL; creatinine, 0.5 mg/dL; Na^+, 137 mmol/L; Cl^-, 105 mmol/L; K^+, 3.8 mmol/L; uric acid, 3.3 mg/dL; calcium, 9.5 mg/dL; phosphorous, 4 mg/dL; total protein, 7.9 g/dL; albumin, 4.9 g/dL; pH, 7.45; PCO_2, 40 mmHg; bicarbonate, 27.4 mEq/L; base excess, 3.2 mEq/L; plasma renin activity, 146 pg/mL (reference: 3 to 16 pg/mL); aldosterone concentration, 62.7 ng/dL (reference: 0.29 to 16.1 ng/dL). The urinalysis and lipid profile were normal. Echocardiography showed concentric left ventricular hypertrophy and a left ventricular mass index (LVMI) of 51.7 g/m²·⁷ (upper limit of normal: 38 g/m²·⁷). The results of the ophthalmologic examination, abdominal ultrasound, renal arterial Doppler ultrasound, Tc-99 m dimercaptosuccinic acid scintigraphy, and renal arterial magnetic resonance angiography were all normal, as were plasma adrenocorticotropic hormone and cortisol levels and 24-hour urinary metanephrine and vanillylmandelic acid levels. Treatment with enalapril (10 mg/day) and amlodipine (10 mg/day) was initiated for severe hypertension. Three months later, the ABPM was completely normal, and after 12 months, the LVMI had decreased to 43.7 $g/m^{2.7}$. The patients voiced no complaints in the 18 months thereafter; periodic ABPMs were performed during the follow-up, and minor drug adjustments were made accordingly. Approximately 2.5 years after the first diagnosis, the patient came to our outpatient department for a routine control. He had no complaints, was on triple antihypertensive therapy (enalapril, amlodipine, and propranolol), and the ABPM was normal. Laboratory tests revealed the following: blood urea nitrogen, 15 mg/dL; creatinine, 0.5 mg/dL; Na^+, 135 mmol/L; Cl^-, 94 mmol/L; K^+, 3 mmol/L. A blood gas analysis was requested following the recognition of hypokalemia; it showed pH, 7.45; PCO_2, 44 mmHg; bicarbonate, 30 mmol/L; base excess, 5.3. The blood K^+ values had ranged from 3.4 to 4 mmol/L. The patient was hospitalized, and treatments with antihypertensive medications were first reduced and then stopped. Renal ultrasound revealed a 3-cm, solid, exophytic mass in the upper pole of the left kidney. Magnetic resonance imaging (MRI) of the abdomen showed a 3.5-cm well-circumscribed mass in the posterolateral upper pole of the left kidney.

What is the MOST likely diagnosis?

    A. Pheochromocytoma
    B. Congenital adrenal hyperplasia
    C. Reninoma
    D. Primary hyperaldosteronism

The correct answer is C
Comment: Our patient presented with hypertension, hypokalemic metabolic alkalosis with elevated plasma renin activity (PRA), aldosterone, and cortisol concentrations.

    Liddle syndrome, congenital adrenal hyperplasia, apparent mineralocorticoid excess, primary aldosteronism, glucocorticoid-remediable aldosteronism, pheochromocytoma, and renovascular disease was ruled out because none of these conditions are associated with elevation of both PRA and serum aldosterone concentration. Diagnosis of renin-secreting tumor (reninoma) was considered as in this condition that hypertension and hypokalemic metabolic alkalosis is associated with the high serum aldosterone and PRA.[1,2] This diagnosis was supported by the findings on renal sonogram and MRI imaging studies.

    Reninoma is a renal juxtaglomerular apparatus tumor (JGA) that produces excessive amounts of renin, resulting in secondary hyperaldosteronism, associated hypokalemia, and hypertension. Other renin-secreting tumors, such as Wilms tumor or rhabdoid tumor of the kidney, should be considered in the differential diagnosis.

    Both MRI and CT scans are highly effective for determining the presence of a JGA. However, in general, only an ultrasound scan is performed during the routine evaluation of hypertensive patients, and this procedure can result in small tumors being missed due to the isoechoic nature of the tumor. A small tumor was most likely present at the first presentation of our patient, but at that time it was not possible to demarcate it from the parenchyma.

    The definitive treatment for reninoma is surgery. Radical nephrectomy or partial nephrectomy can be performed. Tumors are often superficial and can easily be removed by nephron-sparing surgery, such as in our patient.

Case Study 13

A boy presented at the age of 6 months with failure to thrive and constipation. He had not vomited and no drugs had been given. The second child of unrelated parents, his 4-year-old sister had presented with similar symptoms, clinical and biochemical findings at the age of 1 year. On admission his length and head circumference were on the 50th percentiles but he was below the 3rd percentile for weight. His blood pressure was 90/60 mmHg. Venous serum sodium was 135 mmol/L, potassium 2.0 mmol/L, bicarbonate 42.5 mmol/L, chloride 76 mmol/L, creatinine 0.4 mg/dL, calcium 2.83 8.5 mg/dL, phosphate 2.3 mmol/L, albumin 4.1 g/dL. Plasma renin and aldosterone concentrations were fivefold higher than normal. Renal biopsy showed no glomerular, tubular, or interstitial abnormality. On treatment with spironolactone, sodium chloride and potassium chloride, he grew poorly and the hypokalemic alkalosis persisted. When he was 5.5 years old further investigations confirmed the diagnosis and a change of treatment improved his growth rate dramatically.

What is he MOST Likely diagnosis?

    A. Liddle syndrome
    B. Bartter syndrome
    C. Cystic fibrosis
    D. Chloride diarrhea

The correct answer is B
Comment: The raised plasma renin showed that the hypokalemic alkalosis was associated with secondary hyperaldosteronism, thus excluding an adrenal tumor and Liddle syndrome.[1,2] The differential diagnosis included Bartter syndrome and the causes of isolated sodium or chloride depletion: chloride diarrhea, surreptitious administration of laxatives or diuretics (as in Meadow's syndrome), cystic fibrosis, and other causes of continued vomiting or diarrhea. The urinary excretion of prostaglandins (PGE 2) and (PGF 2) was increased 2- to 3-fold above the normal for his age, suggesting Bartter syndrome. However, this is not the primary abnormality in Bartter syndrome and other causes of hypokalemia may increase the urinary prostaglandins. The diagnosis of Bartter syndrome was confirmed by showing that during 5% dextrose infusion the fractional distal chloride reabsorption was less than 62 mL/100 mL glomerular filtration rate (GFR) and that the fractional chloride excretion was greater than 1.5 mL/100 mL GFR. In other causes of secondary hyperaldosteronism, including diuretic abuse, renal chloride reabsorption is not impaired. The demonstration of a reduced rate of erythrocyte sodium efflux and a reduced number of Na^+-K^+ pump receptor sites would also have confirmed Bartter syndrome. Renal biopsy may be normal in young patients with Bartter syndrome, as in this case.

    In the 1st year of treatment with indomethacin, 3 mg/kg/day in divided doses, his growth rate increased from 5 to 13 cm/year. Although the prostaglandin synthetase inhibitors often fail to fully correct the hypokalemia, they do usually abolish the clinical manifestations of Bartter syndrome. Treatment needs to be continued throughout childhood, but it is not yet known for how long it should be continued once growth has ceased.

Case Study 14

A 14-year-old Caucasian female presented to her pediatrician for repair of a laceration and was found to have a blood pressure of 140/90 mmHg. On follow-up her blood pressure had risen to 205/120 mmHg. She was subsequently admitted for blood pressure management. She had no history of systemic symptomatology, including malaise, weakness, headache, visual changes, joint pain, rash, edema, or gross hematuria. She denied the use of illicit drugs or medications such as birth control pills or appetite suppressants. Her past medical history was essentially negative. She had no history of urinary tract infections. She had achieved normal growth and developmental milestones, including puberty. Her most recent blood pressure determination was at 9 years of age and was normal at that time. Her family history was positive only for hypothyroidism involving her mother and her maternal grandmother.

On physical examination, she was well developed with normal cardiac, skin, fundoscopic, and genitourinary examinations. Her blood pressure was symmetrical in all four extremities. Her height and weight were between the 75th and 90th percentiles. Her initial work-up included a normal urinalysis, serum sodium 147 mmol/L, potassium 2.6 mmol/L, bicarbonate 32 mmol/L, blood urea nitrogen 20 mg/dL, creatinine 0.7 mg/dL, calcium 9.6 mg/dL, and a normal complete blood count. In addition, she had a normal thyroxin and thyroid-stimulating hormone. A urine pregnancy and toxicology screen were negative. The serum renin level was measured. A renal ultrasound examination revealed normal-sized kidneys with normal echo texture. A 99m technetium-dimercaptosuccinic acid renal scan showed symmetric uptake and differential function without evidence of scar or other parenchymal defect. The patient had mild left ventricular hypertrophy on echocardiogram. This patient's blood pressure was extremely difficult to control despite aggressive therapy with an angiotensin converting enzyme inhibitor and a calcium channel blocker. She continued to have baseline diastolic blood pressures greater than 90 mmHg. Her serum potassium remained low (3.4 mmol/L) on KC1 supplementation at 40 mmol/day. Her plasma renin activity was suppressed, with a serum renin level of less than 0.2 ng/mL/h (normal range 0.2 to 2.3). Because of this finding associated with her metabolic abnormalities (hypokalemia and metabolic alkalosis), a diagnosis of primary hyperaldosteronism was considered. The patient was followed closely on a liberalized sodium diet (3.5 g/24 h) for 5 days, when a 24-hour urine collection was performed for aldosterone and cortisol. Blood was also drawn for measurement of serum aldosterone and 18-hydroxycorticosterone levels. Results of the above work-up were inconsistent with the diagnosis of primary hyperaldosteronism and included: serum aldosterone 3.0 ng/dL (reference: 1 to 22), 18-hydroxycorticosterone 24 ng/dL (reference: 5 to 80), urine aldosterone 4.6 kg/24 h (reference: 2.3 to 21), and urine cortisol 31 ktg/24 h (reference: 1 to 55).

What is the MOST likely diagnosis of hypertension in this patient with the above electrolyte disorders?

    A. Apparent mineralocorticoid excess (AME)
    B. Liddle syndrome
    C. Congenital adrenal hyperplasia
    D. Primary aldosteronism

The correct answer is A
Comment: The differential diagnosis in this patient with hypertension, hypokalemia, metabolic alkalosis, low plasma renin activity, and low serum and urine aldosterone levels is limited and includes such disorders as Cushing syndrome, congenital adrenal hyperplasia, aldosterone precursor secreting adrenal tumors, exogenous mineralocorticoid, Liddle syndrome, and syndrome of AME.[1-4] This patient had a normal genital examination and normal pubertal development. She had no physical stigmata to suggest Cushing syndrome. She had no history of exposure to exogenous mineralocorticoid (i.e., glycyrrhetinic acid contained in licorice or prescription preparations such as Florinef). The family history was not consistent with Liddle syndrome, which is an autosomal dominant condition.

Based on her laboratory findings the patient was subsequently diagnosed with AME.

This syndrome is an inheritable disorder of cortisol metabolism and clearance due to 1 1 β-hydroxysteroid dehydrogenase enzyme deficiency resulting in excessive, uninhibited stimulation by cortisol of the mineralocorticoid receptor in the kidney. As a result the urinary steroid profile of these patients reveals an abnormally high ratio of cortisol to cortisone metabolites.

AME is clinical picture, which is analogous to patients with primary or secondary hyperaldosteronism but differs in that both renin and aldosterone secretions are suppressed. These patients often present with other associated findings, including failure to thrive or short stature, muscle weakness, ileus, or polyuria/polydipsia secondary to an impaired renal concentrating ability.

There is also an increased incidence of hypercalciuria in these patients. The mode of inheritance remains unclear. The age at the time of diagnosis has varied from 9 months to 27 years.

The therapy for patients with AME varies with the type. Patients with type I disease respond very nicely to mineralocorticoid receptor blockade with spironolactone with lowering of blood pressure and normalization of serum K^+ levels. Patients with type II AME fail to respond to spironolactone but can be effectively treated with dexamethasone. All patients should be maintained on a sodium-restricted diet.

References

Case Study 1

1. Rose BD, Post TW. *Clinical Physiology of Acid-Base and Electrolyte Disorders.* 5th ed. New York, NY: McGraw-Hill; 2001:748–767.

Case Study 2

1. Thomas D, Dubose J. Disorders of acid-base balance. In: Skorecki K, Chertow GM, Marsden PA, Taal MW, Yu AS, eds. *Brenner & Rector's The Kidney.* 10th ed. Philadelphia, PA: Elsevier; 2016:511–558.
2. Schroeder ET. Alkalosis resulting from combined administration of a "nonsystemic" antacid and a cation-exchange resin. *Gastroenterology.* 1969;56:868–874.
3. Fernandez PC, Kovnat PJ. Metabolic acidosis reversed by the combination of magnesium hydroxide and a cation-exchange resin. *N Engl J Med.* 1972;286:23–24.
4. Ziessman HA. Aklalosis and seizure due to a cation-exchange resin and magnesium hydroxide. *South Med J.* 1976;69:497–499.
5. Madias NE, Levey AS. Metabolic aklalosis due to absorption of "nonabsorbable" antacids. *Am J Med.* 1983;74:155–158.
6. Garimella PS, Jaber BL. Patiromer for hyperkalemia in diabetic CKD: a new kid on the block. *Am J Kidney Dis.* 2016;67(4):545–547.8.
7. Galla JH. Metabolic alkalosis. *J Am Soc Nephrol.* 2000;11:369–375.

Case Study 3

1. Rose BD, Post TW. *Clinical Physiology of Acid-Base and Electrolyte Disorders.* 5th ed. New York, NY: McGraw-Hill, Inc; 2001:551–571. chap 18.
2. Assadi F. *Clinical Decisions in Pediatric Nephrology: A Problem Solving Approach to Clinical Cases.* New York: Springer; 2008:69–98. chap 2.

Case Study 4

1. Rose BD, Post TW. *Clinical Physiology of Acid-Base and Electrolyte Disorders.* 5th ed. New York, NY: McGraw-Hill, Inc; 2001:551–571. chap 18.
2. Assadi F. *Clinical Decisions in Pediatric Nephrology: A Problem Solving Approach to Clinical Cases.* New York: Springer; 2008:69–98. chap 2.

Case Study 5

1. Rose BD, Post TW. *Clinical Physiology of Acid-Base and Electrolyte Disorders.* 5th ed. New York, NY: McGraw-Hill, Inc; 2001:551–571. chap 18.
2. Assadi F. *Clinical Decisions in Pediatric Nephrology: A Problem-Solving Approach to Clinical Cases.* New York: Springer; 2008:69–98. chap 2.
3. Pru C, Kjellstrand CM. The FeNa test is of no prognostic value in acute renal failure. *Nephron.* 1984;37:39–42.
4. Anderson RJ. Urinary chloride concentration in acute renal failure. *Miner Electrolyte Metab.* 1982;10:92–97.

Case Study 6

1. Raina R, Krishnappa V, Das A, et al. Overview of monogenic or Mendelian forms of hypertension. *Front Pediatr.* 2019;7:1–13. https://doi.org/10.3389/fped.2019.00263.
2. Yang K, Xiao Y, Tian T, et al. Molecular genetics of Liddle's syndrome. *Clin Chim Acta.* 2014;436:202–206.

3. Palmer BF, Alpern RJ. Liddle's syndrome. *Am J Med.* 1998;104:301–309. https://doi.org/10.1016/s0002-9343(98)00018-7.
4. Salih M, Gautschi I, van Bemmelen MX, et al. Missense mutation in the extracellular domain of αENaC causes Liddle syndrome. *J Am Soc Nephrol.* 2017;28:3291–3299. https://doi.org/10.1681/ASN.2016111163.

Case Study 7

1. Soares SBM, de Menezes Silva LAW, de Carvalho Mrad FC, et al. Distal renal tubular acidosis: genetic causes and management. *World J Pediatr.* 2019;15:422–431.
2. Finer G, Landau D. Clinical approach to proximal renal tubular acidosis in children. *Adv Chronic Kidney Dis.* 2018;25:351–357.
3. Watanabe T. Renal Fanconi syndrome in distal renal tubular acidosis. *Pediatr Nephrol.* 2017;32:1093.
4. Naik SV, Ghousia S, Shashibushan KK, Poornima S. Amelogenesis imperfecta—a case report. *J Oral Health Res.* 2011;2:106–110.

Case Study 8

1. Pessler F, Emery H, Dai L, et al. The spectrum of renal tubular acidosis in pediatric Sjogren syndrome. *Rheumatology (Oxford).* 2006;45:85–91.
2. Zhao J, Chen Q, Zhu Y, et al. Nephrological disorders and neurological involvement in pediatric primary Sjogren syndrome: a case report and review of literature. *Pediatr. Rheumatol.* 2000;18:39 [Online J].

Case Study 9

1. Prosser JD, Cohen AP, Greinwald JH. Diagnostic evaluation of children with sensorineural hearing loss. *Otolaryngol Clin N Am.* 2015;8:975–982. https://doi.org/10.1016/j.otc.2015.07.004.
2. Fulchiero R, Seo-Mayer P. Bartter syndrome and Gitelman syndrome. *Pediatr Clin N Am.* 2019;66:121–134. https://doi.org/10.1016/j.pcl.2018.08.010.
3. Janssen AG, Scholl U, Domeyer C, et al. Disease-causing dysfunctions of barttin in Bartter syndrome type IV. *J Am Soc Nephrol.* 2009;20:145–153. https://doi.org/10.1681/ASN.2008010102.
4. García-Nieto V, Flores C, Luis-Yanes MI, et al. Mutation G47R in the BSNC gene causes Bartter syndrome with deafness in two Spanish families. *Pediatr Nephrol.* 2006;21:643–648. https://doi.org/10.1007/s00467-006-0062-1.
5. Aksoy OY, Cayci FS, Ceylaner S, et al. Hypokalemia and hearing loss in a 3-year-old boy: answers. *Pediatr Nephrol.* 2020;35:617–618. https://doi.org/10.1007/s00467-019-04383-8.

Case Study 10

1. Seyberth HW, Schlingmann KP. Bartter- and Gitelman-like syndromes: salt-losing tubulopathies with loop or DCT defects. *Pediatr Nephrol.* 2011;26:1789–1802.
2. Che R, Yuan Y, Huang S, et al. Mitochondrial dysfunction in the pathophysiology of renal diseases. *Am J Physiol Renal Physiol.* 2014;306:F367–F378.
3. Martin-Hernández E, Garcia-Silva MT, Vara J, et al. Renal pathology in children with mitochondrial diseases. *Pediatr Nephrol.* 2005;20:1299–1305.

Case Study 11

1. Heinz-Erian P, Oberauer M, Neu N, et al. A novel homozygous SLC26A3 nonsense mutation in a Tyrolean girl with congenital chloride diarrhea. *J Pediatr Gastroenterol Nutr.* 2008;47:363–366.
2. Wedenoja S, Hoglund P, Holmberg C. Review article: the clinical management of congenital chloride diarrhoea. *Aliment Pharmacol Ther.* 2010;31:477–485.

Case Study 12

1. Wong L, Hsu THS, Perlroth MG, et al. Reninoma: case report and literature review. *J Hypertens.* 2008;26:368–373.
2. Regolisti G, Cabassi A, Parenti E, et al. Long-standing high-renin hypertension and hypokalemia: renin-secreting tumor of the juxtaglomerular apparatus. *Am J Kidney Dis.* 2009;54:A41–A44.

Case Study 13

1. Winterborn MH, Hewitt GJ, Mitchell MD. The role of prostaglandins in Bartter's syndrome. *Int J Pediatr Nephrol.* 1984;5:31–38.
2. Rodriguez Portales JA, Delea CS. Renal tubular reabsorption of chloride in Bartter's syndrome and other conditions with hypokalemia. *Clin Nephrol.* 1986;26:269–272.

Case Study 14

1. Ulick S, Chan CK, Rao KN, Edassery J, Mantero F. A new form of the syndrome of apparent mineralocorticoid excess. *J Steroid Biochem.* 1989;32:209–212.
2. Shacldeton CHL, Rodriguez J, Arteaga E, Lopez JM, Winter JSD. Congenital 11B-hydroxysteroid dehydrogenase deficiency associated with juvenile hypertension: corticosteroid metabolite profiles of four patients and their families. *Clin Endocrinol (Oxf).* 1985;22:701–712.
3. Ulick S, Tedde R, Wang JZ. Defective ring—a reduction of cortisol as the major metabolic error in the syndrome of apparent mineralocorticoid excess. *J Clin Endocrinol Metab.* 1992;74:593–599.
4. Mantero F, Tedde R, Opocher G, et al. Apparent mineralocorticoid excess type II. *Steroids.* 1994;59:80–83.

CHAPTER 6

Metabolic Acidosis

Case Study 1

A 15-year-old woman with a medical history of diabetes mellitus, obesity, compensated cirrhosis, and nonalcoholic steatohepatitis had right first distal phalanx osteomyelitis diagnosed 4 weeks before presentation and underwent right below-knee amputation. She was admitted to the hospital with abdominal pain and hematemesis.

On admission, the patient denied chest pain, shortness of breath, nausea, vomiting, diarrhea, or urinary symptoms. She also denied using over-the-counter medications. Home medications included aspirin, 81 mg, daily; furosemide, 20 mg, daily; insulin glargine, 10 units, daily; levofloxacin, 500 mg, daily; and linezolid, 600 mg, twice a day.

On physical examination, the patient's body temperature was 36.5°C, heart rate was 86 beats/min, blood pressure was 105/53 mmHg, respiration rate was 14 breaths/min, and oxygen saturation was 98% while breathing room air. Cardiopulmonary examination findings were unremarkable. Her abdomen was distended with mild epigastric tenderness to palpation. There was no lower extremity edema. Neurologic examination was positive for asterixis.

Patient's initial laboratory studies were hemoglobin 6.9 g/dL, white blood cell count 2500/μL, platelet count $24 \times 10^3/\mu L$, sodium 131 mmol/L, potassium 5.5 mmol/L, chloride 94 mmol/L, bicarbonate 10 mmol/L, serum creatinine 0.7 mg/dL, BUN 29 mg/dL, calcium 7.9 mg/dL, albumin 2.3 g/dL, glucose 170 mg/dL, alanine aminotransferase 7 U/L (reference: 0 to 45), aspartase aminotransferase 16 U/L (reference: 7 to 40), alkaline phosphatase 256 U/L (reference: 40 to 150), bilirubin total 0.3 (reference: 0 to 1.5), partial thromboplastin time (PTT) 50 seconds, international normalized ratio (INR) 1.2, lactate dehydrogenase 125 U/L (reference: 0 to 249), lactate 11.5 mol/L, β-hydroxybutyrate 287 mOsm/L. β-Hydroxybutyrate 0.3 mg/dL (reference: 0 to 3), serum osmolality 287 mOsm/kg, serum acetaminophen less than 5.0 μg/mL serum salicylate level less than 0.3 mg/dL, serum ethanol level 2 mg/dL. Arterial blood gas revealed a pH 7.34, PCO_2 19 mmHg, PO_2 116 mmHg, bicarbonate 10 mmol/L. Urinalysis results were benign and blood and urine cultures were negative.

Computed tomography of the abdomen demonstrated moderate ascites and suggested liver cirrhosis. Chest x-ray revealed no acute cardiopulmonary process.

What is the acid-base disturbance in this case?

    A. High anion-gap metabolic acidosis with respiratory alkalosis
    B. High anion-gap metabolic acidosis
    C. Respiratory alkalosis
    D. Distal renal tubular acidosis

The correct answer is A

Comment: This patient has a high–anion gap (AG) metabolic acidosis; corrected for hypoalbuminemia, the AG equals 31. The increase in AG was essentially matched by a decrease in serum bicarbonate concentration $[HCO_3^-]$ according to the delta ratio, $(AG - 12)/(24 - [HCO_3^-])$, which is 1.35 in this case. A delta ratio between 1 and 2 suggests that the patient may not have an additional acid-base disorder. However, this equation assumes that all buffering is extracellular and by bicarbonate, neither of which is correct. The calculated $PaCO_2$ by Winter's formula, that is, $PCO_2 = (1.5 \times [HCO_3^-] + 8) \pm 2$, is 23 mmHg, which is above the arterial blood gas–measured PCO_2 of 19 mmHg, indicating that the patient also has a respiratory alkalosis. In summary, our patient has a high-AG metabolic acidosis with mild respiratory alkalosis.[1,2]

What is the most likely cause of this patient's acid-base disturbance?

Comment: Patient's acid-base disturbance can be further investigated through calculation of her osmolar gap (OG). The calculated osmolality, equivalent to {[2 × (sodium in mmol/L)] + [glucose in mg/dL]}/{18 + [(serum urea nitrogen in mg/dL)/2.8] + [ethanol/3.7]}, is 282 mOsm/kg in our patient. The OG is calculated by taking the difference between measured and calculated serum osmolality, and a normal OG is ≤ 10 mOsm/kg. Our patient had an OG of 5 mOsm/kg so it is unlikely that she had intoxication with glycols or methanol.[3]

The elevated lactate level in this setting indicates the presence of lactic acidosis. The patient does not have signs of shock or hypovolemia. We need to account for our patient's lactic acidosis in the setting of normotension.[4] Salicylate toxicity can cause respiratory alkalosis with high-AG metabolic acidosis. However, it does not explain the patient's lactic acidosis. Moreover, serum salicylate level was undetectable. Ethylene glycol can lead to a false elevation in L-lactate level due to cross-reactivity of its metabolites with the oxidase enzyme that is commonly used to measure ethylene glycol level. However, the normal OG in this patient makes ethylene glycol and methanol toxicity less likely. Also, the patient has no history of any other toxic alcohol exposure. Pyroglutamic acid can be associated with lactic acidosis; however, this patient did not have a history of acetaminophen use. The normal β-hydroxybutyrate level and lack of ketonuria exclude ketoacidosis.

Linezolid is an oxazolidinone antibiotic that inhibits bacterial protein synthesis. It can also impair mitochondrial ribosomal function, leading to severe lactic acidosis, liver toxicity, and myelosuppression.

Nucleoside analogue reverse transcriptase inhibitors, propofol, and metformin can also lead to mitochondrial dysfunction and metabolic acidosis. Major risk factors for linezolid toxicity include prolonged exposure, administration of relatively higher doses, and baseline chronic liver or kidney disease.

This patient's high-AG lactic acidosis is most likely explained by linezolid toxicity. The patient's respiratory alkalosis was thought to be due to her cirrhosis, which is associated with an increased level of progesterone, leading to hyperventilation.

What is the BEST treatment for this patient's metabolic abnormalities?

Comment: Lactic acidosis often resolves rapidly following discontinuation of linezolid therapy.[4] The medication was stopped and repeat laboratory measurements at 72 hours demonstrated significant improvement and normalization of the patient's bicarbonate and lactate values.

Case Study 2

A 15-year-old male was admitted to the hospital with myalgias and generalized weakness. Two weeks before, he had abdominal pain, decreased oral intake, nausea, and vomiting. He denied diarrhea. One week before admission, he developed muscle weakness that worsened until he was unable to get out of bed without assistance. His medical history was unremarkable. His only reported medication was over the-counter ibuprofen for chronic back pain, 2400 to 3200 mg daily for several months. He denied alcohol or solvent abuse. On physical examination, he was alert and oriented. His vital signs were normal. He was unable to raise his upper or lower extremities against gravity and had decreased deep tendon reflexes with intact superficial sensations. The rest of his examination findings were unremarkable. Initial laboratory workup showed normal blood cell counts. Patient's basic metabolic panel were: sodium 142 mmol/L, potassium 1.7 mmol/L, chloride 113 mmol/L, bicarbonate 20 mmol/L, anion gap 9 mmol/L, blood urea nitrogen (BUN) 18 mg/dL, creatinine 1.0 mg/dL, glucose 122 mg/dL, calcium 9.3 mg/dL, phosphorous 1.8 mg/dL, total protein 6.8 g/dL, albumin 4.3 g/dL, magnesium 2.7 mg/dL, creatine kinase 430 U/L (reference: 34 to 294). Venous blood gas revealed pH 7.32, PCO_2 31 mmHg, PO_2 158 mmHg, bicarbonate 15 mmol/L. Antinuclear antibody (ANA), anti-Sjögren syndrome antigen A and B antibodies were 5 U/mL (reference: 0 to 100). The 24-hour urine volume was 5750 mL containing sodium 466 mmol/L, potassium 112 mmol/L, chloride 552 mmol/L, and creatinine 2.25 g mg/dL with osmolality 281 mOsm/kg H_2O. Urinalysis was normal with a pH of 7.0.

The electrocardiogram showed flattened T waves in lateral leads. He received 120 mmol of potassium overnight, and 12 hours after admission, his serum potassium level increased to 2.1 mmol/L.

What is the MOST likely diagnosis in this patient?

A. Hypokalemia secondary to reversible type 2 proximal renal tubular acidosis likely from ibuprofen

B. Hypokalemia secondary to reversible type 1 renal tubular acidosis, likely from ibuprofen

C. Sjögren syndrome

D. Pseudohyperaldosteronism

The correct answer is B

Comment: A systematic approach to hypokalemia can help narrow the differential diagnosis in this case. Hypokalemia can result from shifts of potassium from the extracellular to the intracellular space (internal balance) or from potassium depletion due to losses into the gastrointestinal tract or urine (external balance).[1] Severe hypokalemia with paralysis due to an intracellular potassium shift can be due to hypokalemic periodic paralysis (hereditary or thyrotoxic) or exogenous insulin or catecholamines. In this patient, the relatively high urinary potassium excretion and need for large doses of potassium during replacement as well as the clinical course makes us conclude that he was potassium depleted. The causes of potassium depletion include vomiting, diarrhea, renal tubular acidosis (RTA), toluene toxicity, diuretic use, Bartter and Gitelman syndromes, and acquired or hereditary hypertensive renal potassium wasting disorders.[2-5]

The expected renal response to hypokalemia would be to limit urinary potassium excretion. A patient has abnormal urinary losses during hypokalemia if potassium excretion surpasses 30 mEq in a 24-hour urine collection or a random urine potassium-creatinine ratio is greater than 13 mmol/g. This patient had 30 mmol of potassium per gram of creatinine in the urine on admission and 112 mmol of potassium in the 24-hour urine collection (while getting potassium repletion). The cause of renal potassium wasting can be determined from the associated acid-base disturbance and blood pressure. Patient had a normal anion gap metabolic acidosis. Therefore, there is no need to consider the various causes of hypertensive or normotensive renal potassium wasting with metabolic alkalosis. RTA, toluene toxicity, or diarrhea could cause normal anion gap metabolic acidosis and potassium wasting. RTA with hypokalemia can be seen in type 1 (distal) or type 2 (proximal) RTA. Proximal RTA typically has mild hypokalemia, an acid urine pH (unless treated), and other proximal tubular abnormalities (Fanconi syndrome) that were absent in this patient. Severe hypokalemia and alkaline urine pH are features of distal RTA. Inhaling solvent fumes, such as glue sniffing or paint huffing, results in systemic absorption of toluene, which is oxidized to benzoic acid and then conjugated with glycine to form hippuric acid. These hippurate anions are then secreted into the tubular lumen with sodium and potassium (along with ammonium, which raises the urine pH) causing a very similar picture to distal RTA. In addition to urine potassium and pH, other relevant urine parameters include the urinary osmoles (sodium, potassium, urea, and glucose), which enable us to calculate the urinary osmolar gap, the difference between measured urine osmolarity and calculated urine osmolarity ($2 \times [Na^+ + K^+]$) + [urea ÷ 2.8] + [glucose ÷ 18]), which serves as a surrogate of ammonium excretion.

A normal anion gap metabolic acidosis caused by diarrhea or solvent abuse is associated with high rates of urine ammonium excretion; the rate of urine ammonium excretion is not high in RTA. Urine ammonium is not routinely measured by clinical laboratory tests, but it can be estimated from the gap between measured and calculated urine osmolality; urine ammonium excretion is approximately equal to half the urine osmolar gap. In this patient, the 24-hour urine osmolar gap was not high and hippuric acid was not found in urine. The elevated urine pH without an increase in urinary osmolar gap is consistent with a diagnosis of distal RTA.

The acute onset of distal RTA without nephrocalcinosis makes an acquired rather than a congenital form more likely. Autoimmune disease, most often Sjögren syndrome, is the most common cause of acquired distal RTA. Serologic testing was negative for autoimmune causes, so we should consider additional causes. Although ibuprofen has typically been associated with hyperkalemia, there have been several case reports of severe hypokalemia and transient distal RTA due to abuse of a combination drug containing ibuprofen and codeine. The pathogenesis is unclear but inhibition of carbonic anhydrase, which is present in the proximal and distal tubules, has been suggested. Consistent with the suspicion of ibuprofen being the etiologic agent, after the patient stopped treatment with the medication, his serum potassium level increased dramatically and renal losses decreased. He was discharged with a normal potassium level, normal bicarbonate level, and had no subsequent recurrences.

Case Study 3

A 13-year-old boy with a medical history of type 2 diabetes mellitus and hyperlipidemia was admitted to the hospital for elective surgery to resect an enlarging kidney cyst. His home medications included canagliflozin, 300 mg, daily; rosuvastatin, 20 mg, daily; glipizide, 5 mg, twice daily; and sitagliptin/metformin, 50/1000 mg, twice daily. The patient tolerated the procedure well and was transferred postoperatively to a surgical floor with unremarkable laboratory values. He did well in the immediate postoperative period and was tolerating clear liquids by postoperative day 3. His blood glucose level was regulated by short-acting insulin doses. His outpatient medications were not administered in the hospital. On postoperative day 4, the patient was noted to be tachypneic and tachycardic.

At that time, serum sodium was 136 mmol/L, potassium 5 mmol/L, chloride 108 mmol/L, and bicarbonate 9 mmol/L.

Serum urea nitrogen 22 mg/dL, creatinine 1.0 mg/dL, calcium 8.5 mg/dL, magnesium 2.2 mg/dL, phosphorous 3.8 mg/dL, albumin 3.8 g/dL, glucose 136 mg/dL, lactate 1.7 mmol/L, β-hydroxybutyrate 5.92 mmol/L. Urine glucose was 1000 mg/dL, ketones greater than 150 mg/dL. Arterial blood gas showed pH 7.13, PCO_2 13 mmHg, PO_2 103 mmHg, and bicarbonate 8.5 mmol/L.

Patient received multiple ampules of sodium bicarbonate and a continuous sodium bicarbonate infusion. Nephrology service was consulted for management of metabolic acidosis.

What is the cause of this patient's metabolic acidosis and how should this condition managed?

    A. Canagliflozin (SGLT2 inhibitor) associated euglycemic ketoacidosis
    B. Lactic acidosis
    C. Hypoglycemic ketoacidosis
    D. Glycol intoxication

The correct answer is A

Comment: This patient has high anion gap metabolic acidosis due to ketoacidosis, despite the near-normal blood glucose concentration. He has normal plasma lactate levels but elevated urinary and blood ketone levels. Euglycemic ketoacidosis is an uncommon complication associated with sodium-glucose cotransporter 2 (SGLT2) inhibitor therapy.[1-4] In SGLT2 inhibitor-treated patients with type 2 diabetes, a lower insulin to glucagon ratio leads to nearly 40% higher lipolysis after a meal, 20% higher fat oxidation, 60% lower carbohydrate oxidation, 15% lower glycogen synthesis, and 2-fold higher ketogenesis. The exact mechanism for the development of the more serious euglycemic ketoacidosis associated with SGLT2 inhibitor therapy is not clearly understood, though various theories have been postulated. These include a decrease in insulin levels as a result of insulin-independent hypoglycemia leading to increased lipolysis and enhanced ketogenesis, and a primary increase in glucagon secretion via direct effects on SGLT2 transporters expressed in pancreatic alpha cells leading to increased ketogenesis. Overall, it appears that similar to severe starvation ketoacidosis, SGLT2 inhibitors via various metabolic effects can lead to a low-insulin and high-glucagon state favoring ketogenesis, particularly in the presence of "stressors" such as surgery, excess alcohol consumption, pancreatitis, or severe injury.

SGLT2 inhibitors act by promoting glucose excretion in urine via inhibition of the SGLT2 cotransporter located in the proximal tubule. These drugs lower maximum renal glucose reabsorptive capacity and the renal threshold for glucosuria. There is also evidence that these agents may have beneficial effects by lowering intraglomerular pressure through increasing sodium chloride delivery to the juxtaglomerular apparatus and activating the tubulo-glomerular feedback pathway.[2] These agents have relatively modest hypoglycemic efficacy, but are reported to have beneficial effects on blood pressure, weight, and insulin sensitivity, as well as improved cardiovascular and renal outcomes in patients with type 2 diabetes.[2] Three SGLT2 inhibitors (dapagliflozin, canagliflozin, and empagliflozin) are currently FDA-approved for use in patients with type 2 diabetes. The pharmacokinetic profile of these agents is similar in patients with and without diabetes, and age, race, sex, body weight, food intake, or mildly decreased kidney function does not affect the pharmacokinetic characteristics of the drugs. However, dose reductions are required for moderately decreased kidney function.

Genital mycotic infections (more common in women), urinary tract infections, and orthostatic hypotension due to extracellular fluid volume depletion are the most commonly reported side effects.[3,4] The true frequency of euglycemic ketoacidosis has not been established.

Early recognition of ketoacidosis is the key to successful therapy, but the relatively normal blood glucose levels and a predominance of β-hydroxybutyrate ketone bodies, which are not detected on urine dipsticks, can present a diagnostic challenge. Intravenous bicarbonate therapy alone does not address the underlying pathophysiology. Discontinuing the offending medication, early initiation of intravenous insulin therapy to suppress lipolysis and ketogenesis, and monitoring β-hydroxybutyrate level, as well as other metabolic and acid-base parameters, are all required. In addition, dextrose-containing fluids may be needed to avoid hypoglycemia. An interesting observation in this case is that although the pharmacokinetic half-life of SGLT2 inhibitors is approximately 12 hours, delayed reversibility of the drug's action as manifested by ongoing glycosuria led to persisting metabolic acidosis for several days after cessation of the drug. Although the mechanism of a prolonged action is uncertain, it may reflect continued drug binding to renal transport proteins despite elimination from plasma. Intravenous insulin therapy in this patient was continued along with glucose infusions until postoperative day 11, at which point his serum electrolyte levels normalized and glycosuria was diminished to 300 mg/dL. On postoperative day 11, he was successfully converted to a subcutaneous insulin regimen and discharged on postoperative day 14 on insulin and metformin therapy. Thus, the persistent action of these drugs several days after discontinuation may require prolonged dextrose and insulin therapy to treat SGLT2 inhibitor therapy-associated ketoacidosis.

Case Study 4

A 19-year-old female with a history of depression presented to the emergency department after drinking three-fourth of a gallon of antifreeze over 2 days in a suicide attempt. She reported feeling as if she were "drunk." She also noted nausea and vomiting. On physical examination, the patient appeared comfortable, alert, and oriented. Temperature was 36.5°C, heart rate was 110 beats/min, blood pressure was 100/70 mmHg, respiratory rate was 20 breaths/min, and pulse oximetry was 99% on room air. There was no papilledema. The remainder of the examination had normal findings. Laboratory analysis showed the following values: sodium, 136 mmol/L; potassium, 4.2 mmol/L; chloride, 104 mmol/L; bicarbonate, 17 mmol/L; blood urea nitrogen (BUN), 17 mg/dL; creatinine, 3.0 mg/dL; glucose, 147 mg/dL; corrected anion gap, 18.5; measured serum osmolality, 342 mOsm/kg; lactate, 9.9 mmol/L; pH 7.27; and PCO_2, 36 mmHg. Urinalysis showed specific gravity of 1.010 and trace protein and was negative for blood and ketones. Sediment evaluation showed 0 to 2 red blood cells/high-power field, 0 to 2 white blood cells/high-power field, rare granular casts, and no crystals.

What is the MOST likely cause of metabolic acidosis in this patient?

- A. Propylene glycol intoxication
- B. Ethanol intoxication
- C. Methanol intoxication
- D. Salicylate overdose

The correct answer is A

Although the differential diagnosis of anion gap metabolic acidosis is broad, it is important to rapidly diagnose disorders that require prompt treatment to prevent morbidity and mortality. In individuals who present with altered sensorium or who report ingestions, the clinician must consider consumption of a toxic alcohol.[1-3] These agents are rapidly absorbed from the gastrointestinal tract and initially will increase serum osmolality. Their presence can be ascertained quickly by measuring the osmolar gap: the difference between measured osmolality and calculated osmolality. Calculated osmolality is determined by multiplying the major extracellular cation, sodium (Na^+) ion, by 2 and converting the predominant extracellular solutes, glucose and BUN, from their traditionally reported units (mg/dL) to mOsm/kg by dividing by one-tenth of their molecular weight ($2Na^+$ + Glucose ÷ 18 + BUN ÷ 2.8). In this case, the osmolar gap is 56. A gap greater than 15 suggests the presence of a small-molecular-weight substance. Ethanol and isopropyl alcohol ingestions will present with an osmolar gap but do not cause metabolic acidosis. However, because isopropyl alcohol is metabolized to acetone, ketones may be noted if the nitroprusside reaction is used. Three alcohols—methanol, ethylene glycol, and propylene glycol—are associated with both an osmolar gap and an anion gap metabolic acidosis. Ethylene glycol and methanol are highly toxic. As these two alcohols are metabolized into glycolic/oxalic acid and formic acid, respectively, the osmolar gap will decrease while the anion gap increases. Propylene glycol, used to solubilize numerous medications, is metabolized to lactic acid and is an increasingly recognized cause of anion gap acidosis.[3-6] Medications using this diluent, such as benzodiazepines, if infused rapidly enough can cause an osmolar gap and lactic acidosis.

There are several clues to the correct diagnosis in this case. Both ethylene glycol and methanol are extremely toxic, with 1 mL/kg usually resulting in death. Even if exaggerated, the quantity the patient claimed to have ingested should have been rapidly fatal. Methanol ingestions are associated with visual disturbances through inflammation of the optic nerve, which was not noted. The lack of oxalate crystals in the urine makes ethylene glycol toxicity less likely. Finally, although lactic acidosis can be seen in cases of ethylene glycol toxicity, the level present in this case would be very unusual. Although propylene glycol toxicity is most often noted in hospitalized patients receiving intravenous medications, there has been an increase in the use of propylene glycol as a substitute for ethylene glycol in commercial antifreeze because of its relative lack of toxicity. These agents are advertised as being pet friendly and less toxic. The US Food and Drug Administration considers pharmaceutical-grade propylene glycol as generally safe. However, prolonged high-dose infusions of medications containing propylene glycol can produce significant lactic acidosis through its metabolism. Although no lethal dose has been established in humans, in animals, the LD_{50} is 18 to 20 mL/kg.

Two days after admission, this patient's initial ethylene glycol level returned as undetectable and family members brought in the ingested substance, Sierra antifreeze (Safe Brands Corp), containing 94% propylene glycol.

Toxic alcohol ingestions need to be treated rapidly to avoid toxicity. Often treatment must start prior to confirmation of the substance ingested. Because the toxicity of these alcohols is mediated by their metabolites, treatment is aimed at blocking their enzymatic conversion by alcohol dehydrogenase. This is accomplished by the administration of fomepizole, a potent inhibitor of alcohol dehydrogenase. Dialysis then can be considered to remove the alcohol and treat the acidosis. Propylene glycol is far less toxic than ethylene glycol. Toxicity usually manifests as confusion and kidney failure. Although deaths from propylene glycol toxicity are extremely rare, fomepizole has been used in treatment. Although in retrospect ethylene glycol toxicity was unlikely, in view of the morbidity associated with its ingestion, this patient was treated with fomepizole.

Case Study 5

An 18-year-old woman with a 4-year history of recurrent dyspnea was evaluated for 4 days of worsening shortness of breath and anorexia. One month before admission, fasting hyperglycemia was diagnosed and she was prescribed a low-carbohydrate and a high-protein diet. On examination, blood pressure was 112/71 mmHg and heart rate was 141 beats/min. She weighed 42 kg and was 162 cm tall; body mass index was 16 kg/m^2. She was alert, but afebrile and emaciated and had dry skin. Initial laboratory findings showed metabolic acidosis and ketosis. Intravenous hydration with normal saline solution was started, and nutritional supplements with protein and amino acids were given. Despite these measures, the patient developed blurred vision and confusion on hospital day 4. Neurologic examination showed normal cranial nerves, including no ophthalmic paresis or facial diplegia, but decreased visual acuity. Computed tomography of the brain showed an area of decreased attenuation within the bilateral basal ganglia. Admission blood biochemistry and arterial blood gas results are as follows: serum sodium 138 mmol/L, potassium 3.1 mmol/L, chloride 116 mmol/L, bicarbonate 9.0 mmol/L, anion gap 15 mmol/L, BUN 15 mg/dL, creatinine 1.3 mg/dL, estimate glomerular filtration rate (eGFR) 48 mL/min/1.72 m^2, albumin 3.2 g/dL, ketone 6.0 mmol/L, glucose 110 g/dL, osmolality 285 mOsm/kg, pH 7.36, PCO$_2$ 16.2 mmHg. Of note is the development of profound hyperammonemia with an ammonia level of 327 g/dL (192 mmol/L).

What is the most likely cause of this patient's metabolic acidosis and how might this patient be managed?

    A. Starvation ketoacidosis
    B. Lactic acidosis
    C. Methylmalonic acidemia complicated with toxic amblyopia.
    D. Methanol intoxication

The correct answer is C
Comment: In the setting of a low serum albumin level, the patient's serum anion gap of 13 mEq/L (13 mmol/L) represents an expanded anion-gap metabolic acidosis. According to the clinical

course and original laboratory data, a tentative diagnosis of starvation ketoacidosis was made; however, initial management with intravenous fluids failed to correct the metabolic acidosis. There was no clinical evidence of lactic acidosis, methanol intoxication (19 mg/L; toxic level, 200 mg/L), or acetaminophen overdose (0.12 g/mL; toxic level, 75 g/mL at 12 hours). Upon recognition of acute hyperammonemia, an occult metabolic disorder was suspected after acute liver failure, drug toxicity, and infectious complications were excluded. The constellation of metabolic acidosis, ketoacidosis, and hyperammonemia could be ascribed to an organic acidemia.[1-4] These conditions are characterized by the excretion of non-amino organic acids in urine and disrupted serum amino acid metabolism, particularly of branched-chain amino acids. Methylmalonic and propionic acidemia are the most frequent forms of branched-chain organic acidemias. Affected patients typically present in the neonatal period or early infancy with signs of life-threatening metabolic acidosis and increased anion gap. A few are detected at an older age. Organic acidemias typically present with poor feeding, protein intolerance, vomiting, increasing lethargy that progresses to coma, and muscular hypotonia.

Serum amino acid analysis showed hyperglycinemia, and urine chromatography/mass spectrometry organic acid analysis indicated increased concentrations of methylmalonic, 2-oxooctanoic, and 1,2-benzenedicarboxylic acids. This picture is consistent with methylmalonic acidemia. *MUT, MMAA,* and *MMAB* are the 3 genes (encoding methylmalonyl coenzyme A mutase, methylmalonic aciduria type A protein, and methylmalonic aciduria type B protein, respectively) and there are at least eight different complementation groups associated with methylmalonic academia. Patients in whom residual enzymatic activity is present tend to have later and more variable presentations and a better prognosis. Affected individuals may appear well, but be prone to acute metabolic decompensation after excessive protein intake or metabolic stressors, as seen in our patient. Although genetic analysis was not performed in our patient, the constellation of urine and serum organic acid analysis, radiologic features, and the mentioned clinical findings should raise the suspicion of this under-recognized disease.

Because of the patient's refractory hyperammonemia and worsening visual disturbance, continuous venovenous hemodialysis (CVVHD) therapy was initiated promptly before results of the urine organic-acid analysis were available. The patient's consciousness cleared in the sixth hour of CVVHD, and she experienced gradual improvement in visual acuity in the following days. CVVHD therapy was halted after 60 hours because of resolution of hyperammonemia (ammonia, 58 μg/dL). Continuous renal replacement therapies are effective in the rapid clearance of these low-molecular-weight toxic metabolites, particularly in patients with inborn errors of metabolism, such as organic acidemia or urea cycle disorders. Prolonged latencies in the flashlight visual evoked potentials test were noticed initially, consistent with optic neuropathy (also termed toxic amblyopia). Methylmalonic acidemia complicated with optic neuropathy is rare and insidious and can progress to optic atrophy and irreversible visual deficits. After CVVHD therapy, visual disturbance and repeated visual evoked potentials testing showed a major recovery from the initial presentation.

In conclusion, this case highlights the use of dialysis for severe hyperammonemia in patients with underlying organic acidemia and acute neurologic manifestations. Prompt initiation is critical to avoid irreversible brain damage.

Case Study 6

A 14-year-old girl was seen for recurrent fractures. At the age of 2 weeks, she had been hospitalized because of failure to thrive and hyperchloremic metabolic acidosis. Laboratory findings at that time were as follows: pH, 7.15; PCO_2, 48 mmHg; bicarbonate, 16.2 mmol/L; serum sodium, 139 mmol/L; potassium, 5.0 mmol/L; chloride, 114 mmol/L; and anion gap, 9 mmol/L. Her urinary pH was 7.8, with a urinary sodium level of 33 mmol/L, potassium level of 10 mmol/L, and chloride level of 17 mmol/L, giving a urinary anion gap of 26 mmol/L. Bicarbonate supplementation for renal tubular acidosis (RTA) was started, but over the years, it was decreased from 8 to 2 mEq/kg/day. The patient was of Mediterranean descent, and her parents were consanguineous in the second degree. Two brothers and four sisters were healthy. She had been evaluated for developmental delay and growth retardation, but no definitive diagnosis had been made. In addition, her dentition had required surgical intervention because of dental caries and misalignment. One and a half years before presentation, she fractured the first toe of her right foot after minor trauma. Two months before presentation, she fractured her first cervical vertebra from minor trauma. On physical examination, she was 1.46 m tall and 3 standard deviations (SDs) less than the mean for age, with a normal weight for height. Laboratory results were as follows: calcium, 9.0 mg/dL; phosphate, 4.83 mg/dL; alkaline phosphatase, 91 U/L; intact parathyroid hormone, 18.9 pg/mL (reference: 15 to 65 pg/mL); and 25-hydroxyvitamin D, 10 ng/mL (reference: 8 to 32 ng/mL). Capillary blood gas pH was 7.27, and bicarbonate level was 22.1 mmol/L. Urinary calcium excretion was 3.5 mg/ kg/day (reference: 4 mg/kg/day). During bicarbonate loading, maximum increase in urinary PCO_2 was 77 mmHg (reference: 80 mmHg), with a urinary-blood PCO_2 difference of 32 mmHg (reference: 40 mmHg). Urinary pH increased from 5.96 to 8.3 during the test. Urinary citrate-creatinine ratio increased from 0.05 to 0.65 mmol/mmol. Ultrasound showed bilateral nephrocalcinosis.

Radiograph of the left hand showed increased cortical thickness and density of the bones of the hand and wrist, with bone-in-bone appearance in the metacarpal bones suggestive of osteopetrosis. In addition, there is an old avulsion fracture of the base of the proximal phalanx. The dual-energy x-ray absorptiometry scan of the lumbar spine revealed increased bone mineral density of the lumbar vertebrae.

What is the MOST likely diagnosis?

   A. Renal tubular acidosis type 1 (RTA-1)
   B. Renal tubular acidosis type 2 (RTA-2)
   C. Carbonic anhydrase II deficiency
   D. Renal tubular acidosis type 4

The correct answer is C

Comment: Based on hyperchloremic metabolic acidosis with a positive urinary anion gap, type 1 (distal) RTA was diagnosed in this patient. This was supported further by the bicarbonate-loading test, in which defective distal H+ excretion was shown. Hypocitraturia, hypercalciuria (in our case, borderline), and nephrocalcinosis are also typical features of type 1 RTA. As expected, her bicarbonate needs decreased with time from 8 to 2 mmol/kg/day. Still, despite correction of acidosis, she showed poor height gain. In addition, she had developmental delay and dental decay, neither of which typically is encountered in patients with RTA. When she developed several fractures after minor trauma, osteopenia secondary to renal acidosis combined with hypercalciuria were first suspected. However, radiographs showed osteopetrosis, which was confirmed by means of dual-energy x-ray absorptiometry. The combination of RTA and osteopetrosis is suggestive of carbonic anhydrase II deficiency.[1,2] This diagnosis was further supported by intracranial calcifications. Carbonic anhydrase II enzymatic activity in erythrocyte lysates was found to be deficient, and a novel homozygote *c.2321GT* mutation was identified in the patient. Her parents were heterozygous. This is the same nucleotide involved in the far more common "Arabic mutation," but in the latter, the mutation is c.2321GA. Computed tomographic scan of the head revealed intracranial calcifications in the caudate nucleus typical for carbonic anhydrase type II deficiency.

Carbonic anhydrase II deficiency is inherited in an autosomal recessive mode. The underlying gene is mapped to chromosome 8q22, and several mutations have been described.

Carbonic anhydrase II is involved in proximal renal tubular bicarbonate reclamation and distal renal tubular acidification. Therefore, many patients with carbonic anhydrase II deficiency show characteristics of both proximal and distal RTA. Some patients develop nephrocalcinosis, as did our patient, in whose phenotype type 1 RTA predominated. Deficiency of carbonic anhydrase II disrupts the balance between osteoclast and osteoblast activity in favor of bone deposition. This causes excessive, but brittle, bone formation (osteopetrosis) that leads to an increased fracture risk. The function of carbonic anhydrase II in oligodendrocytes and astrocytes in the brain is unknown. However, most patients with carbonic anhydrase II deficiency develop intracranial calcifications involving the basal ganglia and periventricular and subcortical white matter. Calcification usually is not present at birth, but appears after the second year of life.

In contrast to other forms of osteopetrosis, cranial nerve entrapment and hematologic complications caused by bone marrow compression are relatively rare. There is no curative treatment for carbonic anhydrase II deficiency, and therapy is restricted to symptomatic correction of metabolic acidosis.

Case Study 7

A 17-year-old woman with a history of hypertension was admitted to the hospital for generalized weakness and muscle cramping with a greater than 2 packs per day smoking history for the past 2 years. She had been hospitalized 4 months prior with similar presenting symptoms, which were attributed to severe hypokalemia 2.0 mmol/L. She denied diarrhea, vomiting, laxative use, diuretic use, or alcohol abuse. Her home medications included potassium chloride, 40 mEq twice per day, and ibuprofen. Her vital signs at admission showed she was hypotensive (89/55 mmHg). The physical examination was significant for 4- or 5-muscle strength of upper and lower extremities. The admission laboratory findings were sodium 134 mmol/L, potassium 1.6 mmol/L, chloride 103 mmol/L, bicarbonate 20 mmol/L, calcium 10.0 mg/dL, magnesium 1.8 mg/dL, phosphorous 1.1 mg/dL, creatinine 1.0 mg/dL, glucose 132 mg/dL, albumin 3.9 mg/dL, and 25-hydroxyvitamin D 25 ng/mL.

The random urine electrolytes showed sodium 11 mmol/L, potassium 10 mmol/L, chloride 13 mmol/L, and anion gap 9 mmol/L. Urinary potassium-creatinine ratio (mmol/g) was 130 (> 13 suggestive of renal potassium wasting). 24-Hour urine potassium was 108 mmol (> 30 suggestive of renal potassium wasting), β_2-microglobulin, greater than 20,000 µg/L (reference: < 300), retinol-binding protein-creatinine ratio 143,200 µg/g (reference: < 172), and glucose (dipstick) negative.

The electrocardiogram showed sinus arrhythmia, flattened T waves, and prolonged QT interval of 667 ms.

What is the Most Likely diagnosis and how should this patient be treated?

    A. Lowe syndrome
    B. Congenital Fanconi syndrome
    C. Acquired Fanconi syndrome
    D. Dent disease

The correct answer is C

Comment: The patient's admission laboratory findings revealed a normal anion gap metabolic acidosis with positive urine anion gap-suggestive of renal tubular acidosis (RTA).[1-4] The differential diagnosis includes proximal and distal RTA, given this patient's hypokalemia with renal potassium wasting. Markedly elevated urinary excretions of β_2-microglobulin and retinol-binding protein support a proximal tubulopathy.

Proximal RTA is caused by reduced reabsorption of filtered bicarbonate in the proximal convoluted tubule, which leads to renal bicarbonate wasting. In addition to decreased bicarbonate reabsorption, proximal RTA is commonly associated with other solute reabsorption impairments including phosphate, glucose, and amino acids. This generalized proximal tubulopathy is called Fanconi syndrome.

Most causes of proximal RTA are acquired, but inheritable causes of primary isolated proximal RTA can occur, as well as secondary proximal RTA with familial Fanconi syndrome in certain hereditary diseases (Wilson disease, cystinosis, Lowe syndrome, Fanconi-Bickel syndrome, Dent disease, etc.). Acquired proximal RTA is commonly caused by injury to the proximal tubule secondary to paraprotein disease, autoimmune disease (Sjögren syndrome), medication toxicity, or heavy metal toxicity. Severe vitamin D deficiency can also cause proximal RTA.[5–10]

Given the patient's proximal tubulopathy and absence of any known family history of potential hereditary causes, the patient was evaluated for acquired causes of proximal tubulopathy. Testing for paraprotein disease with serum protein electrophoresis with immunofixation, serum free light chains, and urine protein electrophoresis with immunofixation was unremarkable. Likewise, testing for autoimmune disease with antibodies against antinuclear and extractable nuclear antigens was unremarkable. Her 25-hydroxyvitamin D level was within normal limits. The review of this patient's current and past prescriptions and over-the-counter medications did not identify any offending agent. A heavy metals screen was ordered to evaluate for potential heavy metal toxicity, including arsenic, cadmium, mercury, lead, copper, and zinc. The patient was found to have severe cadmium toxicity, with 4.4 µg in a 24-hour urine collection, corresponding to a cadmium-creatinine ratio of 6.24 µg/g.

Cadmium is a heavy metal that can cause both severe acute and chronic toxicity. The kidneys are the primary target organ for chronic cadmium toxicity. Sources of cadmium exposure include smoking cigarettes, eating contaminated foods (rice and grains farmed with cadmium-containing fertilizer), and occupational exposure.

The main source of cadmium exposure in smokers is inhalation of tobacco smoke, as opposed to ingestion of contaminated foods in never-smokers. Smoking doubles the lifetime body burden of cadmium.

Daily intake of cadmium through contaminated food is around 30 µg, of which only 1% to 10% is absorbed. A single cigarette has around 2 µg of cadmium, of which up to 10% is inhaled through smoking. Inhalation from smoking 1 pack (20 cigarettes) daily is between 1 and 3 µg.

The critical urinary cadmium-creatinine ratio associated with onset of renal tubular injury is 2 to 10 µg/g. This patient had a ratio of 6.2 µg/g.

After systemic absorption by inhalation or ingestion, cadmium is freely filtered across the glomerulus and reabsorbed by proximal tubular cells while bound to metallothionein. Metallothionein is degraded by lysosomes within tubular cells, releasing free cadmium that generates reactive oxygen species, which result in proximal tubulopathy and RTA.

Chronic cadmium toxicity can progress to Fanconi syndrome. Progressive loss of kidney function from cadmium toxicity does not commonly occur.[11–14] Unfortunately, tubular injury from chronic cadmium toxicity is typically irreversible, even after cessation of exposure.

Management of this patient's proximal tubulopathy and RTA starts with avoiding the offending agent: in this case, smoking cessation is required. This patient reported smoking 2 packs per day—exposure to approximately 2 to 6 µg of inhaled cadmium daily. The patient received education on the cause of her proximal tubulopathy and the link between cigarette smoking and cadmium toxicity.

After correction of this patient's severe hypokalemia using intravenous potassium, she was prescribed potassium citrate with split dosing throughout the day for treatment of her proximal RTA and to maintain normokalemia. Bicarbonate supplementation in patients with proximal RTA can result in increased urinary bicarbonate excretion with resultant worsening of hypokalemia. Potassium levels must be monitored closely with alkali therapy; concurrent potassium supplementation is often required.

Case Study 8

A 13-year-old male with a history of epilepsy has a grand mal seizure. Laboratory tests taken immediately after the seizure has stopped reveal arterial pH 7.14, PCO_2 45 mmHg, serum sodium 140 mmol/L, K 5.5 mmol/L, chloride 98 mmol/L, and bicarbonate 17 mmol/L.

What is the acid-base disturbance and what will happen to his plasma potassium after correction of acidosis?

    A. Mixed metabolic and respiratory acidosis
    B. Simple metabolic acidosis

The correct answer is A
Comment: This patient has a combined respiratory and high anion gap metabolic acidosis, most likely due to seizure-induced lactic acidosis. There is likely to be no change, since neither lactic acidosis nor its correction seem to affect the internal distribution of potassium.[1,2]

Case Study 9

An 18-year-old man (80 kg) with a history of chronic bronchitis develops severe diarrhea caused by pseudomembranous colitis. It is noted that the volume of diarrheal fluid is approximately 1 L/h. Results of the initial laboratory tests are: serum sodium 138 mmol/L, potassium 3.8 mmol/L, chloride 115 mmol/L, bicarbonate 9 mmol/L, arterial pH 6.07, and PCO_2 40 mmHg.

What is the most likely acid-base disorder and how much bicarbonate should be given to raise the plasma pH to 7.20?

    A. Simple metabolic acidosis
    B. Mixed metabolic acidosis and respiratory acidosis
    C. Mixed metabolic acidosis and respiratory alkalosis
    D. Mixed metabolic alkalosis and respiratory acidosis

The correct answer is B
Comment: This patient has a mixed metabolic and respiratory acidosis, since a PCO_2 of 40 mmHg is inappropriately high in a patient with a plasma bicarbonate concentration of 9 mmol/L. The expected value is about 22 mmHg, since the PCO_2 normally falls by about 1.2 mmHg for every 1 mmol/L reduction in the plasma bicarbonate concentration.

    The H^+ concentration at a pH of 7.20 is 63 mmol/L. Thus,
    $[H^+] = 24 \times [PCO_2] \div [HCO_3^-]$ or $63 = 24 \times 46/[HCO_3^-]$ or $[HCO_3^-] = 15$ mmol/L. At this degree of acidemia, the initial distribution of the excess acid is 50% to 70% of lean body weight. Thus,
    HCO_3^- deficit $= 0.6 \times 80 \times (15 - 9)$ or 288 mmol is needed to raise plasma pH to 7.20.[1,2]

Case Study 10

A 15-year-old female has severe chronic renal failure. The following laboratory data are obtained: serum sodium 137 mmol/L, potassium 5.4 mmol/L, chloride 102 mmol/L, bicarbonate 10 mmol/L, arterial pH 7.22, PCO_2 25 mmHg.

Why does metabolic acidosis develop in renal failure?

    A. Uremia
    B. Reduced glomerular filtration rate

    C. Decreased NH_4^+ excretion

    D. Reduced bicarbonate reabsorption

The correct answer is C

Comment: The metabolic acidosis in renal failure is primarily due to reduced NH_4^+ excretion, which prevents the urinary excretion of all of dietary acid load.[1,2]

Case Study 11

A 19-year-old woman with type 1, insulin-dependent diabetes is admitted to the hospital with a soft-tissue infection of the palate. The initial laboratory data include the following: serum sodium 140 mmol/L, potassium 3.8 mmol/L, chloride 110 mmol/L, bicarbonate 23 mmol/L, and glucose 147 mg/dL.

    The patient eats sparingly because of pain on swallowing. To minimize the risk of hypoglycemia, her insulin is withheld. Repeat blood tests are obtained 36 hours later: serum sodium 135 mmol/L, potassium 5.0 mmol/L, chloride 105 mmol/L, bicarbonate 15 mmol/L, glucose 270 mg/dL, anion gap 15 mmol/L, ketone 4 + arterial pH 7.32, and PCO_2 30 mmHg.

Why is the anion gap only slightly elevated despite the presence of ketoacidosis?

    A. β-Hydroxybutyrate and acetoacetate excretion in urine

    B. Laboratory error

    C. Increased serum sulfates and phosphates concentration

    D. Ethylene glycol ingestion

The correct answer is A

Comment: The acidemia is due to retention of H^+ ions from the ketoacids; the associated anions (β-hydroxybutyrate and acetoacetate) were presumably excreted in the urine, resulting in only a minor elevation in the anion gap.[1,2] The patient should be given insulin with glucose. This will correct the ketoacidosis without the risk of hypoglycemia.

Case Study 12

A 12-year-old girl was rushed into the Emergency Department following a motor vehicle accident and was found to have stroke as a result of left parietal hemorrhage. Her medical history was uneventful except for a history of chronic asthma diagnosed 2 years earlier. Physical examination revealed a well-nourished and developed child for her age. She was stuporous, disoriented, and did not follow commands. She was breathing comfortably in room air with deep respirations. The blood pressure was 120/78 mmHg, pulse 71 beats/min, and respiratory rate 29 breaths/min. Her chest was clear to auscultation and percussion. Examination of the eyes, ears, nose, and throat was unremarkable. The remaining physical examination was unremarkable. She was transferred to the neurosurgery intensive care unit for monitoring. She remained stable and repeated imaging demonstrated a resolving brain hemorrhage. Arterial blood gas (ABG) showed a blood pH of 7.44, PCO_2 24 mmHg, PO_2 90 mmHg, and bicarbonate 15 mmol/L.

What is the MOST likely acid-base disturbance in this patient?

    A. Proximal renal tubular acidosis (RTA-2)

    B. Distal renal tubular acidosis (RTA-1)

    C. Chronic respiratory acidosis

    D. Mixed metabolic acidosis and respiratory acidosis

The correct answer is C

Comment: A low plasma bicarbonate concentration due to CRA is often misdiagnosed as a metabolic acidosis and mistreated with the administration of alkali therapy especially when blood pH and PCO_2 are unavailable.

Our patient presented with a low serum bicarbonate concentration, hypocapnia, and positive UAG, which suggest the diagnosis of chronic respiratory alkalosis (CRA), distal renal tubular acidosis (dRTA), or mixed CRA and dRTA.[1-3] The constellation of hyperventilation as a result of stroke and history of chronic asthma, blood pH in the upper range of normal, and positive urine anion gap (UAG) in the absence of chronic renal disease in our patient are consistent with the diagnosis of primary CRA rather than the presumed dRTA.[4,5] The positive UAG is the result of suppressed ammonium (NH_4) excretion, which is a compensatory response to chronic alkalemia.[6-8] The urine pH of 6.1 in our patient does not necessarily suggest a defect in hydrogen ion (H^+) secretion, as in the setting of chronic alkalemia; distal ammonia (NH_3) excretion increases to the extent that the secreted H^+ is almost completely buffered as ammonium (NH_4). This may result in a very low free H^+ in the lumen to lower the urine pH below 5.5, as was the case in our patient. However, the expected serum bicarbonate is 15 mEq/L for a PCO_2 of 24 mmHg in our patient, which closely approximates the expected renal compensation, satisfying the diagnosis of CRA and distinguishing CRA from mixed metabolic acidosis and CRA.

In CRA, UAG is increased (positive) on account of suppressed ammonium (NH_4) excretion, which is a compensatory response to chronic alkalemia.[9-12] Because dRTA is relatively rare and CRA is frequently observed in hospitalized patients, UAG helps distinguish metabolic acidosis from CRA in the initial evaluation of hypocarbonatemia.

UAG can help in evaluating the cause of a low plasma bicarbonate concentration, as our teaching case illustrates. The UAG, calculated as urine $(Na^+ + K^+) - (Cl^-)$ is a useful diagnostic index to estimate kidney ability to excrete ammonium in patients with metabolic acidosis, when urine ammonium is not measured.

There is a strong relationship between UAG and urine ammonium excretion; that is to say, the more ammonium in the urine, the lower the UAG is with a value ranging from 0 to 200 mEq/L during metabolic acidosis. In patients with dRTA, the UAG is positive, because of the impaired H^+ secretion in the distal nephron leading to reduced ammonium excretion.

In CRA, the UAG is also positive secondary to low ammonium excretion, which is a compensatory response to chronic alkalemia. In the present case, the diagnosis of CRA as the cause of the low plasma bicarbonate concentration was suspected before ABG evaluation because the patient had hyperventilation on physical examination and the UAG was positive. Moreover, there were no clinical features to suspect metabolic acidosis caused by dRTA and the patient did not have CKD to explain the low bicarbonate concentration and positive UAG.

In CRA, the renal adaptation involves suppression of ammonium excretion and decreasing bicarbonate reabsorption. This results in a net reduction in acid excretion that helps attenuate the increase in blood pH. The compensatory renal response to CRA is so efficient in lowering plasma bicarbonate concentrations that blood pH is close to normal.

It is worth noting that the ability of the UAG as a surrogate for ammonium excretion in patients with chronic kidney disease (CKD) is limited because urine ammonium excretion falls as glomerular filtration rate (GFR) declines. In addition, the quantity of unmeasured anions in the urine such as sulfate and phosphate, which are not included in the typical UAG calculation, critically influences the ability of UAG to estimate NH4 concentration in CKD patients.

Case Study 13

A 5-year-old white male with a history of bronchospasm was admitted to the hospital for treatment of status asthmaticus. Physical examination revealed a well-developed male in respiratory distress. Blood pressure was 115/59 mmHg, heart rate was 92 beats/min, respiratory rate was 18 breaths/min, and temperature was 38°C. Expiratory wheezing was heard bilaterally. Laboratory data on admission were blood pH 7.41, PCO_2 58 mmHg, sodium 141 mmol/L, potassium 4.6 mmol/L, chloride 100 mmol/L, and bicarbonate 29 mmol/L. The patient was treated with repeated doses of albuterol sulfate and intravenous infusion of theophylline and methylprednisolone. Oxygen was administered by nasal prongs at a flow rate of 4 L/min. After 36 hours, repeated laboratory studies revealed: serum sodium 142 mmol/L, potassium 3.1 mmol/L, chloride 93 mmol/L, bicarbonate 29 mmol/L, creatinine 0.5 mg/dL, and urea nitrogen 15 mg/dL. The arterial blood pH was 7.37, PCO_2 36 mmHg, and PO_2 88 mmHg.

What acid-base disturbance is present at this time?

A. Respiratory acidosis
B. Mixed metabolic alkalosis and metabolic acidosis
C. Mixed reparatory acidosis and metabolic acidosis
D. Mixed respiratory acidosis and metabolic alkalosis

The correct diagnosis is B

Comment: The initial blood gas values, with the pH of 7.41 and a PCO_2 of 58 mmHg, are consistent with the pattern of respiratory failure. The elevated serum bicarbonate (29 mmol/L) suggests that the respiratory acidosis had been proceeding for a sufficient time to permit some degree of renal compensation.[1,2] As a rule, serum bicarbonate will increase by 3.5 mmol/L for each 10 mmHg rise in PCO_2 in chronic respiratory acidosis (Δ bicarbonate = 0.35 Δ PCO_2).[3,4]

Therapy with bronchodilators normalized the blood pH but reduced blood PCO_2. Moreover, the anion increased by 14 mmol/L, while blood bicarbonate concentration reduced by no more than 6 mmol/L. The increased anion gap and the low blood bicarbonate concentration signify the presence of metabolic acidosis. A diagnosis of pure metabolic acidosis could not be made in this patient since the fall in blood bicarbonate concentration is not matched by a commensurate rise in the unmeasured anion concentration. As a rule, with metabolic acidosis of the high anion gap variety, there should be a 1:1 correspondence between decreasing serum bicarbonate and increasing AG (Δ bicarbonate/ AG = 1). Whenever the anion gap is elevated but serum bicarbonate is not reduced reciprocally, a mixed metabolic acidosis and alkalosis must be strongly considered. In this patient, the reciprocity between the decrement in blood bicarbonate and increment in anion gap is lost by 8 mEq/L, providing evidence for a coexisting metabolic alkalosis. The presence of hypochloremia favors this interpretation.

The increased anion gap metabolic acidosis in this patient is the result of lactic acidosis owing to the therapy of bronchospasm. The finding of a blood lactate level of 6.1 mmol/L supports this diagnosis during albuterol therapy. With cessation of albuterol, the patient's blood lactate fell within 24 hours to 0.7 mmol/L. During this period, his blood bicarbonate concentration increased, and his anion gap fell to 13 mmol/L. Increased work of breathing could not account for the rise in the blood lactate level in this patient, since the initial respiratory rate of 18 breaths/min argues against such a possibility. Furthermore, the patient never had hypotension, sepsis, signs of tissue hypoxia, or any of the other known causes of lactic acidosis. The cellular mechanism by which β2-adrenergic stimulation causes lactic acidosis is related to 13 z-receptor activation and subsequent stimulation of adenylate cyclase. Adenylate cyclase, in turn, enhances cyclic AMP-mediated activation of glycogenolysis, lipolysis, and Na^+-K^+-ATPase. As muscle lacks glucose-6-phosphatase, lactate is the end product of muscle glycogenolysis. Increased free fatty acids from lipolysis inhibit pyruvate oxidation, which also results in lactic production. Activation of Na^+-K^+ in the cell membrane results in sodium efflux and potassium influx.

Theophylline is known to potentiate the β2-adrenergic effects by increasing the cellular cyclic AMP levels through inhibition of 5′-phosphodiesterase. Glucocorticoids also might enhance the sensitivity of β-receptors to β-adrenergic agents. The metabolic alkalosis in the patient is most likely the result of both hypokalemia and the state of posthypercapnia.

Case Study 14

A 16-year-old white male was found unconscious in the street and was brought into the emergency room. The patient was stuporous, without focal neurological signs. Blood pressure was 120/80 mmHg and his pulse 80 beats/min. Examination of the head, eyes, ears, nose, and throat was unremarkable. His chest was clear to auscultation and percussion. The remainder of the physical examination was unremarkable. Laboratory investigations showed: serum sodium 137 mmol/L, potassium 4.6 mmol/L, chloride 102 mmol/L, bicarbonate 15 mmol/L, urea nitrogen 43 mg/dL, creatinine 1.0 mg/dL, and glucose 200 mg/dL. Serum ketones were trace positive and serum osmolality was 330 mOsm/kg. Blood pH was 7.32 and PCO_2 was 28 mmHg. Urinalysis was negative with a pH of 5.1.

What acid-base disorder is present?

    A. Simple anion gap metabolic acidosis
    B. Mixed anion gap metabolic acidosis and respiratory acidosis
    C. Mixed anion gap metabolic acidosis and respiratory alkalosis
    D. Lactic acidosis

The correct answer is A

Comment: A low plasma bicarbonate concentration and a low pH signify the presence of metabolic acidosis.[1] The PCO_2 is depressed by 10 mmHg and the plasma bicarbonate concentration by 9 mmol/L. This level of respiratory compensation is appropriate for the steady-state level of bicarbonate. The fall in plasma bicarbonate concentration is matched by a commensurate rise in the unmeasured anion concentration; thus, this is a pure high anion gap type of metabolic acidosis.

Under normal conditions, the osmolar gap, difference between the measured and the estimated serum osmolality [2 (sodium concentration (mEq/L)] + [BUN (mg/dL) + 2.8] + [glucose concentration (mg/dL)+18], is less than 10 mOsm/kg H_2O. As a general rule, a value greater than this indicates the presence of an additional osmotically active substance in the circulation. Methanol intoxication, ethylene glycol intoxication, and alcohol ketoacidosis are disorders associated with high anion gap metabolic acidosis and increased serum osmolality.[2,3] The measured serum osmolality in this patient was 330 mOsm/kg H_2O, giving an osmolar gap of 30 mOsm/kg H_2O. The patient had no oxalate crystals in the urine, as found in ethylene glycol intoxication, and there was no evidence of optic papillitis on funduscopic examination, as might be anticipated in a patient with methanol intoxication. Blood alcohol levels were very high, indicating the diagnosis of alcoholic ketoacidosis.

Case Study 15

A 2-year-old male child was admitted with shortness of breath and drowsiness for 1 day. He had suffered from acute intermittent diarrhea treated with loperamide and dioctahedral smectite and was fed with glucose water recently for 1 week. He had a pertinent history of midgut volvulus status post bowel resection at the age of 1 month. His pulse rate was 140 beats/min, blood pressure 70/46 mmHg, respiratory rate 40 breaths/min, and body temperature 37.0°C. Physical examination showed drowsy consciousness, suprasternal and intercostal retraction, and delayed capillary refill time. Laboratory studies were notable for profound, high anion gap (AG) metabolic acidosis (HCO_3^- 7.0 mmol/L, AG 25 mmol/L), hyperammonemia (ammonia 220 µg/dL), and hypokalemia (3.0 mmol/L). Urine analysis revealed Na^+ 69 mmol/L, K^+ 15 mmol/L, Cl^- 58 mmol/L, and osmolality 420 mOsm/kg. Routine stool analysis did not show pus cells. His severe metabolic acidosis and hyperammonemia were unresponsive to intravenous high-dose sodium bicarbonate ($NaHCO_3$ 20 mmol/kg/day) administration for 2 days.

What is the MOST likely cause of this patient's metabolic acidosis and hyperammonemia?

A. D-lactic acidosis with hyperammonemia
B. Ketoacidosis
C. Uremic acidosis
D. Lactic acidosis

The correct answer is A

Comment: Patient presented with high AG metabolic acidosis and normal serum osmolal gap, kidney function, glucose, ketone bodies, and L-lactate, thus eliminating ethanol intoxication, uremic acidosis, ketoacidosis, and lactic acidosis as possible causes.[1,2] In addition, he had a triad of the history of short bowel disease, diarrhea, and neurological features (altered mentality) suggesting D-lactic acidosis generated from gastrointestinal bacterial overgrowth in the colon. Higher serum D-lactate level (9.6 mmol/L) measured by spectrophotometric assay confirmed this diagnosis. Oral neomycin to eradicate the bacterial overgrowth led to normalization of serum D-lactate with correction of metabolic acidosis and rapid recovery of neurological features. Of note, hyperammonemia was also evident and could result from the failure of ammonia disposal in the liver and overproduction of ammonia. His liver function was normal. Defects in the urea cycle usually have normal acid-base state or an accompanied ketoacidosis (organic acidemia).

The overproduction of ammonia was highly responsible for his hyperammonemia and could originate from systemic ammonia generated by kidneys and skeletal muscle, and portal ammonia produced by gut microflora. Hypokalemia and metabolic acidosis as observed in our patient are two well-known factors to stimulate the systemic ammoniagenesis of kidneys and muscle. Ammoniagenesis by overgrown bacteria might also have been contributory. Gut ammonia production was completely resolved with the correction of D-lactic acidosis and hypokalemia.

Removal of the offending agents and elimination of the bacterial overgrowth in colon and repletion of volume with alkalization by sodium bicarbonate are the mainstay treatment of D-lactic acidosis. The offending agents, including carbohydrates and D-lactate-containing crystalloids, should be withdrawn. Probiotics containing D-lactate-producing *Lactobacillus* spp. commonly prescribed for gastroenteritis should be avoided. Oral non-absorbable antibiotics such as neomycin are absolutely "Sine Qua Non" to completely eradicate the overgrown bacterial flora in the colon, as shown in this case. Rarely, hemodialysis is indicated for refractory severe acidosis with compromised hemodynamics. For recurrent and severe D-lactic acidosis, cyclic antibiotic treatment and/or non-D-lactate-producing probiotics for alteration of intestinal microbiota could be considered.

Case Study 16

A 15-year-old Chinese girl presented to the emergency department with muscle paralysis of bilateral lower extremities over the course of 1 day. She had a 2-year history of polyuria, nocturia, and rampant dental caries and calculi. She denied vomiting, diarrhea, or use of alcohol, laxatives, or diuretics, and her family history was unremarkable.

Her pulse rate was 90 breaths/min, blood pressure 112/72 mmHg, and body temperature 36.4°C. Physical examination revealed severe dental caries and calculi with dry oral mucosa. Her thyroid gland was not enlarged. Neurologic examination disclosed symmetric flaccid paralysis with areflexia of both lower extremities. The remainder of the physical examination was unremarkable. The most striking biochemical abnormalities were profound hypokalemia (1.8 mmol/L) and hyperchloremic metabolic acidosis (pH 7.28, bicarbonate 16.6 mmol/L, Na^+ 141 mmol/L, and Cl^- 114 mmol/L). Her renal, liver, and thyroid function were all normal (creatinine 0.9 mg/dL).

Urinalysis revealed proteinuria (1+), low urine specific gravity (1.010), high K^+ excretion (transtubular K^+ gradient 5, 24-hour urine K^+ 38 mmol/day), positive urine anion gap (Na^+ 43 mmol/L, K^+ 16 mmol/L and Cl^- 39 mEq/L), and persistent alkaline urine (pH 7 to 7.5). Electrocardiogram revealed prolonged PR interval with flattened T wave. Abdominal ultrasonography showed bilaterally medullary nephrocalcinosis.

What is the MOST likely diagnosis in this patient?

    A. Hypokalemic familial periodic paralysis
    B. Systemic lupus erythematous
    C. Sjögren syndrome
    D. Fanconi syndrome

The correct answer is C
Comment: This 15-year-old girl presented with hypokalemic paralysis, which can result from hypokalemic periodic paralysis (HPP) due to acute K^+ shift into cells or non-HypoPP due to a large total body K^+ deficit. Measurements of urinary K^+ excretion and blood acid-base status can help in the differential diagnosis. Her high urinary K^+ excretion, reflected by an elevated transtubular potassium gradient (TTKG), suggested renal K^+ wasting and non-HypoPP. Her concurrent hyperchloremic metabolic acidosis suggested a condition with both K^+ depletion and direct or indirect bicarbonate loss (renal tubular acidosis). The assessment of urine $NH4^+$ excretion by urine anion gap and/or urine osmolal gap separates renal tubular acidosis (RTA) from non-RTA. A positive urine anion gap indicated defective $NH4^+$ excretion associated with RTA. Her persistently alkaline urine (pH > 7.0) pointed to a diagnosis of distal RTA. In fact, hypokalemia is a common finding in distal RTA and results from the combination of renal Na^+ wasting, secondary hyperaldosteronism, and bicarbonaturia.

Nevertheless, the underlying cause of distal RTA must be identified. Upon review of her history, she had been experiencing dry mouth for the past 3 months despite normal Schirmer's test for dry eye. An exhaustive work-up demonstrated elevated anti-Ro antibody, rheumatoid factor, antinuclear antibody (> 1:1280), polyclonal IgG, typical delayed salivary secretion on salivary scintigraphy and sialo duct ectasia and typical periductal lymphocytic infiltration (focus score 3) in the salivary gland biopsy. Renal histology showed chronic tubulointerstitial nephritis with predominant lymphocytic infiltration. After ruling out other autoimmune diseases, like systemic lupus erythematous or juvenile arthritis, primary SS was diagnosed.[1-4]

Sjögren syndrome is a chronic autoimmune disease characterized by progressive lymphocytic infiltration of exocrine glands with typical features of keratoconjunctivitis, sicca, and xerostomia. Various degrees of extraglandular involvement, like arthritis, RTA, and lymphoma may develop before or after glandular damage. SS is most prevalent in women in their fourth and fifth decades and uncommon in children or adolescents. The clinical presentations of juvenile Sjögren syndrome are diverse. Dry eye and dry mouth sensation are the most common presenting complaints in adults, but usually develop later in juveniles, reflecting the atypical presentations of juvenile Sjögren syndrome at the outset. The nonspecific clinical picture and lack of universal diagnostic criteria mean that most patients are under-diagnosed until they experience complications. Profound hypokalemia with paralysis is a rare primary manifestation of SS in children.

Impaired distal tubular H^+ secretion is by far the most common renal manifestation of Sjögren syndrome. It takes time to progress from impaired distal tubular H^+ secretion to full-blown RTA. Therefore, defective renal acidification (pH > 5.5) in response to the acid-load test and low urine citrate excretion are the earliest indices to suggest renal involvement in Sjögren syndrome. Impaired ability to concentrate (hyposthenuria) is also another marker of early primary Sjögren syndrome.

Hypokalemia and nephrocalcinosis (or nephrolithiasis) are common but late manifestations in distal RTA, because they are nearly asymptomatic (> 90%) in the early stages. The combination of renal Na^+ wasting, secondary hyperaldosteronism, and bicarbonaturia in distal RTA contribute to hypokalemia. Metabolic acidosis, per se, can induce bone resorption and reduce renal tubular calcium and phosphate reabsorption, leading to increased urine calcium and phosphate excretion. This, in combination with hypocitraturia, as a result of metabolic acidosis and hypokalemia, precipitates the formation of nephrocalcinosis or nephrolithiasis.

With respect to therapy, K^+ citrate must be used to correct hypokalemia and metabolic acidosis and prevent further nephrocalcinosis. Care for oral involvement includes mechanical stimulation of the salivary glands, diet modification, regular oral hygiene, and topical fluoride. Prompt recognition and management of Sjögren syndrome achieves a good prognosis by preventing glandular and extraglandular complications. Corticosteroids are the drugs of choice for Sjögren syndrome with visceral involvement. In life-threatening cases, mycophenolate mofetil and novel biological therapies like rituximab and infliximab can be attempted.

Case Study 17

A 10-week-old female infant developed hypertension. The elevated blood pressure was associated with metabolic alkalosis and urinary chloride wastage. The family history was unremarkable. Her urinalysis, blood urea nitrogen (BUN), and serum creatinine concentrations were all normal. A renal ultrasound was normal. A technetium-99m diethylenetriaminepentaacetic acid (DTPA) renal scans with captopril showed normal blood flow bilaterally. The head ultrasound and echocardiogram were normal. Blood epinephrine, norepinephrine, catecholamines, thyroxin, and steroid levels were also normal. Treatment with various combinations of labetalol, hydralazine, captopril, methyldopa, nifedipine, and spironolactone, all at high doses, failed to control the elevated blood pressure. Serum aldosterone level and peripheral plasma renin activity were low.

What is the MOST likely diagnosis?

    A. Apparent mineralocorticoid excess
    B. Congenital adrenal hyperplasia
    C. Primary hyperaldosteronism
    D. Liddle syndrome

The correct answer is D
Comment: Our patient had normal renal function and structure. In addition, her normal physical examination, baseline laboratory data, including the low plasma renin activity and aldosterone secretion, and the findings on echocardiogram, renal ultrasound, and renal scan excluded the possibility of coarctation of aorta, congenital heart disease, adrenogenital syndrome, and infectious, neurologic, endocrine, and renovascular causes of hypertension. The constellation of hypertension, metabolic alkalosis, and low plasma renin activity and aldosterone level in our patient prompted us to consider other diagnostic possibilities. The lack of therapeutic response to spironolactone, with good response to amiloride, strongly suggested the diagnosis of Liddle syndrome.[1,2] The recurrence of hypertension and metabolic alkalosis after cessation of amiloride that was subsequently treated with amiloride confirmed the diagnosis of Liddle syndrome.

Liddle syndrome classically presents with the concurrent triad of hypertension, hypokalemia, and metabolic alkalosis similar to disorders caused by mineralocorticoid excess. The consistent finding among patients with Liddle syndrome is decreased aldosterone and renin secretion. However, not all patients with Liddle syndrome are hypokalemic at presentation, similar to our case.

The differential diagnosis of Liddle syndrome includes some forms of congenital adrenal hyperplasia including 11β-HSD, the syndrome of apparent mineralocorticoid excess, familial cortisol resistance, and a deoxycorticosterone-producing tumor. If a diagnosis is not firmly established, a therapeutic response to dexamethasone should lead to the suspicion of possible 11β-HSD. CT or magnetic resonance imaging can usually detect deoxycorticosterone-producing tumor.

The primary abnormality in Liddle syndrome is a distal renal tubular transport defect characterized by increased rate of sodium reabsorption and, in most cases, increased rate of potassium and hydrogen ion secretion resulting in fluid retention, hypertension, suppression of renin and aldosterone secretion and hypokalemic metabolic alkalosis. Data derived from cloned sodium channel genes indicate that the site of the enhanced activity of the sodium channel, in Liddle syndrome, is the late distal tubule and cortical outer medullary portions of the collecting tubule. The genetic abnormality involves the beta or gamma subunit of the collecting tubule sodium channel.

Therapy in Liddle syndrome consists of prescribing amiloride or triamterene, which directly close the sodium channels. The mineralocorticoid antagonist spironolactone activity is not mediated in this disorder.

Case Study 18

A 25-day-old male infant was admitted to the hospital because of diarrhea and dehydration. His mother was a 22-year-old black female, who had an uncomplicated pregnancy and delivery. His birth weight was 2.4 kg. He was discharged from the premature nursery at 2 weeks of age, weighing 2.32 kg. A routine urinalysis at 1 week of age was normal. At home he did well initially but then began to feed poorly. When seen in the emergency room he was severely dehydrated, cachectic, and tremulous. His weight was 2.20 kg, temperature 38.7°C, pulse 140 beats/min, and respiratory rate 30 breaths/min. Physical examination was otherwise unremarkable. Laboratory data on admission included the following: hematocrit 50%, blood urea 19 mg/dL, Na^+ 159 mmol/L, Cl^- 138 mmol/L, and bicarbonate 14.8 mmol/L. Urinalysis revealed the following: pH 5, trace of protein, and no cells. Blood, stool, and urine cultures were negative. On admission the diagnosis of sepsis was suspected; antibiotics were given for 10 days in addition to conventional intravenous fluids. After 3 days of therapy the infant was markedly improved, having gained 320 g in weight. On the 6th hospital day, hyperchloremic acidosis was still present despite complete correction of the dehydration. The laboratory findings were blood pH 7.17, Na^+ 132 mmol/L, Cl^- 120 mmol/L, K^+ 5.2 mmol/L, bicarbonate 10.0 mmol/L, urea 21 mg/dL, calcium 19.1 mg/dL. The urine pH was 5.5 and the urinary molar ratio of calcium to creatinine was 0.96. The acidosis persisted and he was started on an oral citrate mixture (10 mEq/day) and calcium gluconate. On the 10th hospital day, the blood pH was 7.18, bicarbonate 12.5 mmol/L, and Cl^- 115 mmol/L. The dose of citrate was increased to 40 mEq/day (16 mEq/kg) with gradual and complete correction of the acidemia. The effect of this therapy was remarkable in that the baby gained 2 kg in the following 2 months. While receiving citrate, the urine pH was consistently above 7, and the Ca/Cr ratio decreased to 0.45. At 3 months of age inulin clearance was 86 mL/min/1.73 m². Citrate therapy was stopped, with immediate reappearance of the hyperchloremic acidosis, which, however, disappeared promptly with reinstitution of therapy. The infant was discharged at 3.5 months of age, in good health, weighing 4.96 kg. He received a regular diet plus 40 mEq/day sodium citrate.

What is the MOST likely diagnosis?

    A. Proximal renal tubular acidosis
    B. Distal renal tubular acidosis
    C. Tubulointerstitial disease
    D. Fanconi syndrome

The correct answer is D

Comment: The persistence of hyperchloremic acidosis, with no apparent cause, combined with normal renal function, suggests the diagnosis of renal tubular acidosis (RTA). The ability to acidify the urine maximally and, during acidosis, to excrete titratable acid and ammonium at normal rates excludes the diagnosis of distal RTA.[1,2]

Most commonly proximal RTA is one abnormality in a complex of renal tubular dysfunction, as encountered in the Fanconi syndrome. These disorders are excluded by examinations for abnormalities other than RTA, including polyuria, aminoaciduria, glucosuria, phosphaturia, nephrocalcinosis, bone disease, and serum abnormalities other than hyperchloremic acidosis.

The diagnosis of proximal RTA, in which there is a large ongoing loss of bicarbonate in the urine, often exceeding 10% to 15% of the filtered load, is supported by the need to provide citrate at a rate of 10 or more mEq/kg/24 h in order to maintain the serum bicarbonate within the normal range.

The diagnosis of proximal RTA is confirmed by the demonstration of a renal bicarbonate threshold below normal for age. Some infants with distal RTA are "bicarbonate wasters," but they usually do not excrete more than 5% of their filtered bicarbonate.

Patients with isolated proximal RTA do not waste potassium and, therefore, can be treated exclusively with sodium salts (usually sodium bicarbonate or sodium citrate). Their dosage requirement, however, must be adjusted to maintain the blood bicarbonate within normal limits. The most important evidence of adequacy of treatment is acceleration in the rate of growth to achieve catch-up and then maintenance of a normal growth velocity.

Case Study 19

A 16-year-old white male was found unconscious in the street and was brought into the emergency room. The patient was stuporous, without focal neurological signs. Blood pressure was 120/80 mmHg and his pulse 80 beats/min. Examination of the head, eyes, ears, nose, and throat was unremarkable. His chest was clear to auscultation and percussion. The remainder of the physical examination was unremarkable. Laboratory investigations showed: serum sodium 137 mmol/L, potassium 4.6 mmol/L, chloride 102 mmol/L, bicarbonate 15 mmol/L, urea nitrogen 43 mg/dL, creatinine 1.0 mg/dL, and glucose 200 mg/dL. Serum ketones were trace positive and serum osmolality was 330 mOsm/kg H_2O. Blood pH was 7.32 and PCO_2 was 28 mmHg. Urinalysis was negative with a pH of 5.1.

What acid-base disorder is present?

  A. High anion gap metabolic acidosis
  B. Mixed reparatory acidosis and high anion gap metabolic acidosis
  C. Mixed reparatory alkalosis and high anion gap metabolic acidosis
  D. Chronic respiratory alkalosis

The correct answer is A

Comment: A low plasma bicarbonate concentration and a low pH signify the presence of metabolic acidosis. The PCO_2 is depressed by 10 mmHg and the plasma bicarbonate concentration by 9 mEq/L. This level of respiratory compensation is appropriate for the steady state level of bicarbonate. The fall in plasma bicarbonate concentration is matched by a commensurate rise in the unmeasured anion concentration; thus, this is a pure high anion gap type of metabolic acidosis.

Under normal conditions, the osmolar gap, difference between the measured and the estimated serum osmolality (2 × sodium concentration, mEq/L) + (BUN, 2.8 mg/dL) + (glucose concentration, 18 mg/dL), is less than 10 mOsm/kg H_2O. As a general rule, a value greater than this indicates the presence of an additional osmotically active substance in the circulation. Methanol intoxication, ethylene glycol intoxication, and alcohol ketoacidosis are disorders associated with high anion gap metabolic acidosis and increased serum osmolality. The measured serum osmolality in this patient was 330 mOsm/kg/H_2O, giving an osmolal gap of 30 mOsm/kg H_2O. The patient had no oxalate crystals in the urine, as found in ethylene glycol intoxication, and there was no evidence of optic papillitis on funduscopic examination, as might be anticipated in a patient with methanol intoxication. Blood alcohol levels were very high, indicating the diagnosis of alcoholic ketoacidosis.

Disorders producing metabolic acidosis and elevated anion gap include methanol intoxication, ethylene glycol intoxication, and alcohol ketoacidosis, and one must utilize the history, physical examination, and supporting laboratory data to identify the specific cause when it is not apparent.[1-3] Patients should be questioned specifically about a history of diabetes, renal disease, and alcohol or other drug ingestions. The physical examination provides important information regarding tissue perfusion and mental status. The presence of acidosis and an increased anion gap in a patient in shock most often is due to lactic acidosis. In a patient with unexplained metabolic acidosis, the degree to which the anion gap is elevated can be helpful in identifying the cause. Patients who have sniffed solvents or who are intoxicated with salicylates commonly have anion gaps of 17 to 19 mEq/L. Patients with the other disorders listed usually have anion gaps between 20 and 30 mEq/L. Severe acidemia, a pH less than 7.00, occurs most commonly in diabetic ketoacidosis, lactic acidosis, and methanol or ethylene glycol intoxication. Hyperglycemia signifies diabetic ketoacidosis or hyperglycemic hyperosmolar coma. Hyperglycemia and glycosuria also can occur in salicylate intoxication. Conversely, hypoglycemia should suggest alcoholic ketoacidosis, because serum glucose levels are lower than 50 mg/dL in about 13% of patients with this disorder. Ketonuria occurs almost invariably in diabetic ketoacidosis, commonly in alcoholic ketoacidosis and in approximately 25% of patients with salicylic intoxication. In patients with ethylene glycol intoxication, the urine sediment can contain many calcium oxalate crystals. In addition to the value of finding an elevated anion gap, the relationship between the increase in the anion gap and the fall in plasma bicarbonate concentration may also be helpful diagnostically. As a rule, with metabolic acidosis of the high anion gap variety, there should be 1:1 correspondence between decreasing serum bicarbonate and increasing anion gap. Whenever the anion gap is elevated but serum bicarbonate is not reduced reciprocally, a mixed metabolic acidosis and alkalosis must be strongly considered.

Calculation of the osmolar gap may be helpful, particularly if methanol and ethylene glycol levels cannot be determined rapidly. The osmolar gap is defined as the difference between the measured and the calculated osmolality. A discrepancy of 10 mOsmol or more between measured and calculated osmolality suggests the presence of an osmotically active substance in the plasma that is not measured and, thus, not included in the calculation. Such an elevation of the osmolar gap occurs in methanol, ethanol, and ethylene glycol intoxication.[4-8]

Case Study 20

A 12-year-old girl was rushed to the emergency department following a motor vehicle accident and was found to have stroke as a result of left parietal hemorrhage. Her weight was 45 kg (50th percentile), height 139 cm (10th percentile). The vital signs were temperature 38.6°C, blood pressure 120/78 mmHg (90th percentile), pulse 71 beats/min, and respiratory rates 29 breaths/min. Her breathing was rapid and deep. Her chest was clear to auscultation and percussion. Abdomen was soft and non-tender. The Glasgow coma scale estimated between 9 and 12. The remainder of the physical examination was normal.

Serum Na^+ was 140 mmol/L (reference: 135 to 145 mmol/L), K^+ 3.0 mmol/L (reference: 4 to 5 mmol/L), Cl^- 113 mmol/L (reference: 105 to 110 mmol/L), bicarbonate 18 mEq/L normal range 22 to 26 mEq/L), and anion gap 9.0 mmol/L [(Na^+) − (Cl^- + HCO_3^-)] (normal range 8 to 16 mmol/L). Urinalysis revealed a pH of 5.5, specific gravity 1.018 without protein or blood. Urine pH was 5.7, Na⁺ 52 mmol/L, K⁺ 41 mmol/L, Cl⁻ 77 mmol/L, and UAG 16 mmol/L (Na⁺ + K⁺) − (Cl⁻).

Serum creatinine was 0.8 mg/dL (normal range 0.5 to 1.0 mg/dL) and eGFR was 101 mL/min/1.73 m² (normal 95 to 101 mL/min/1.72 m²). The positive UAG in the clinical setting of hyperventilation suggested CRA as the likely diagnosis. The diagnosis was later confirmed by obtaining capillary blood gas, which showed a decrease in PCO_2 and high normal pH values.

What acid-base disturbance is present and what is the MOST likely explanation for the development of positive UAG?

    A. Chronic respiratory alkalosis (CRA)
    B. Type-1 distal renal tubular acidosis (dRTA-1)
    C. Mixed respiratory alkalosis and dRTA
    D. None of the above

The correct answer is A

Comment: In evaluation of patients with low serum bicarbonate concentration, CRA and dRTA-1 are often within the spectrum of differential diagnoses.[1-6] CRA can present with a picture that is similar to dRTA-1. Failure to diagnose CRA can lead to inappropriate alkali therapy, which, in turn, may cause cerebral vasoconstriction and hypocalcemia, both of which could cause seizure and increase the morbidity and mortality of the underlying disease.

In our patient, the constellation of hyperventilation, low serum bicarbonate concentration, and positive UAG helped to distinguish CRA from MA even in the absence of arterial blood gas analysis.

The use of UAG as a surrogate of ammonium (NH_4^+) excretion may differentiate between CRA and MA especially when arterial blood gas is not obtained. When the clinical history (hyperventilation) supports CRA, urine pH above 5.5 in non-gap acidosis does not necessarily suggest a primary defect in H⁺ secretion such as dRTA-1 as CRA also suppresses renal free H⁺ excretion, maintaining a positive UAG and causing urine pH above 5.5 as our patient illustrates.

The UAG represents the differences between the principal cations (Na⁺ + K⁺) and anion (Cl⁻) and is used as a surrogate of renal NH_4 excretion. In the setting of CRA distal ammonia (NH_3) excretion increases to the extent that the secreted H⁺ is almost completely buffered as NH_4^+. This may result in a very low free H⁺ in the lumen to lower the urine pH below 5.5.

In simple respiratory alkalosis, the decline in bicarbonate concentration is a proportional response to the decrement in PCO_2. The expected serum bicarbonate for a PCO_2 between 17 and 25 mmHg among our patients closely approximates the expected renal compensation, signifying the presence of pure CRA, excluding the diagnosis of mixed acid-base disorders.

Although a positive UAG in a setting of low serum bicarbonate concentration may support the diagnosis of CRA, in the absence of blood gas results, history of hyperventilation and clinical findings of hyperpnea are necessary underpinnings to diagnosis and with positive UAG providing support and guidance. Treatment of the underlying illness usually improves CRA and metabolic treatment is generally not indicated. Rebreathing into a closed system, anxiolytic medications, or opioids have been used rarely to slow respiration.

References

Case Study 1

1. Gabow PA. Disorders associated with an altered anion gap. *Kidney Int.* 1985;27:472–483.
2. Madias NE. Lactic acidosis. *Kidney Int.* 1986;29:752–774.
3. Singh R, Arain E, Buth A, et al. Ethelene glycol poisoning: an unusual cause of altered mental status and the lessons learned from management of the disease in the acute setting. *Case Rep Crit Care.* 2016;2016:9157393.
4. Kraleti S, Soultanova I. Pancytopenia and lactic acidosis associated with linezolid use in a patient with empyema. *J Ark Med Soc.* 2013;110:62–63.

Case Study 2

1. Sterns RH, Cox MA, Feig PU, et al. Internal potassium balance and the control of the plasma potassium concentration. *Medicine.* 1981;60(5):339–354.
2. Palmer B, Clegg DJ. Physiology and pathophysiology of potassium homeostasis: core curriculum 2019. *Am J Kidney Dis.* 2019;74(5):682–695.
3. Carlisle EJ, Donnelly SM, Vasuvattakul S, et al. Glue-sniffing and distal renal tubular acidosis: sticking to the facts. *J Am Soc Nephrol.* 1991;1(8):1019–1027.
4. Batlle DC, Hizon M, Cohen E, et al. The use of the urinary anion gap in the diagnosis of hyperchloremic metabolic acidosis. *N Engl J Med.* 1988;318(10):594–599.
5. Ng JL, Morgan DJ, Loh NK, et al. Life-threatening hypokalaemia associated with ibuprofen-induced renal tubular acidosis. *Med J Aust.* 2011;194(6):313–316.

Case Study 3

1. Ferrannini E, Muscelli E, Frascerra S, et al. Metabolic response to sodium-glucose cotransporter 2 inhibition in type 2 diabetic patients. *J Clin Invest.* 2014;124(2):499–508.
2. DeFronzo RA, Norton L, Abdul-Ghani M. Renal, metabolic and cardiovascular considerations of SGLT2 inhibition. *Nat Rev Nephrol.* 2017;13(1):11–26.
3. Stenlof K, Cefalu WT, Kim KA, et al. Efficacy and safety of canagliflozin monotherapy in subjects with type 2 diabetes mellitus inadequately controlled with diet and exercise. *Diabetes Obes Metab.* 2013;15(4):372–382.
4. Monami M, Nardini C, Mannucci E. Efficacy and safety of sodium glucose co-transporter-2 inhibitors in type 2 diabetes: a meta-analysis of randomized clinical trials. *Diabetes Obes Metab.* 2014;16(5):457–466.

Case Study 4

1. Mehta AN, Emmett JB, Emmett M. GOLD MARK: an anion gap mnemonic for the 21st century. *Lancet.* 2008;372(9642):892.
2. Gabow PA. Disorders associated with an altered anion gap. *Kidney Int.* 1985;27(2):472–483.
3. Kraut JA, Kurtz I. Toxic alcohol ingestions: clinical features, diagnosis, and management. *Clin J Am Soc Nephrol.* 2008;3(1):208–225.
4. Miller ON, Bazzano G. Propanediol metabolism and its relation to lactic acid metabolism. *Ann N Y Acad Sci.* 1965;119(3):957–973.
5. Zosel A, Egelhoff E, Heard K. Severe lactic acidosis after an iatrogenic propylene glycol overdose. *Pharmacotherapy.* 2010;30(2):219.
6. Horinek EL, Kiser TH, Fish DN, et al. Propylene glycol accumulation in critically ill patients receiving continuous intravenous lorazepam infusions. *Ann Pharmacother.* 2009;43(12):1964–1971.

Case Study 5

1. Ogier de Baulny H, Saudubray JM. Branched-chain organic acidurias. *Semin Neonatol.* 2002;7(1):65–74.
2. Deodato F, Boenzi S, Santorelli FM, et al. Methylmalonic and propionic aciduria. *Am J Med Genet C Semin Med Genet.* 2006;142C(2):104–112.
3. Venditti CP. Methylmalonic acidemia. In: *Gene Reviews at Gene Tests: Medical Genetics Information Resources (Database Online).* Seattle: University of Washington. www.genetests.org. Accessed January 16, 2010.
4. Ledley FD, Levy HL, Shih VE, et al. Benign methylmalonic aciduria. *N Engl J Med.* 1984;311(16):1015–1018.

Case Study 6

1. Shah GN, Bonapace G, Hu PY, et al. Carbonic anhydrase II deficiency syndrome (osteopetrosis with renal tubular acidosis and brain calcification): novel mutations in CA2 identified by direct sequencing expand the opportunity for genotype-phenotype correlation. *Hum Mutat.* 2004;24(3):272. https://doi.org/10.1002/humu.9266.
2. Bosley TM, Salih MA, Alorainy IA, et al. The neurology of carbonic anhydrase type II deficiency syndrome. *Brain.* 2011;134(Pt 12):3502–3515. https://doi.org/10.1093/brain/awr302.

Case Study 7

1. Soleimani M, Rastegar A. Pathophysiology of renal tubular acidosis: core curriculum 2016. *Am J Kidney Dis.* 2016;68:488–498.
2. Rodriguez Soriano J. Renal tubular acidosis: the clinical entity. *J Am Soc Nephrol.* 2002;13:2160–2170.
3. Ram R, Swarnalatha G, Dakshinamurty KV. Renal tubular acidosis in Sjogren's syndrome: a case series. *Am J Nephrol.* 2014;40:123–130.
4. Ali Y, Parekh A, Baig M, et al. Renal tubular acidosis type II associated with vitamin D deficiency presenting as chronic weakness. *Ther Adv Endocrinol Metab.* 2014;5:86–89.
5. World Health Organization. *Exposure to Cadmium: A major public health concern. Preventing disease through healthy environments.* WHO; 2010. https://www.who.int/ipcs/features/cadmium.pdf. Accessed June 2, 2021.
6. Waalkes MP. Carcinogenesis. *Mutat Res.* 2003;533:107–120.
7. Roels H, Djubgang J, Buchet JP, et al. Evolution of cadmium-induced renal dysfunction in workers removed from exposure. *Scand J Work Environ Health.* 1982;8:191–200.
8. Johri N, Jacquillet G, Unwin R. Heavy metal poisoning: the effects of cadmium on the kidney. *Biometals.* 2010;23:783–792.
9. International Program on Chemical Safety Cadmium. *Environmental Health Criteria 134.* World Health Organization; 1992. http://www.inchem.org/documents/ehc/ehc/ehc134.htm.
10. Agency for Toxic Substances and Disease Registry. *Case Studies in Environmental Medicine (CSEM). Cadmium Toxicity.* U.S. Department of Health and Human Services; 2008. https://www.atsdr.cdc.gov/csem/cadmium/docs/cadmium.pdf.
11. Mannino DM, Holguin F, Greves HM, et al. Urinary cadmium levels predict lower lung function in current and former smokers: data from the Third National Health and Nutrition Examination Survey. *Thorax.* 2004;59:194–198.
12. Horiguchi H, Oguma E, Sasaki S, et al. Comprehensive study of the effects of age, iron deficiency, diabetes mellitus, and cadmium burden on dietary cadmium absorption in cadmium-exposed female Japanese farmers. *Toxicol Appl Pharmacol.* 2004;196:114–123.
13. Ashraf MW. Levels of heavy metals in popular cigarette brands and exposure to these metals via smoking. *Sci World J.* 2012;2012:729430.
14. Prozialeck WC, Edwards JR. Mechanisms of cadmium-induced proximal tubule injury: new insights with implications for biomonitoring and therapeutic interventions. *J Pharmacol Exp Ther.* 2012;343:2–12.

Case Study 8

1. Rose BD, Post TW. *Clinical Physiology of Acid-Base and Electrolyte Disorders.* 5th ed. New York: McGraw-Hill, Inc.; 2001. [chap 18, 551–571].
2. Assadi F. *Clinical Decisions in Pediatric Nephrology: A Problem Solving Approach to Clinical Cases.* New York: Springer; 2008. [chap 2, 69–98].

Case Study 9

1. Rose BD, Post TW. *Clinical Physiology of Acid-Base and Electrolyte Disorders.* 5th ed. New York: McGraw-Hill, Inc.; 2001. [chap 18, 551–571].
2. Assadi F. *Clinical Decisions in Pediatric Nephrology: A Problem Solving Approach to Clinical Cases.* New York: Springer; 2008. [chap 2, 69–98].

Case Study 10

1. Rose BD, Post TW. *Clinical Physiology of Acid-Base and Electrolyte Disorders.* 5th ed. New York: McGraw-Hill, Inc.; 2001. [chap 18, 551–571].
2. Assadi F. *Clinical Decisions in Pediatric Nephrology: A Problem Solving Approach to Clinical Cases.* New York: Springer; 2008. [chap 2, 69–98].

Case Study 11

1. Rose BD, Post TW. *Clinical Physiology of Acid-Base and Electrolyte Disorders.* 5th ed. New York: McGraw-Hill, Inc.; 2001. [chap 18, 551–571].

2. Assadi F. *Clinical Decisions in Pediatric Nephrology: A Problem Solving Approach to Clinical Cases.* New York: Springer; 2008. [chap 2, 69–98].

Case Study 12

1. Narines RG, Emmett M. Simple and mixed acid-base disorders: practical approach. *Medicine (Baltimore).* 1980;59:151–187.
2. Krapf R, Beeler I, Hertner D, et al. Chronic respiratory alkalosis. The effect of sustained hyperventilation on renal regulation of acid-base equilibrium. *N Engl J Med.* 1991;324(20):1394–1401.
3. Muppidi V, Kolli S, Dandu V, et al. Severe respiratory alkalosis in acute ischemic stroke: a rare presentation. *Cureus.* 2020;12(4):e7747. https://doi.org/10.7759/cureus.7747.
4. Vasileiadis I, Alevrakis E, Ampelioti S, et al. Acid-base disturbances in patients with asthma: a literature review and comments on their pathophysiology. *J Clin Med.* 2019;8:563. https://doi.org/10.3390/jcm8040563.
5. Carlisle EJ, Donnelly SM, Halperin ML. Renal tubular acidosis (RTA): recognize the ammonium defect and the pHorget the urine pH. *Pediatr Nephrol.* 1991;5(2):242–248.
6. Madison LL, Seldin DW. Ammonia excretion and enzymatic adaptation in human subjects, as disclosed by administration of precursor amino acids. *J Clin Invest.* 1958;37(11):1615–1627.
7. Goldstein MB, Bear R, Richardson RM, et al. The urine anion gap: a clinically useful index of ammonium excretion. *Am J Med Sci.* 1986;292:198–202.
8. Batlle DC, Hizon M, Cohen E, et al. The use of the urinary anion gap in the diagnosis of hyperchloremic metabolic acidosis. *N Engl J Med.* 1988;318(10):594–599.
9. Seifter JL. Integration of acid-base and electrolyte disorders. *N Engl J Med.* 2015;372(4):391–392.
10. Batlle D, Saleem K, Nithin R. The use of bedside urinary parameters in the evaluation of metabolic acidosis. In: Wesson D, ed. *Metabolic Acidosis.* New York: Springer Science; 2016:39–51.
11. Raphael KL, Gilligan S, Ix JH. Urine anion gap to predict urine ammonium and related outcomes in kidney disease. *Clin J Am Soc Nephrol.* 2018;13:205–212.
12. Battlle D, Chin-Theodorou J, Tucker MB. Metabolic acidosis or respiratory alkalosis? Evaluation of low plasma bicarbonate using the urine anion gap. *Am J Kidney Dis.* 2017;70:440–444.

Case Study 13

1. Assadi F. Clinical quizzes on acid-base problems. *Pediatr Nephrol.* 1993;7(3):321–325. https://doi.org/10.1007/BF00853235.
2. Assadi FK. Therapy of acute bronchospasm: complicated by lactic acidosis and hypokalemia. *Clin Pediatr (Phila).* 1989;28:258–260.
3. Rosa RM, Silva P, Young JB, et al. Adrenergic modulation of extrarenal potassium disposal. *N Engl J Med.* 1980;302:431–434.
4. Narins RG, Emmett M. Simple and mixed acid-base disorders: practical approach. *Medicine (Baltimore).* 1980;59:161–187.

Case Study 14

1. Assadi F. Clinical quizzes on acid-base problems. *Pediatr Nephrol.* 1993;7(3):321–325. https://doi.org/10.1007/BF00853235.
2. Gabow PA. Disorders associated with an altered anion gap. *Kidney Int.* 1985;27:472–483.
3. Gabow PA. Ethylene glycol intoxication. *Am J Kidney Dis.* 1988;11:277–279.

Case Study 15

1. Kowlgi NG, Chhabra L. D-lactic acidosis: an underrecognized complication of short bowel syndrome. *Gastroenterol Res Pract.* 2015;476215. https://doi.org/10.1155/2015/476215.
2. Yilmaz B, Schibli S, Macpherson AJ, et al. D-lactic acidosis: successful suppression of D-lactate-producing Lactobacillus by probiotics. *Pediatrics.* 2018;142:e20180337. https://doi.org/10.1542/peds.2018-0337.

Case Study 16

1. Fox RI. Sjögren's syndrome. *Lancet.* 2005;366:321–331.
2. Ohlsson V, Strike H, James-Ellison M, et al. Renal tubular acidosis, arthritis and autoantibodies: primary Sjogren syndrome in childhood. *Rheumatology.* 2006;45:238–240.

3. Skalova S, Minxova L, Slezak R. Hypokalaemic paralysis revealing Sjogren's syndrome in a 16-year old girl. *Ghana Med J.* 2008;42:124–128.
4. Houghton K, Malleson P, Cabral D, Petty R, Tucker L. Primary Sjögren's syndrome in children and adolescents: are proposed diagnostic criteria applicable? *J Rheumatol.* 2005;32:2225–2232.

Case Study 17

1. Assadi F, Kimura RE, Subramanian U, et al. Liddle syndrome in a newborn infant. *Pediatr Nephrol.* 2002;17:609–611. https://doi.org/10.1007/s00467-002-0897-z.
2. Palmmer BF, Alpern RJ. Liddle syndrome. *Am J Med.* 1998;104. 310–309.

Case Study 18

1. Edelmann CM Jr. Isolated proximal (type 2) renal tubular acidosis. In: Gonick HC, Buckalew VM Jr, eds. *Renal Tubular Disorders; Pathophysiology, Diagnosis, and Management.* New York: Dekker; 1985:261–279.
2. Rodriguez-Soriano J, Boichis H, Stark H, et al. Proximal renal tubular acidosis. A defect in bicarbonate reabsorption with normal urinary acidification. *Pediatr Res.* 1967;1:81–98.

Case Study 19

1. Kappy M, Morrow G. A diagnostic approach to metabolic acidosis in children. *Pediatrics.* 1980;65:351–356.
2. Assadi F. Clinical quizzes on acid-base problems. *Pediatr Nephrol.* 1993;7:321–325. https://doi.org/10.1007/BF00853235.
3. Gabow PA. Disorders associated with an altered anion gap. *Kidney Int.* 1985;27:472–483.
4. Gennari JF, Serum osmolality. Uses and limitations. *N Engl J Med.* 1984;310:102–105.
5. Smithline N, Gardner K. Gaps—amniotic and osmolal. *JAMA.* 1976;236:1594–1597.
6. Gabow PA. Ethylene glycol intoxication. *Am J Kidney Dis.* 1988;11:277–279.
7. Emmett M, Narins RG. Clinical use of the anion gap. *Medicine (Baltimore).* 1977;65:38–54.
8. Narins RG, Emmett M. Simple and mixed acid-base disorders: practical approach. *Medicine (Baltimore).* 1980;59:161–187.

Case Study 20

1. Brened K, de Vries AP, Gans PO. Physiological approach to assessment of acid-base disturbances. *N Engl J Med.* 2014;371:1434–1445.
2. Battle D, Ba Aqeel SH, Marquez A. Urine anion gap in context. *Clin J Am Soc Nephrol.* 2018;13:195–197.
3. Raphael KL, Gilligan S, Ix JH. Urine anion gap to predict urine ammonium and related outcomes in kidney disease. *Clin J Am Soc Nephrol.* 2018;13:205–212.
4. Battle D, Chin-Theodorou J, Tucker MB. Metabolic acidosis or respiratory alkalosis? Evaluation of low plasma bicarbonate using the urine Anion gap. *Am J Kidney Dis.* 2017;70:440–444.
5. Krapf R, Beeler I, Hertner D, et al. Chronic respiratory alkalosis: the effect of sustained hyperventilation on renal regulation of acid-base equilibrium. *N Engl J Med.* 1991;324:1394–1401.
6. Muppidi V, Kolli S, Dandu V, et al. Severe respiratory alkalosis in acute ischemic stroke: a rare presentation. *Cureus.* 2020;12:e7747. https://doi.org/10.7759/cureus.7747.

CHAPTER 7

Hypocalcemia

Case Study 1

A patient with recurrent diarrhea complains of severe muscle weakness. There is no history of carpopedal spasm, or physical findings of Trousseau or Chvostek sign, consistent with hypocalcemia. The electrocardiogram reveals ST-segment and T-wave changes with premature ventricular beats, which are felt to be compatible with hypokalemia. The following laboratory data are obtained: serum sodium 140 mmol/L, potassium 1.3 mmol/L, chloride 110 mmol/L, bicarbonate 10 mmol/L, albumin 4.1 g/dL, calcium 6.3 mg/dL, arterial pH 7.26, PCO_2 23 mmHg.

How would you correct this patient's electrolyte disorders?

    A. Treatment of hypokalemia should proceed the correction of hypocalcemia
    B. Treatment of hypocalcemia should proceed the correction of hypokalemia
    C. Treatment of acidosis should proceed before the correction of hypokalemia
    D. Treatment of acidosis should proceed before the correction of hypocalcemia

The correct answer is A

Comment: Correction of the acidemia will drive potassium into the cells, further reducing the plasma potassium concentration. In this setting, in which the acidemia is not severe, alkali therapy should be withheld until potassium supplements have partially corrected the hypokalemia.[1,2]

    Hypocalcemia protects against the effects of hypokalemia via an uncertain mechanism. Thus, treatment of the hypokalemia should precede correction of the hypocalcemia. It should be noted that, for the same reasons, hypokalemia protects against the neuromuscular effects of hypocalcemia. Thus, increasing the plasma potassium concentration in this setting may precipitate hypocalcemic tetany. However, this risk is generally less serious.[1,2]

Case Study 2

An 8-year-old girl presented with two episodes of generalized tonic-clonic seizures lasting less than 5 minutes, aborted with intravenous midazolam bolus. There was no history of fever, headache, vomiting, blurring of vision, deafness, or head trauma. There was no history of muscle cramps, abnormal sensations like tingling, burning or numbness of hands, or stridor. There was no history of polyuria. There was no family history of epilepsy or any neurological disorders in parents or siblings. Her development and scholastic performance were appropriate for age. There was no history of learning disabilities or behavioral problems. At presentation, the child was conscious, oriented, and afebrile. At admission, pulse rate was 94 beats/min, and blood pressure was 108/78 mmHg (50th to 90th percentile). The weight (26.5 kg), height (124 cm), and head circumference (51 cm) were appropriate for age. There were no neurocutaneous markers or dysmorphic facies. No cleft palate or dental anomalies were noted. Meningeal signs were absent. Neurological examination revealed positive Chvostek sign (twitching of facial muscles in response to tapping over the facial nerve) and positive Trousseau sign (carpopedal spasm induced by pressure applied to the arm by an inflated sphygmomanometer cuff). Examination of the other systems was unremarkable. Investigations showed capillary blood glucose of 124 mg/dL. Serum sodium (139 mmol/L) and potassium (4.4 mmol/L) were normal; however, serum calcium (6.1 mg/dL) and ionized calcium (0.54 mmol/L) were low, and serum phosphorus (10.5 mg/dL) was high. The blood urea (31 mg/dL), serum creatinine (0.3 mg/dL), magnesium (1.9 mg/dL), serum albumin (4.7 g/dL), and uric acid (2.8 mg/dL) were normal. Blood gas analysis (pH 7.39, bicarbonate 22 mEq/L) was normal. Serum 25 (OH) vitamin D level was 33 ng/mL, and iPTH level was 0.01 pg/mL (reference: 15 to 30 pg/mL). Spot urine calcium/creatinine ratio was 0.42, consistent with hypercalciuria. The 24-hour urine calcium levels were 90 mg/24 h (> 4 mg/kg/24 h). The skeletal survey was normal, with no evidence of osteosclerosis or cortical thickening. Kidney ultrasonogram (USG) revealed homogeneous diffusely hyperechoic medullary pyramids with acoustic shadowing in both kidneys suggestive of grade 3 nephrocalcinosis. Contrast-enhanced computed tomography (CECT) of brain revealed symmetrical, dense calcification in bilateral basal ganglia and bilateral frontal lobes. There was no evidence of cataract, microphthalmia, papilledema, or hyperopia. There were no corneal and retinal calcifications on ophthalmological evaluation. Echocardiogram was normal. Electrocardiogram showed prolonged QTc interval.

The past medical history was notable. She was the first-born child of third-degree consanguineous parents. She had a smooth perinatal transition with normal birth weight (3 kg) and length (50 cm). There was normal postnatal growth period with age-appropriate developmental milestones. At 3 months of age, she presented with two episodes of multifocal clonic seizures to another hospital. There was no evidence of hypoglycemia. Meningitis was ruled out by cerebrospinal fluid analysis. However, her serum calcium (5.3 mg/dL) was low, and serum phosphorus (12.2 mg/dL) was high similar to the current episode. She had not been evaluated with urine calcium levels or kidney USG at that time. The blood urea (22 mg/dL), serum creatinine (0.12 mg/dL), magnesium (2.6 mg/dL), sodium (136 mmol/L), potassium (4.8 mmol/L), serum albumin (4.2 g/dL), uric acid (2.8 mg/dL), and alkaline phosphatase (276 U/L) were normal. Ultrasonogram of the cranium did not show any abnormality. Serum 25 (OH) vitamin D level was normal (reference: 24.3 ng/mL), and iPTH level was less than 2.5 pg/mL (reference: 15 to 30 pg/mL). She had been treated with intravenous calcium gluconate at that time for 2 days. There were no further episodes of seizures, and she was discharged from the hospital with oral calcium carbonate and calcitriol supplements. However, she was on irregular follow-up. On probing, it was revealed that she had recurrent episodes of tetany requiring intravenous calcium administration at another institution.

During the current admission at our hospital, the child was managed with intravenous calcium gluconate for 48 hours. Oral calcium carbonate and oral calcitriol doses were titrated to achieve near normal serum calcium levels. Therapy with oral hydrochlorothiazide and potassium citrate was initiated in view of hypercalciuria and nephrocalcinosis. Sevelamer was prescribed for hyperphosphatemia, which led to a decrease in serum phosphorus levels. A targeted genetic analysis by clinical exome sequencing was performed.

What is the MOST likely diagnosis and how would you treat it?

    A. Pseudohypoparathyroidism
    B. Familial isolated hypoparathyroidism (FIH)
    C. DiGeorge syndrome
    D. CHARGE syndrome

The correct answer is B
Comment: This child presented with recurrent episodes of tetany and seizures, in association with grade 3 nephrocalcinosis, who was confirmed to have hypoparathyroidism due to heterozygous

missense variation in the *GCM2* gene (autosomal dominant inheritance). Nephrocalcinosis can complicate hypoparathyroidism in a significant proportion of cases.

The differential diagnoses for hypocalcemia with nephrocalcinosis are familial isolated hypoparathyroidism (FIH), syndromic hypoparathyroidism, calcium-sensing receptor (CaSR)-activating mutations (sporadic and autosomal dominant), pseudohypoparathyroidism (insensitivity to PTH), and acquired causes of hypoparathyroidism (HPT). Familial hypoparathyroidism has autosomal recessive (*GCM2*, *PTH* gene mutations), autosomal dominant (*CaSR* gene mutation and some cases of *GCM2* mutations), or X-linked (*SOX3* gene mutation) inheritance.[1-3] DiGeorge syndrome type 1 and type 2, CHARGE syndrome, autoimmune polyendocrine syndrome type 1, Kenny-Caffey syndrome type 1 and type 2, Sanjad-Sakati syndrome, Barakat syndrome, Kearns-Sayre syndrome, MELAS syndrome, mitochondrial trifunctional protein deficiency syndrome, Gracile bone dysplasia, and Pearson syndrome are the syndromic causes of hypoparathyroidism. Activating mutations of the *CaSR* gene cause autosomal dominant hypocalcemia type 1. Pseudohypoparathyroidism is caused by insensitivity to the PTH hormone due to mutations in genes *PTHR1*, *GNAS*, *PRKAR1A*, and hypomagnesemia.[1] The acquired causes of hypoparathyroidism include activating antibodies to the *CasR*, maternal hyperparathyroidism, post-surgical and radiation-induced damage to the parathyroid glands, deposition of iron or copper (thalassemia, hemochromatosis, Wilson disease), or infiltration (neoplastic invasion, sarcoidosis, amyloidosis).

Our patient had tetany, convulsions with hypocalcemia, hyperphosphatemia, low serum PTH, nephrocalcinosis, and calcifications in basal ganglia and frontal lobes. Hence, a provisional diagnosis of hypoparathyroidism was considered. Syndromic and acquired causes of hypoparathyroidism were considered unlikely, as there were no features or history suggestive of the same. Pseudohypoparathyroidism was ruled out, as serum PTH was low. A targeted genetic analysis by clinical exome sequencing was performed in our case which revealed a heterozygous missense variation *c.1151C > T* in exon 5 of the *GCM2* gene *(Chr 6: 10874598G > A)*, confirming the diagnosis of familial isolated hypoparathyroidism-type 2 (autosomal dominant inheritance).

Management of such cases includes evaluation, treatment of acute hypocalcemia, and long-term follow-up. The index case presented with seizures to our pediatric emergency unit. At admission, there were no features suggestive of meningitis, and the blood glucose was normal. The index case had hypocalcemia, hyperphosphatemia with low PTH levels, and normal serum creatinine, confirming hypoparathyroidism. Another condition with similar clinical manifestations (tetany, seizures), hypocalcemia, hyperphosphatemia, and ectopic calcifications in brain and kidneys is pseudohypoparathyroidism. However, specific clinical features (short stature, obesity, rounded face, and brachydactyly mostly affecting the 4th and 5th metacarpals and metatarsals in Albright hereditary osteodystrophy) and high serum PTH levels in pseudohypoparathyroidism differentiate it from hypoparathyroidism.

Hypoparathyroidism is associated with ectopic calcifications. Hence, screening for calcifications in the kidney and brain is recommended. This includes urinary calcium/creatinine ratio and renal ultrasonogram to look for nephrocalcinosis and computed tomography (CT) of cranium for basal ganglia and intracerebral calcifications. Ophthalmological evaluation for posterior subcapsular cataract should be done which can occur due to elevated calcium-phosphorus products accumulating in the lens of the eyes.[2,3] Our index case had elevated urinary calcium/creatinine ratio (0.42) and grade 3 nephrocalcinosis with bilateral symmetrical calcification in basal ganglia and frontal lobes.

Treatment of acute hypocalcemia aims at control of seizures and correction of hypocalcemia to prevent further seizures. Intravenous calcium gluconate (elemental calcium 9.3 mg/mL) 1 to 2 mL/kg (total dose should not exceed 10 mL) diluted with an equal amount of dextrose should be given slowly at the rate of 0.5 to 1 mL/min under strict cardiac monitoring, followed by infusion of the same solution every 4 to 6 hours until calcium is normalized. Long-term goals in the management of hypoparathyroidism are to achieve a near normal range of serum calcium (8 to 9 mg/dL) to prevent seizures and tetany and decrease calcium–phosphate products to prevent ectopic calcifications. Targeting higher serum calcium levels and overzealous treatment with oral calcium and calcitriol should be avoided which can result in hypercalciuria and nephrocalcinosis leading to renal impairment or chronic kidney disease in some cases. To achieve this, oral calcium (calcium carbonate or calcium citrate) and active form of vitamin D3 (calcitriol) or vitamin D2 should be supplemented. Severe hyperphosphatemia needs to be treated with phosphate binders such as sevelamer. Thiazide diuretics (hydrochlorothiazide) effectively reduce urinary calcium excretion and are often used in cases where normocalcemia (lower normal) is not achieved with adequate calcium and calcitriol doses; they are also used in cases with nephrocalcinosis. On follow-up, serum calcium and phosphate levels, 6-monthly urinary calcium/creatinine ratio, and renal ultrasonogram (for nephrocalcinosis) should be done to titrate the doses of oral calcium and calcitriol supplementations. The newer treatment regimens for hypoparathyroidism are teriparatide and recombinant human PTH. Recent trials with teriparatide (recombinant human PTH1-34 [rhPTH1-34]) in children with hypoparathyroidism showed promising results with a decrease in the requirement of oral calcium and calcitriol supplementation, steady serum calcium concentration, and decrease in urinary calcium excretion. Our patient responded well to calcitriol and calcium supplements, along with hydrochlorothiazide and sevelamer, resulting in an increase in serum calcium levels and decrease in serum phosphorus levels on follow-up. Therefore, teriparatide was not prescribed.

Case Study 3

The patient was a 12-year-old girl, who had been born after 36 weeks of gestation by cesarean section after an uneventful pregnancy with birth weight of 2450 g, height of 47 cm, and head circumference of 37 cm. She was the first-born infant of healthy parents (24-year-old mother and 28-year-old father); however, the patient was consanguineous as the parents were second-degree cousins.

The patient was first brought to another center with afebrile seizures at the age of 5 months. During investigation of the cause of the seizures, her serum calcium level was found to be 6.8 mg/dL. Two doses of oral vitamin D injection and oral calcium lactate were given to treat the hypocalcemia. However, oral calcium lactate treatment was ineffective, and she had two more afebrile seizures by the age of 8 months. In addition to hypocalcemic seizures, there was a history of recurrent febrile urinary tract infections up to the age of 1 year.

The patient was admitted to the hospital with a diagnosis of acute pyelonephritis at the age of 14 months. The patient's height was 66 cm (< 3rd percentile), weight was 6700 g (3rd to 10th percentile), and head circumference was 42.5 cm (< 3rd percentile) at admission. The patient was first able to hold her head up at 6 months and was able to sit without support at the age of 1 year. The patient could not walk at admission. She had a syndromic facial appearance characterized by trigonocephaly with square head, hypertrophy of the right cheek, broad forehead, hypertelorism, low nasal bridge, micrognathia, and underdeveloped and low-set ears.

The patient had hypernatremic dehydration. Laboratory investigations revealed a hemoglobin level of 8.6 g/dL, mean erythrocyte corpuscular volume of 84 fL, total leukocyte count of 12 × 10^9/L, platelet count of 299 × 10^9/L, urine density of 1025, pH 6, and abundant leukocytes in urine sediment examination. The results of serum analysis were as follows: blood urea nitrogen (BUN), 85 mg/dL; creatinine, 1.3 mg/dL; sodium, 153 mmol/L; potassium, 4.6 mmol/L; albumin, 4.8 g/dL; alkaline phosphatase, 206 U/L; calcium, 8.3 mg/dL; phosphorus, 7.2 mg/dL; magnesium, 2 mg/dL; 25-hydroxy vitamin D, 36 ng/mL; C-reactive protein, 46 mg/L; parathyroid hormone (PTH), 10.5 pg/mL (reference: 15 to 65 pg/mL); and spot urine calcium/creatinine ratio, 0.33. On blood gas analysis, pH was 7.30 and bicarbonate level was 13.5 mEq/L. The patient was treated with appropriate antibiotic therapy and intravenous hydration. Ultrasonography revealed dilation in the left proximal ureter, hydronephrosis in the left kidney, and right renal hypoplasia. Voiding cystourethrography (VCUG) showed left-grade IV vesicoureteral reflux (VUR). Dimercaptosuccinic acid scan showed absence of right kidney activity and multiple scars in the left kidney.

In post-discharge follow-up, serum analysis showed an average urea level of 62 mg/dL, creatinine level of 1.2 mg/dL, metabolic acidosis, anemia (mean 8.5 g/dL), hypocalcemia (mean 8.5 mg/dL), and hyperphosphatemia (mean 6.9 mg/dL). Therefore, calcium acetate, Shohl solution, calcitriol, and erythropoietin treatments were started with the diagnosis of chronic kidney disease. Despite the presence of hypocalcemia and hyperphosphatemia, the mean serum PTH level was 11.7 pg/mL (range: 5.7 to 13 pg/mL).

Two STING (subureteral transurethral injection) procedures for VUR were performed at the age of 2 years, and ureteroneocystostomy was performed at the age of 4 years, and VUR was not detected in repeated VCUG.

Bilateral sensorineural hearing loss requiring cochlear implantation was diagnosed at 3 years. Auditory brainstem response testing revealed that the patient had moderate sensorineural deafness, with hearing loss of 70 dB at mid and higher frequencies in both ears.

Hypomagnesemia (1.4 mg/dL) began to develop at 5 years. The patient showed increased fractional excretion of magnesium (11%; N: < 2%), and, therefore, oral magnesium supplementation was started.

The father, mother, and brother were healthy and had no kidney or auditory problems; their serum magnesium, calcium, and phosphorus levels were normal.

What is the MOST likely diagnosis?

A. Barakat syndrome
B. Hypoparathyroidism
C. Pseudohypoparathyroidism
D. Renal osteodystrophy

The correct answer is A

Comment: The patient was diagnosed with Barakat syndrome due to the triad of the presence of hypoparathyroidism, deafness, and renal anomalies (HDR).[1] Barakat syndrome is characterized by mutations or deletions in the *GATA3* gene.[2] The serum PTH levels did not increase despite chronic kidney disease due to hypoparathyroidism. As in this case, hypomagnesemia along with hypermagnesuria have been reported in patients with HDR syndrome, but no relationship has been demonstrated between the *GATA3* gene and hypomagnesemia.

In a chromosomal karyotype study (GTG-banding analysis) performed because of the syndromic facial appearance, de novo 46 XX, deletion (p13–14) was detected. The GATA binding protein 3 (*GATA3*) gene is located at 10p14, and our patient had a deletion in this region. Treatment of HDR syndrome is symptomatic. The condition that most requires treatment is hypocalcemia. Depending on the severity of hypocalcemia, oral calcium or calcitriol is given, with severe cases receiving intravenous calcium gluconate. Deafness can be detected at an early stage in routine newborn screening programs, which is important for language and educational development.

The prognosis of the disease is generally related to the severity of the kidney disease. When chronic kidney disease develops, it should be detected in the early stages and should be prevented from progressing to stage 5, kidney failure, although successful kidney transplantation has been reported in this syndrome.

Case Study 4

You are asked to see a 7-year-old boy because of hypokalemia during a hospitalization for the evaluation of a recent seizure disorder, which occurred 3 days ago. Phenytoin has been given for his seizure. Past medical history is significant for chronic kidney disease of unknown etiology. He has been taking sevelamer hydrochloride for the control of mild hyperphosphatemia, and he has received no vitamin D products. Shortly after admission, he undergoes a magnetic resonance imaging scan of the brain with gadolinium contrast that shows signs of a small, healed, left-sided cerebral infarct. The patient feels well. His vital signs are BP 110/70 mmHg, pulse 80 beats/min, respirations 15 breaths/min, temperature 37°C. The remainder of physical examination is unremarkable and includes the absence of Chvostek and Trousseau signs. His laboratory data include the following: calcium 5.8 mg/dL, phosphate 4.1 mg/dL, albumin 3.8 g/dL, sodium 139 mmol/L, potassium 4.2 mmol/L, chloride 105 mmol/L, bicarbonate 22 mmol/L, BUN 33 mg/dL, and creatinine 1.3 mg/dL.

Which ONE of the following is the MOST likely cause of hypocalcemia in this patient?

 A. Hypoparathyroidism
 B. Gadolinium-induced pseudohypocalcemia
 C. Hypomagnesemia
 D. Vitamin D deficiency
 E. Sevelamer administration

The correct answer is B
Comment: Macrocyclic gadolinium complexes used in MR scanning are known to interfere with the colorimetric determination of calcium by binding with the test reagents.[1] Patients with renal insufficiency can have spuriously low serum calcium.

Case Study 5

You are called for a curbside consult about a 3-year-old child who has developed growth failure, muscle weakness, and bone pain. Radiographic studies indicate the presence of rickets, including bowed legs, thick fuzzy growth plates, and widened knee joints. Laboratory data reveal serum sodium 140 mmol/L, potassium 3.9 mmol/L, chloride 104 mmol/L, bicarbonate 29 mmol/L, BUN 12 mg/dL, creatinine 0.4 mg/dL, calcium 8.1 mg/dL, phosphate 2.5 mg/dL, magnesium 1.9 mg/dL, albumin 3.9 g/dL, PTH 87 pg/mL, calcidiol 45 ng/mL, calcitriol 98 pg/mL, hemoglobin 14.0 g/dL, and white blood count 5600 cell/µL. Urinalysis was normal.

What is the correct diagnosis?

 A. Pseudo-vitamin D-deficient rickets (1-alpha hydroxylase deficiency, vitamin D-dependent rickets type 1)
 B. Vitamin D deficiency
 C. Hypoparathyroidism
 D. Pseudohypoparathyroidism
 E. Hereditary vitamin D-resistant rickets (HVDRR)

The correct answer is E
Comment: Hereditary resistance to vitamin D is an autosomal recessive disorder. It is associated with end-organ resistance to calcitriol usually caused by mutations in the gene encoding the vitamin D receptor; the defect in the receptor interferes with binding of the hormone-receptor complex to DNA, thereby preventing calcitriol action and leading to hypocalcemia and secondary hyperparathyroidism.[1]

Case Study 6

A 2-year-old North African boy was brought to our hospital because of absent teeth development and failure to walk. The patient appeared to be well nourished and content. His body mass index was 19.1 kg/m (90th percentile), he was 86 cm long (25th percentile), and he weighed 13.6 kg (75th percentile). Palpation of the patient's extremities revealed prominent, flared distal radii, humeral and femurs. The result of a total serum calcium test was 1.4 mmol/L (normal 2.1 to 2.6).

What is the MOST likely diagnosis?

    A. Hyperparathyroidism
    B. Hypoparathyroidism
    C. Vitamin D-deficiency rickets
    D. X-linked hypophosphatemia rickets

The correct answer is C
Comment: This patient was found to have low serum calcium, phosphate, and 25-hydroxyvitamin D, as well as high levels of parathyroid hormone.

    A combination of factors, including the patient's low milk intake and the results of his physical examination, raised the likelihood of vitamin D-deficiency rickets.[1-3] The results of laboratory tests confirmed this diagnosis.

Case Study 7

A 6-year-old boy presented with hard, nodular skin lesions on his torso. The patient was short (< 3rd percentile), and he had mild developmental delays and obesity. Because a skin biopsy demonstrated subcutaneous calcification, his total serum calcium level was measured and found to be 7.6 mg/dL.

What is the MOST likely diagnosis? (Select all that apply)

    A. Pseudohypothyroidism
    B. Hypoparathyroidism
    C. Vitamin D efficiency rickets
    D. Albright hereditary osteodystrophy

The correct answers are B and D
Comment: This patient had high levels of phosphate and very high levels of parathyroid hormone. Test results also revealed normal 25-hydroxyvitamin D levels and a high ratio of calcium to creatinine in his urine.

    A laboratory profile that is consistent with hypoparathyroidism except for a high level of parathyroid hormone supports a diagnosis of pseudohypoparathyroidism.[1-4] This patient also had a short stature, obesity, a round face and brachydactyly of his fourth and fifth fingers. These are all features of Albright hereditary osteodystrophy, a disorder in which a maternally inherited mutated copy of the *GNAS1* gene leads to parathyroid-hormone resistance.[1-3]

Case Study 8

A 12-year-old boy presented with concerns about intermittent numbness of his extremities. He reported having had one episode where he "lost control" of his right leg and fell. A computed tomography (CT) scan showed calcification of the basal ganglia. His total serum calcium level was 7.1 mg/dL.

What is the MOST likely diagnosis?

A. Vitamin D deficiency rickets
B. Hypoparathyroidism
C. X-linked hypophosphatemia rickets
D. Pseudohypoparathyroidism

The correct answer is B
Comment: This patient had high levels of phosphate but normal levels of magnesium and parathyroid hormone. The results of laboratory investigations supported a diagnosis of hypoparathyroidism. A subsequent genetic workup identified a rare activating mutation of the calcium receptor. This mutation causes the receptor to inappropriately sense low calcium levels as being normal.[1-5]

Hypocalcemia in children may be asymptomatic or there may be a wide range of signs and symptoms such as laryngospasm, tetany, muscle cramps, seizures, paresthesia, numbness, Chvostek sign, Trousseau sign, and prolonged QTc intervals (> 450 ms). Because very young patients cannot accurately verbalize symptoms, they are more likely to present with signs such as weakness, feeding problems, facial spasms, jitteriness, or seizures. In addition, features of conditions known to be associated with hypocalcemia may be identified, including growth failure, developmental delay, lymphadenopathy, hepatosplenomegaly, bone abnormality, and facial deformity.

There are multiple causes of hypocalcemia in children; thus, diagnosis must follow a systematic approach.

Since pediatric hypocalcemia can represent the first manifestation of a genetic disorder, a definitive diagnosis may eventually require further testing at a specialized center.

Under normal circumstances, calcium homeostasis maintains total calcium levels within the narrow range of 2.1 to 2.6 mmol/L (ionized calcium 1.0 to 1.3 mmol/L). The first step in maintaining a healthy calcium balance is adequate dietary intake of calcium. Normal intake of breast milk or infant formula supplies age-appropriate amounts of calcium. Older children require a balanced diet that provides 500 mg (children aged 1 to 3 years), 800 mg (4 to 8 years), or 1300 mg (> 8 years) of calcium daily. One cup of milk contains about 300 mg of calcium.

Calcium homeostasis depends on multiple interacting organ systems. The parathyroid glands sense hypocalcemia via membrane-bound receptors and rapidly generate parathyroid hormone. (Release of parathyroid hormone requires adequate magnesium levels.) Once released, the hormone promotes a shift from net bone formation to calcium-liberating bone resorption. In the kidneys, parathyroid hormone up regulates retention of urinary calcium and enhances renal activation of potent 1,25-dihydroxy vitamin D, whose major role is to increase intestinal calcium absorption. Formation of 1,25-dihydroxy vitamin D requires adequate amounts of precursor vitamin D from diet or exposure to UV light. Finally, normalization of calcium feeds back to inhibit parathyroid hormone secretion.

Case Study 9

A 15-year-old man that showed symptoms and signs of severe and prolonged hypocalcemia due to unrecognized vitamin D deficiency. He presented at the emergency room reporting abdominal pain and vomiting since the evening before. Blood tests showed increased levels of rhabdomyolysis markers, severe hypocalcemia, hypophosphatemia, hypomagnesemia, normal renal function, elevated levels of alkaline phosphatase, extremely high levels of parathyroid hormone, and hypovitaminosis D. Radiological skeletal features of bone demineralization and bone abnormalities suggestive of osteomalacia were additionally detected. Other secondary causes of hypocalcemia were excluded. Clinical and biochemical resolution were progressively obtained only after an intramuscular loading dose of cholecalciferol was added to the standard calcium intravenous replacement therapy.

How would you treat this patient's severe hypocalcemia?

A. Intramuscular loading dose of cholecalciferol

B. Intravenous calcium replacement therapy

C. Combination of vitamin D and calcium administration

D. None of the above

The correct answer is C

Comment: This case report shows that osteomalacia consequent to a severe vitamin D deficiency can present with acute symptoms and signs of severe hypocalcemia requiring hospital admission. In such cases, vitamin D administration, and not intensive calcium supplementation alone, is essential to achieve clinical resolution of symptoms and normalization of mineral metabolism parameters.[1-4]

Case Study 10

A 19-year-old female was hospitalized to the intensive care unit for the management of severe preeclampsia during her 17th week of gestation. Her past medical history was unremarkable. She presented with symptoms of headache, palpitations, abdominal pain, nausea, and vomiting of 1 week duration. Upon initial evaluation, she was noted to have severe hypertension, BP 173/114 mmHg. The rest of the vital signs were pulse 98 beats/min, temperature 36.5°C, and oxygen saturation of 99% in room air. Physical examination revealed mild, diffuse abdominal tenderness to palpation and mild, symmetric peripheral edema. The remainder of the systemic examination was normal. Laboratory investigations were significant for marked proteinuria, bland urine sediment examination, and mild elevation of hepatic enzymes, elevated serum uric acid, and a normal renal function. Her admission blood gas showed a nonanion gap metabolic acidosis with mild respiratory alkalosis (pH: 7.37, bicarbonate: 15 mmol/L, PCO_2: 27 mmHg and PO_2: 106 mmHg, anion gap: 8 mmol/L).

An obstetric ultrasound was done revealing holoprosencephaly, enlarged anterior placenta with extremely elevated βHCG levels (2,285,500 mIU/mL), suggesting partial molar pregnancy.

A diagnosis of early severe preeclampsia was made and the patient was managed with antihypertensive therapy; she was given three doses of intravenous (IV) hydralazine (total 25 mg), one dose of IV Labetalol 20 mg, and then was started on nicardipine infusion with a mean arterial pressure goal of 120 mmHg. She was also given multiple doses of furosemide to manage her volume status. One dose of sodium polystyrene sulfonate (Kayexalate) suspension (15 g) was given to manage her mild hyperkalemia. Infusion of magnesium sulfate in Lactate Ringer (40 g/500 mL) was started at a rate of 25 mL/h for seizure prophylaxis; the infusion was continued for the first 3 days of hospitalization with close neurologic and electrolytes monitoring. An urgent delivery of the fetus was indicated due to severe preeclampsia and fetal ultrasound findings incompatible with life, so a cesarean section was performed as per patient's preference. Chromosomal examination of the fetal tissue led to a diagnosis of fetal triploid.

After delivery, the patient's blood pressure started to improve gradually over the following few days. However, she was noted to have significant changes in serum calcium (6.5 mg/dL) and potassium (5.7 mEq/L) levels during that period, corresponding to high serum magnesium levels.

Work up for etiology of hyperkalemia included plasma aldosterone concentration (PAC) (19.2 ng/dL), plasma renin activity (PRA) (9.6 ng/mL/h), and a trans-tubular potassium gradient (TTKG) of 4.6. There was no evidence of hemolysis, acute decline in renal function, or administration of medications known to affect serum potassium levels such as NSAIDs, beta blockers, heparin, etc. Additionally, the patient was tested negative for HIV, hepatitis serology, and serum antinuclear antibodies (ANA). Also, her serum thyroid stimulating hormone (TSH) level was normal.

What is the etiology of hypocalcemia and hyperkalemia in this patient?

A. Hypermagnesemia-induced hyperkalemia

B. Pseudohypocalcemia

C. Hypoparathyroidism

D. Vitamin D deficiency

The correct answer is A

Comment: Iatrogenic hypermagnesemia should be considered in the differential diagnoses of hypocalcemia and hyperkalemia whenever magnesium infusions are used, especially for obstetric indications. Stopping the magnesium infusion will likely reverse the electrolyte changes, if the renal function is intact, but sometimes temporary stabilizing measures for management of hypocalcemia and hyperkalemia may be required.

After excluding other causes of hyperkalemia, a diagnosis of hypermagnesemia-induced hyperkalemia was made.[1-3] The serum potassium level started to decline after the discontinuation of magnesium infusion on day 3 of hospitalization. Patient was noted to have slight hypokalemia after normalization of serum magnesium levels, which was attributed to administration of IV furosemide (utilized for management of volume overload and hypertension). The calcium level started to decline, corresponding to increasing magnesium levels. Serum parathyroid hormone (PTH) was obtained and was 86 pg/mL (normal). Serum calcium normalized after normalization of serum magnesium levels.

References

Case Study 1

1. Engel FL, Martin SP, Taylor H. On the relation of potassium to the neurological manifestations of hypocalcemic tetany. *Bull Johns Hopkins Hosp.* 1949;84:295.
2. Assadi F. *Clinical Decisions in Pediatric Nephrology: A Problem Solving Approach to Clinical Cases.* New York: Springer; 2008. [chap 2, 69–98].

Case Study 2

1. Mannstadt M, Bilezikian JP, Thakker RV, et al. Hypoparathyroidism. *Nat Rev Dis Primers.* 2017;3:17055.
2. Bilezikian JP, Brandi ML, Cusano NE, et al. Management of hypoparathyroidism: present and future. *J Clin Endocrinol Metab.* 2016;101:2313–2324.
3. Mantovani G, Bastepe M, Monk D, et al. Diagnosis and management of pseudohypoparathyroidism and related disorders: first international consensus statement. *Nat Rev Endocrinol.* 2018;14:476–500.

Case Study 3

1. Barakat AJ, Raygada M, Rennert OM. Barakat syndrome revisited. *Am J Med Genet.* 2018;176:1341–1348.
2. Muroya K, Hasegawa T, Ito Y, et al. GATA3 abnormalities and the phenotypic spectrum of HDR syndrome. *J Med Genet.* 2001;38:374–380.

Case Study 4

1. Prince MR, Erel HE, Lent RW, et al. Gadodiamide administration causes spurious hypocalcemia. *Radiology.* 2003;227:639–646.

Case Study 5

1. Malloy PJ, Pike JW, Feldman D. The vitamin D receptor and the syndrome of hereditary 1,25-dihydroxyvitamin D-resistant rickets. *Endocrine Rev.* 1999;20:156–188.

Case Study 6

1. Kruse K. Vitamin D and parathyroid. In: Ranke MB, ed. *Diagnostics of Endocrine Function in Children and Adolescents.* 3rd ed. Basel, Switzerland: Karger; 2003:240.
2. Primary vitamin D deficiency in children. *Drug Ther Bull.* 2006;44:12–16. https://doi.org/10.1136/dtb.2006.44212.
3. Health Canada. Food and nutrition. In: *Dietary Reference Intakes: Reference Values for Elements.* Health Canada: Ottawa; 2005. www.hc-sc.gc.ca/fn-an/nutrition/reference/table/ref_elements_tbl_e.html. Accessed October 15, 2021.

Case Study 7

1. Kruse K. Vitamin D and parathyroid. In: Ranke MB, ed. *Diagnostics of Endocrine Function in Children and Adolescents.* 3rd ed. Basel, Switzerland: Karger; 2003:240.
2. Diamond FB Jr, Root AW. Pediatric endocrinology. In: Sperling MA, ed. *Pediatric Endocrinology.* 2nd ed. Philadelphia: Saunders; 2002:97.
3. Primary vitamin D deficiency in children. *Drug Ther Bull.* 2006;44:12–16. https://doi.org/10.1136/dtb.2006.44212.
4. Health Canada. Food and nutrition. In: *Dietary Reference Intakes: Reference Values for Elements.* Health Canada: Ottawa; 2005. www.hc-sc.gc.ca/fn-an/nutrition/reference/table/ref_elements_tbl_e.html. Accessed October 15, 2021.

Case Study 8

1. Kruse K. Vitamin D and parathyroid. In: Ranke MB, ed. *Diagnostics of Endocrine Function in Children and Adolescents.* 3rd ed. Basel, Switzerland: Karger; 2003:240.
2. Diamond Jr FB, Root AW. Pediatric endocrinology. In: Sperling MA, ed. *Pediatric Endocrinology.* 2nd ed. Philadelphia: Saunders; 2002:97.
3. Primary vitamin D deficiency in children. *Drug Ther Bull.* 2006;44:12–16. https://doi.org/10.1136/dtb.2006.44212.
4. Health Canada. Food and nutrition. In: *Dietary Reference Intakes: Reference Values for Elements.* Health Canada: Ottawa; 2005. www.hc-sc.gc.ca/fn-an/nutrition/reference/table/ref_elements_tbl_e.html. Accessed October 15, 2007.
5. Spiegel AM. The parathryoid glands, hypercalcemia and hypocalcemia. In: Goldman L, Ausiello D, eds. *Cecil Texbook of Medicine.* 22nd ed. Philadelphia: W.B. Saunders; 2004.

Case Study 9

1. Bhan A, Rao AD, Rao DS. Osteomalacia as a result of vitamin D deficiency. *Endocrinol Metab Clin North Am.* 2010;39:321–331.
2. Reuss-Borst MA. Metabolic bone disease osteomalacia [in German]. *Z Rheumatol.* 2014;73:316–322.
3. Reginato AJ, Coquia JA. Musculoskeletal manifestations of osteomalacia and rickets. *Best Pract Res Clin Rheumatol.* 2003;17:1063–1080.
4. Diamond TH, Ho KW, Rohl PG, et al. Annual intramuscular injection of a megadose of cholecalciferol for treatment of vitamin D deficiency: efficacy and safety data. *Med J Aust.* 2005;183:10–12.

Case Study 10

1. Iglesias M-H, Giesbrecht EM, von Dadelszen P, et al. Postpartum hyperkalemia associated with magnesium sulfate. *Hypertens Pregnancy.* 2011;30:481–484.
2. Nassar AH, Salti I, Makarem NN, et al. Marked hypocalcemia after tocolytic magnesium sulphate therapy. *Am J Perinatol.* 2007;24:481–482.
3. Cholst IN, Steinberg SF, Tropper PJ, et al. The influence of hypermagnesemia on serum calcium and parathyroid hormone levels in human subjects. *N Engl J Med.* 1984;310:1221–1225.

CHAPTER 8

Hypercalcemia

Case Study 1

A 19-year-old male was admitted to a local hospital with lethargy. His medical history was most notable for major depressive disorder complicated by two previous suicide attempts, and poorly controlled insulin-dependent diabetes mellitus. On arrival to the emergency department, he was afebrile and hemodynamically stable and had a respiratory rate of 18 breaths/min. On examination, he was lethargic and oriented to self-only and had dry mucous membranes. Routine laboratory tests showed sodium of 144 mmol/L, potassium 3.8 mmol/L, chloride 98 mmol/L, bicarbonate 34 mmol/L, blood urea nitrogen (BUN) 24 mg/dL, creatinine 1.2 mg/dL, glucose 231 mg/dL, calcium (corrected) 13.4 mg/dL, magnesium 0.9 mg/dL, phosphorous 3.6 mg/dL, and albumin 3.5 g/dL. Urine toxicology screen and serum overdose panel results were negative; findings from computed tomography (CT) of the head were unremarkable.

What is the MOST likely cause of this patient's lethargy and what studies should be undertaken to evaluate further his condition?

A. Hyperparathyroidism
B. Sarcoidosis
C. Multiple myeloma
D. Calcium-alkali syndrome

The correct answer is D

Comment: In this patient, there are several life-threatening diagnoses that should be excluded, including a drug overdose, hypoglycemia, diabetic ketoacidosis, seizure, and head trauma. With a preliminary evaluation that is completely negative for these conditions, hyperkalemia is the likely cause.

Serum calcium level is regulated by parathyroid hormone (PTH), which senses serum calcium level through calcium-sensing receptors. PTH regulates serum calcium level through vitamin D-mediated calcium absorption by the gut, calcium resorption from bone, and calcium absorption by the kidney. The first diagnostic step therefore is to check serum PTH level. If PTH level is elevated, primary hyperparathyroidism (PHP) is likely. If PTH level is low/low normal, hypercalcemia could be due to PTH-related peptide (PTHrp) or vitamin D metabolites. Hypercalcemia due to PTHrp occurs in advanced malignancy, often with widespread metastasis. Therefore, measurement of PTHrp in the absence of clear malignancy should only be done when other causes of hypercalcemia have been ruled out. Granulomatous diseases will typically cause an elevation in 1,25-dihydroxyvitamin D level, whereas vitamin D intoxication presents with elevated 25-hydroxyvitamin D level. PTH-dependent hypercalcemia may be associated with mild hyperchloremic metabolic acidosis, while hypercalcemia due to vitamin D metabolites or excess calcium intake may be associated with mild metabolic alkalosis. If vitamin D metabolite and PTH levels are normal, hypercalcemia due to multiple myeloma should be ruled out. In patients with a personal and familial history of benign hypercalcemia, familial hypocalciuric hypercalcemia (FHH) should be considered. This patient had no family or personal history of hypercalcemia. Rarely, familial hypercalcemia may be caused by a defect in the conversion of 1,25-dihydroxyvitamin D to inactive forms. Finally, other causes such as milk-alkali syndrome should be considered.[1-5]

The patient presented with hypercalcemia (calcium, 13.4 mg/dL), acute kidney injury (AKI; creatinine of 1.3 mg/dL), and metabolic alkalosis (total carbon dioxide of 34 mmol/L). Initial laboratory test results supported a diagnosis of milk-alkali syndrome. Further history revealed that he was ingesting at least one bottle of Tums (calcium carbonate) daily.

In the gut, both a transcellular and a paracellular pathway absorb calcium. Calcium will be poorly absorbed in the intestine if it forms insoluble salts or there is insufficient activated vitamin D, but very large calcium loads may be absorbed even in the absence of vitamin D through the paracellular pathway. Decades ago, the syndrome was seen in patients receiving high doses of sodium bicarbonate and calcinated-magnesia (Sippy Powder) for peptic ulcer disease, but now is often secondary to excessive self-administration of calcium and vitamin D. These supplements are widely used to treat osteoporosis. A more accurate term, as suggested, is calcium-alkali syndrome. Because calcium carbonate is often the trigger for calcium-alkali syndrome, serum phosphorus levels are usually normal, in contrast to classic milk-alkali syndrome, which is associated with hyperphosphatemia. Calcium-alkali syndrome is now the third most common cause of admission for hypercalcemia. The acuity of the patient's presentation may be because hypercalcemia creates a vicious cycle resulting in renal retention of calcium. Calcium causes vasoconstriction in vascular beds, including the kidney, resulting in a decrease in the filtered load of calcium. In addition, hypercalcemia inhibits the sodium/potassium/chloride ($Na^+/K^+/2Cl^-$) cotransporter and aquaporin expression, leading to further volume depletion, AKI, and increased calcium absorption in the proximal and distal nephron. Last, ingestion of alkali leads to production of alkaline urine, which further promotes calcium reabsorption.

To summarize, excessive ingestion of calcium carbonate by the patient resulted in hypercalcemia, AKI, and metabolic alkalosis, a triad that is the hallmark of calcium-alkali syndrome.[1-5]

Case Study 2

You are asked to see a 17-year-old female college student in the emergency room with hypercalcemia and kidney failure. She notes the onset of mild polyuria and nocturia 6 to 8 months earlier. Headache, constipation, and malaise became apparent approximately 6 weeks earlier. She began using a tanning salon 4 weeks before. A day earlier, she visited her mother who noted that she was "not herself" and seemed confused. Past medical history is significant for passing a single kidney calculus 2 years before. She has a 1-year history of mild hypertension for which she was treated with hydrochlorothiazide, 50 mg/day. She does not smoke or drink alcohol. She denies the use of any other medications or over-the-counter supplements. She denies any hormonal therapy and avoids all dairy products. On examination, she appears in no acute distress. Blood pressure is 140/92 mmHg; pulse, 86 beats/min; respiratory rate, 12 breaths/min; body temperature, 37°C; body weight, 62.5 kg; and height, 159 cm. Heart rate is regular with no murmurs, the lungs are clear, the abdomen is soft with no masses, and there is no pitting edema. Neurological examination shows mild depression and some cognitive dysfunction.

Laboratory studies show the following: hematocrit, 46%; leukocyte count, 5.6×10^9/L; BUN, 61 mg/dL; serum creatinine, 3.0 mg/dL; serum sodium, 140 mmol/L; serum potassium, 3.9 mmol/L; serum chloride, 101 mmol/L; serum bicarbonate, 22 mmol/L; serum calcium, 13.8 mg/dL; serum phosphate, 3.9 mg/dL; serum magnesium, 1.9 mg/dL; and serum albumin, 4.2 g/dL. Urinalysis shows trace protein, no glucose, no blood, 2 to 4 hyaline casts per high-power field (HPF), but no erythrocytes or leukocytes.

Which of the following treatment modalities would you like to order now? (Select all that apply)

A. Calcitonin
B. Intravenous saline solution
C. Surgical consult
D. Mithramycin
E. Pamidronate/zoledronate

The correct answer is B
Comment: The initial treatment of symptomatic hypercalcemia should have three elements to provide some efficacy, both initially and several days later. Virtually all patients with significant hypercalcemia have some element of extracellular fluid volume contraction. For this reason, it is important to start therapy with intravenous saline. Calcitonin is effective in approximately 70% of patients. It is safe and relatively nontoxic, and it acts to lower serum calcium within several hours. For this reason, it should be the initial agent of choice to provide some benefit before the more potent bisphosphonates become maximally effective. It typically loses its effectiveness within 48 hours in most patients. For this reason, it is important to begin therapy with a bisphosphonate at this time, as well.

Bisphosphonates block the hypocalciuric effect of PTH. They act by interfering with metabolic activity of osteoclasts; they are cytotoxic to osteoclasts. Pamidronate, zoledronic acid, and etidronate are the currently available agents that are recommended for the treatment of malignancy-associated hypercalcemia. Zoledronate appears to be the most efficacious with a maximum effect occurring in 48 to 72 hours.[1–4]

Case Study 3

Which of the following signs and symptoms are due to the effects of hypercalcemia per se? (Select all that apply)

A. Polyuria
B. Muscle weakness
C. Band keratopathy
D. Shortening of the QT interval
E. Constipation
F. Shortness of breath
G. Cognitive dysfunction
H. Supraventricular tachycardia

The correct answers are A, C, D, E, and G
Comment: Chronic hypercalcemia leads to a defect in concentrating ability that may induce polyuria and polydipsia in up to 20% of patients. This is due to down regulation of aquaporin-2 water channels and activation of the normal calcium-sensing receptor in the loop of Henle, which reduces sodium chloride reabsorption in this segment and thereby impairs the interstitial osmotic gradient.[1]

Hypercalcemia directly shortens the myocardial action potential, which is reflected in a shortened QT interval.[2] Band keratopathy, a reflection of subepithelial calcium phosphate deposits in the cornea, is a very rare finding in patients with hypercalcemia.[3] It extends, as a horizontal band across the cornea in the area that is exposed between the eyelids. Calcium salts probably precipitate in that site because of the higher local pH induced by the evaporation of CO_2.

Constipation is the most common gastrointestinal complaint in patients with hypercalciuria. It is likely related to decreased smooth muscle tone. Personality changes and affective disorders have been described at a serum calcium level above 12 mg/dL. Confusion, organic psychosis, hallucinations, somnolence, and coma are seen until serum calcium concentration is above 16 mg/dL.[4–6]

Case Study 4

Which of the following factors may be contributing to this patient's kidney failure at the initial presentation? (Select all that apply)

   A. Extracellular fluid volume contraction
   B. Hypercalcemia-induced renal vasoconstriction
   C. Nephrocalcinosis
   D. Granulomatous glomerulonephritis

The correct answers are A, B, C, and D
Comment: Mild hypercalcemia is only rarely associated with renal insufficiency. Higher elevations in serum calcium concentration (12 to 15 mg/dL) can lead to a reversible fall in glomerular filtration rate that is mediated by direct renal vasoconstriction and natriuresis-induced volume contraction.

Long-standing hypercalcemia and hypercalciuria lead to the development of chronic hypercalcemic nephropathy, which may be irreversible and continue to progress despite cure of the underlying conditions such as hyperparathyroidism. Calcification, degeneration, and necrosis of the tubular cells lead to cell sloughing and eventual tubular atrophy as well as interstitial fibrosis and calcification. These changes are most prominent in the medulla but can also be seen in the cortex. Interstitial calcium deposition can be detected by radiographic imaging studies. Nephrocalcinosis that can be detected by plain radiography of the abdomen is advanced and reflects severe renal parenchymal involvement. Ultrasonography or CT can detect earlier stages of the disease. An interstitial nephritis with granuloma formations is common in sarcoidosis, but the development of clinical disease manifested by renal insufficiency is unusual.[1–3]

Case Study 5

While the patient is receiving therapy and you are monitoring the serum calcium, it is time to begin ordering diagnostic studies.

Which of the following would you order first? (Select all that apply)

   A. Parathyroid hormone level
   B. Calcitriol level
   C. Calcidiol level
   D. Parathyroid hormone-related peptide level
   E. Abdominal computed tomography
   F. Abdominal flat plate
   G. Bone marrow examination
   H. Serum electrophoresis

The correct answers are A, B, and F
Comment: Diagnosis of PHP is always high on the list in an outpatient presenting with hypercalcemia. Granulomatous disease is certainly a possibility given the hilar adenopathy and hypercalcemia of several years duration. Measurement of calcitriol is therefore a good idea. An abdominal flat plate to look for nephrocalcinosis is reasonable in case of the history of kidney failure.[1–3]

Case Study 6

The PTH level was 2 pg/mL (reference range: 10 to 65 pg/mL) and 1,25-dihydroxyvitamin D (calcitriol) was 72 ng/mL (reference range: 9 to 47 ng/mL). The abdominal flat plate shows bilateral nephrocalcinosis.

Which of the following are the most likely diagnosis? (Select all that apply)

A. Nephrocalcinosis
B. Primary hyperparathyroidism
C. Malignancy
D. Granulomatous disease
E. Milk-alkali syndrome
F. Ultraviolet light toxicity

The correct answers are A, D, and F
Comment: The elevated calcitriol and low PTH levels are consistent with granulomatous disease. There is hilar adenopathy on the radiography image, which makes the diagnosis of sarcoidosis very likely.[1-3] It is very unlikely that exposure to a tanning salon alone would lead to elevated calcitriol level as calcitriol production is normally feedback regulated. However, in a patient with a granulomatous disease where calcitriol production is not feedback regulated, increased production of calcidiol, 25-hydroxyvitamin D, would aggravate hypercalcemia.

Case Study 7

Which of the following would be appropriate as part of the therapeutic regimen for this patient? (Select all that apply)

A. Low calcium diet
B. Low oxalate diet
C. Pamidronate
D. Low-dose corticosteroid therapy
E. Avoidance of tanning salon
F. Furosemide administration

The correct answers are A, B, D, and E
Comment: Treatment of hypercalcemia or hypercalciuria is aimed at reducing intestinal calcium absorption and calcitriol synthesis. This can be achieved by reducing the calcium intake (no more than 400 mg/dL), reducing oxalate intake, elimination of dietary vitamin D supplements, avoidance of sun exposure, and low-dose glucocorticoid therapy (prednisone, 10 to 30 mg/dL).[1-3] Serum calcium concentration typically begins to fall in 2 days, but the full hypocalcemic response may take 7 to 10 days depending upon the prednisone dose. Inhibition of calcitriol synthesis by the activated mononuclear cells is thought to play a major role in this response, although inhibition of intestinal calcium absorption and of osteoclast may also actively contribute.

Concurrent restriction of dietary oxalate is required to prevent a marked increase in oxalate absorption and hyperoxaluria. The latter may increase the risk of kidney calculus formation, even though urinary calcium excretion is reduced.

Oxalate absorption is normally limited by the formation of insoluble calcium oxalate salts in the intestinal lumen.[4] Dietary calcium restriction leads to more free oxalate than can then be absorbed if oxalate intake is unchanged.[5]

Case Study 8

A 15-year-old girl returns for her annual checkup. When seen last year, physical examination and laboratory studies showed no abnormality. Routine bone densitometry revealed low bone density (> 2.5 standard deviations below normal) and she was placed on alendronate. She now returns with no complaints. Laboratory studies show the following: hematocrit, 46%; BUN, 14 mg/dL; serum creatinine, 1.1 mg/dL; serum sodium, 140 mmol/L; serum potassium, 3.9 mmol/L; serum chloride, 105 mmol/L; serum bicarbonate, 26 mmol/L; serum calcium, 11.3 mg/dL; serum phosphate, 3.4 mg/dL; serum magnesium, 1.9 mg/dL; and serum albumin, 4.2 g/dL. Urinalysis shows trace protein, no glucose, no blood, no casts, and no erythrocyte or leukocyte.

The 24-hour urinary calcium excretion is 463 mg. The PTH level is 57 pg/mL (reference: 10 to 65 pg/mL).

What is the most likely diagnosis based upon the laboratory studies?

    A. Familial hypocalciuric hypercalcemia
    B. Primary hyperparathyroidism
    C. Malignancy
    D. Granulomatous disease

The correct answer is B
Comment: A PTH level in the high normal range is inappropriate in a patient with hypercalcemia and indicates the presence of PHP. This occurs in 5% to 20% of patients with this condition.[1-3]

Case Study 9

What would you like to do now?

    A. Order a sestamibi parathyroid scan
    B. Call the surgeon
    C. Follow the patient and schedule follow-up in 6 months

The correct answer is B
Comment: This patient has PHP and fulfills the criteria for surgical removal of parathyroid glands, because her 24-hour urinary calcium excretion is greater than 250 mg and her serum calcium is greater than 1 mg/dL above the normal level.[1-3] The indications for surgery in patients with hyperparathyroidism include (1) a serum calcium concentration of 1.0 mg/dL or more above the upper limit of normal, (2) hypercalciuria (urinary calcium excretion > 400 mg/day) while having a usual diet, (3) a creatinine clearance 30% or more below the age-matched normal level, (4) bone density at the hip, lumbar spine, or distal radius that is more than 2.5 standard deviations below peak bone mass (T score < -2.5), (5) age less than 50 years old, and (6) problem with periodic follow-up.

Case Study 10

A 19-year-old man with a positive human immunodeficiency virus test notes the onset of blurring of vision since several weeks before. Ophthalmology examination reveals white, fluffy retinal lesions, located close to the retinal vessels and associated with hemorrhage. Cytomegalovirus retinitis is diagnosed and he starts on intravenous therapy with foscarnet, 120 mg/kg twice daily, for 2 weeks, to be followed by maintenance therapy with an intravenous dosage of 90 mg/kg, once daily. He complains of several episodes of numbness and tingling, particularly around his mouth with the first several treatment protocols. This morning, he experiences a generalized seizure immediately following completion of his treatment. Laboratory studies show the following: hematocrit, 28%; leukocyte count, $4.6 \times 10^9/L$; BUN, 8 mg/dL; serum creatinine, 1.0 mg/dL; serum sodium, 140 mmol/L; serum potassium, 4.0 mmol/L; serum chloride, 106 mmol/L; serum bicarbonate, 25 mmol/L; serum calcium, 9.9 mg/dL; serum phosphate, 3.5 mg/dL; serum magnesium, 1.9 mg/dL; and serum albumin, 3.7 mg/dL. His physicians are concerned and confused. His symptoms sound like hypocalcemia, but his serum calcium concentration and serum albumin level are within reference ranges.

What would you recommend being done next? (Select all that apply)

A. Measure a PTH level
B. Reduce the foscarnet dose and measure serum-ionized calcium at the end of the next infusion
C. Measure serum calcidiol level
D. Measure serum ionized magnesium level
E. Order computed tomography of the head
F. Check blood gas during the infusion

The correct answers are B, E, and F
Comment: Foscarnet (trisodium phosphonoformate) has been shown to chelate calcium.[1] The plasma-ionized calcium typically falls by 0.4 mg/dL with a 120 mg/kg dose. These changes are clinically significant and can be associated with paresthesia and seizures. Acute respiratory alkalosis associated with hyperventilation due to pain or anxiety can also reduce the ionized calcium concentration. This is because the binding of calcium to protein is pH-dependent.[2,3]

Case Study 11

A 15-year-old boy presents with hypercalcemia and a 6-month history of leukemia.

The pathologic effects of his leukemia that results in hypercalcemia include which of the following mechanisms?

A. Increased bone resorption induced by prostaglandin production
B. Interleukin-6-induced bone resorption
C. Parathyroid hormone-related protein induced increase in bone resorption and reduction in calcium excretion
D. Tumor necrosis factor-induced activation of osteoblast proliferation
E. Transforming growth factor-β-induced increase in osteoclast activity

The correct answer is C
Comment: The pathophysiology underlying hypercalcemia of malignancy can be compared with its counterpart-primary hyperparathyroidism. Both syndromes are humoral in nature, with one being caused by PTH and the other by PTHrp. Both are associated with hypercalcemia, accelerated osteoclastic bone resorption, and reductions in renal phosphate reabsorption; both display increases in nephrogenous cyclic adenosine monophosphate excretion as a result of the interaction of PTH or PTHrp with the proximal tubular PTH/PTHrp receptor/adenyl cyclase complex.[1-5]

Case Study 12

A previously well 14-year-old Caucasian boy presented with initial concerns of short stature and low weight for age compared with his twin sister. He was asymptomatic at presentation. On examination, he was nondysmorphic and appeared well but small, with unremarkable heart, lung, abdominal, skin, and musculoskeletal findings. His growth parameters were as follows: weight 35 kg (< 3rd percentile, World Health Organization [WHO] growth curve, z-score 2.808), and height 148 cm (< 3rd percentile, WHO growth curve, z-score -2.411). He was also hypertensive, with a blood pressure of 154/116 mmHg (> 99th percentile for height), but other vital signs within the normal range. He had elevated creatinine (1.7 mg/dL), urea (43 mg/dL), and total calcium (12.1 mg/dL). Serum albumin was normal at 4.6 g/dL, ionized calcium elevated at 1.67 mmol/L, magnesium normal at 4.0 mg/dL, and alkaline phosphatase decreased at 96 U/L (200 to 630 U/L). He was mildly anemic, with a hemoglobin 10.5 g/dL and normal mean corpuscular volume (MCV) 81.6 pg, white blood cell (WBC) count 3.9×10^9/L, and platelet count 205×10^9/L. He had a mildly elevated C-reactive protein (CRP) of 3.0 mg/L, and erythrocyte sedimentation rate (ESR) of 25 mm/h. The remainder of his electrolytes was unremarkable. The patient was admitted for treatment of hypercalcemia with hyperhydration; amlodipine 5 mg once daily was also started for antihypertensive therapy.

Hypercalcemia workup showed normal 1,25-vitamin D of 166 pmol/L (reference: 48 to 190 pmol/L) and normal phosphate of 1.55 mmol/L (1.18 to 1.98 mmol/L) in the context of low PTH of 7 ng/L (reference: 12 to 78 ng/L), which excluded the diagnosis of hyperparathyroidism. Spot urinary calcium to creatinine ratio (Ca/Cr) was elevated at 1.76 mmol/mmol (< 0.7 mmol/mmol) and associated with nephrocalcinosis on renal ultrasound. Further assessment showed a urinary concentrating defect, with specific gravity less than 1.005 and urine osmolality of 208 mmol/kg H_2O. He underwent chest x-ray and bone marrow aspiration in the context of normocytic anemia, leukopenia, and hypercalcemia; both examinations were normal. Echocardiography showed no evidence of left ventricular hypertrophy and good biventricular function. On ophthalmologic examination, however, bilateral panuveitis and posterior-pole multifocal chorioretinitis leading to inflammation in the anterior segment were found.

What is the cause of hypercalcemia in this patient?

A. Calcium-sensing receptor mutation
B. Sarcoidosis
C. Vitamin D intoxication
D. Milk-alkali syndrome

The correct answer is B

Comment: Many clinical disorders are associated with hypercalcemia including hyperparathyroidism, malignancies, granulomatous disease, tubulointerstitial nephritis with uveitis (TINU), vitamin A and vitamin D intoxications, thiazide diuretic use, excessive calcium supplementation leading to milk-alkali syndrome, prolonged immobilization, and calcium-sensing receptor mutation.

In our patient, diagnosis of hyperparathyroidism was excluded as the blood PTH level was suppressed. Although our patient had normocytic anemia and leukopenia, normal bone marrow aspirate and chest imaging made a diagnosis of malignancy unlikely. In our case, there was no history of excessive vitamin D supplementation and levels of 25(OH)-vitamin D and 1,25(OH)$_2$-vitamin D were normal, so excluding this as a cause. Likewise, there was no history of retinoic acid use in our patient, so this was excluded. There was no history of diuretic use. Our patient was quite active at presentation, with no reported debilitating injury, so immobilization cause was also excluded. Calcium-sensing receptor was excluded, as this mutation is associated with familial hypercalcemia and our patient-appropriate hypercalciuria.

At this point, TINU and sarcoidosis remained on our differentials.[1-3]

To differentiate TINU and various granulomatous diseases such as tuberculosis, cat-scratch disease, and berylliosis, the following investigations were undertaken: angiotensin-converting enzyme (ACE) test, conjunctival biopsy, renal biopsy, Mantoux tuberculosis testing, and *Bartonella henselae* serologies. Results led to a final diagnosis of sarcoidosis.[1-8]

Sarcoidosis is a multisystem granulomatous disease of unknown etiology that rarely presents in childhood. Classically, clinical features of sarcoidosis in older children include pulmonary infiltration and lymphadenopathy. As outlined above, however, our patient presented with renal manifestations including elevated creatinine, hypertension, and associated hypercalcemia, hypercalciuria, and nephrocalcinosis. Renal involvement occurs in approximately 10% to 20% of adult patients with sarcoidosis, and impairment is most commonly a result of disorders of calcium homeostasis, leading to nephrocalcinosis and nephrolithiasis. In children, sarcoidosis-related renal disease occurs with comparable frequency (11%) and can manifest in a variety of similar ways. Like in adults, nephrocalcinosis and nephrolithiasis leading to obstructive uropathy are the most common causes of renal injury in childhood disease.

Sarcoidosis can also affect the kidney directly through inflammatory processes targeting the tubular interstitium and glomerulus, leading to granulomatous interstitial nephritis (GIN), the most common renal lesion on biopsy, and a spectrum of glomerular diseases, respectively. Membranous glomerulonephritis (GN) is the most frequent glomerular disease reported in the setting of sarcoidosis and has curiously been linked to antiphospholipase A2 receptor antibodies (anti-PLA2R), suggesting that perhaps primary and secondary membranous GN share this specific pathophysiologic process. Other reported renal complications of sarcoidosis include proliferative or crescentic GN, focal segmental glomerulosclerosis, and immunoglobulin A (IgA) nephropathy.

Treatment is required when renal manifestations of sarcoidosis are present due to the significant risk of progression to renal failure. To target the disease process, the mainstay of treatment is corticosteroids. Not only do steroids decrease inflammation, they decrease calcium absorption from the intestine and block activity of 1-alpha hydroxylase in macrophages, thereby inhibiting production of 1,25-vitamin D and depressing 24-vitamin D hydroxylase. There is no standard protocol for dose and duration of corticosteroid therapy; however, most studies recommend a starting dose of 0.5 to 1.0 mg/kg, which should be maintained for at least 4 weeks. Both hyperhydration and treatment with steroids were used as initial therapies in our patient and were effective in improving both hypercalcemia and renal function.

Mycophenolate mofetil (MMF) can be used as a steroid-sparing therapy. Although evidence for use of MMF is limited, several case reports and case series demonstrate benefit. Usually MMF is started after approximately 4 weeks of steroid therapy.

Methotrexate has been used for treating some extrarenal manifestations of sarcoidosis; however, importantly, it is not recommended for treatment of renal sarcoidosis due to its exclusive excretion via the kidneys.

Tumor necrosis factor α (TNF-α) is thought to play a significant role in granuloma formation and maintenance in sarcoidosis; therefore, anti-TNF therapy has long been a proposed target for treatment. Efficacy of treatment with infliximab (an anti-TNF-α monoclonal antibody) has been demonstrated (though the evidence is supported by case reports only) and has been shown to improve renal function in the setting of steroid-resistant disease. Conversely, etanercept (a soluble TNF-α receptor blocker) induces sarcoidosis. Although the pathogenesis of sarcoidosis induced by etanercept remains unclear, multiple mechanisms may contribute to granuloma formation, including inability to induce complement-mediated cell lysis, as is accomplished with anti-TNF-α antibodies (infliximab) that inhibit both soluble and membrane forms of TNF-α.

Case Study 13

A 13-month-old boy presented to our pediatric emergency department with failure to gain weight for the past 3 months. He had had excessive irritability, anorexia, polyuria, and polydipsia for the last 20 days. His mother also complained that the child cries excessively during micturition. He had not passed stools for 3 days and had several episodes of nonbilious vomiting 6 hours before admission. He was born at term by cesarean section. Infantile course was uneventful.

The child was exclusively breastfed for 6 months and complementary feeding started at 6 months of age. Total daily milk intake was 500 mL of cow's milk per day along with only two servings of cereals and vegetables. The child had also received intramuscular vitamin D (3,000,000) injections weekly followed along with oral vitamin D supplements (4000 IU) daily for the last 10 weeks for suspected vitamin D-deficient rickets.

On physical examination, the patient was afebrile with a pulse rate 96 beats/min, respiratory rate 24 breaths/min, and blood pressure 92/62 mmHg (50th to 90th percentile for age, sex, and height). His weight was at the 25th centile and height at the 50th centile for his age. The child had decreased skin turgor, sunken eyeballs, and dry oral mucosa (signs of some dehydration). The systemic examination was unremarkable. Laboratory results revealed hemoglobin 11.5 g/dL, total leucocyte count $11.8 \times 10^3/\mu L$, with differential leucocyte count 50% polymorphs, 46% lymphocytes, 3% eosinophils, and 1% monocytes, platelets $200 \times 10^3/\mu L$, erythrocyte sedimentation rate 12 mm/h, random blood sugar 98 mg/dL, BUN 20 mg/dL, serum creatinine 0.5 mg/dL, serum Na^+ 142 mmol/L, K^+ 3.6 mmol/L, serum albumin 4.3 mg/dL. Urine and blood cultures were sterile. Urine pH was 6.0, specific gravity 1.005. Urine microscopy showed 15 to 20 WBCs/HPF and 5 to 10 red blood cells/HPF. Urine volume was 7 mL/kg/h during the first 24 hours of admission. Early morning serum osmolality was 292 mOsm/kg and urine osmolality was 128 mOsm/kg. Arterial blood gases showed pH 7.35, bicarbonate 21, and PCO_2 38. Other laboratory investigations revealed serum calcium of 19 mg/dL (normal 8.5 to 10.3 mg/dL), serum phosphate of 4.21 mg/dL (normal 3.8 to 6.5 mg/dL), serum alkaline phosphatase of 419 U/L (normal 145 to 420 U/L), ionized calcium of 2.47 mmol/L, spot calcium creatinine ratio of 2.85 g/g (normal < 0.53 g/g), and 24-hour urinary calcium of 4.76 mg/kg/day (normal < 4 mg/kg/day). An electrocardiogram showed sinus rhythm, with a regular rate and normal intervals. There was no evidence of band keratopathy on eye examination.

Ultrasound of abdomen at admission revealed a 7-mm calculus in the left kidney. Serum amylase and lipase taken on day 3 of admission in view of persistent vomiting and abdominal pain were 111 and 1631 U/L, respectively, which increased to 367 U/L and 2520 U/L, respectively, over the next 48 hours.

During hospitalization, the child was treated with intravenously administered fluids (vigorous hydration with normal saline initially and then 5% dextrose solution at one-half normal strength at 1.5 times maintenance), furosemide 1 mg/kg/dose, and intravenously administered hydrocortisone at 10 mg/kg/day. For further workup intact parathyroid hormone (iPTH) was undetectable (15 to 65 pg/mL), 25(OH)D, vitamin A and E levels were sent. Despite these therapies, the total calcium level was persistently high and did not decrease until the 5th hospital day, at which time it decreased to 16 mg/dL. Although the patient was symptomatically better, with decreased irritability and normal urine output, calcium levels continued to be alarmingly high. Therefore, the patient was given a single dose of intravenous pamidronate (0.5 mg/kg) as an infusion over 4 hours after premedication with acetaminophen and antihistaminic prophylaxis (as a precaution to prevent fever and hypersensitivity reaction, respectively). Serum calcium levels gradually normalized over the next 4 days. On hospital day 4, vitamin A levels became available, which were normal.

What is the MOST likely cause of this patient's hypercalcemia?

    A. Hyperparathyroidism
    B. Familial benign hypocalciuric hypercalcemia (calcium-sensing receptor gene [CASR])
    C. Vitamin D intoxication
    D. Sarcoidosis

The correct answer is C
Comment: This infant presented with failure to thrive, excessive irritability, polyuria, polydipsia, and severe hypercalcemia. PHP was ruled out as the child had undetectable PTH and normal

serum phosphorus levels. Malignancy as a cause of hypercalcemia was less likely as serum alkaline phosphatase levels were at the upper limit of normal and there was no organomegaly or abdominal mass detected on physical examination or by ultrasonography of the abdomen. There was no contact history of tuberculosis, and a chest x-ray did not reveal any evidence of sarcoidosis or tuberculosis. *CASR* mutation was ruled out, as this condition is associated with low urinary calcium excretion and normal to high serum PTH level.

Finally, the elevated serum 25(OH) vitamin D (> 450 ng/mL) established the diagnosis of vitamin D intoxication as a cause for hypercalcemia.[1-5] Hypercalciuria in this patient is the cause of diabetes insipidus (polyuria). Hypercalciuria can cause polyuria by impairing calcium-sensor receptors on the apical membrane of the collecting duct cells leading to inhibition of aquaporin-2 expression in the collecting duct.

Vitamin D is a fat-soluble vitamin, which can be acquired exogenously from fish, oysters, and fortified dairy products or can be synthesized in the skin from 7-dehydrocholesterol after exposure to ultraviolet radiation. According to the American Academy of Pediatrics, 200 IU/day of vitamin D supplementation is recommended in all breastfed infants or non-breastfed infants on fortified milk of < 500 mL/day. There are limited data on safe upper tolerable limits of vitamin D in children. The stated safe upper limit vitamin D tolerability is 4000 IU/day in adults but varies from 2500 to 4000 IU/day in young children.

Vitamin D intoxication has been reported in infants/children consuming fortified milk products and even in children receiving pharmacological doses of vitamin D for treatment of documented or suspected vitamin D-deficient rickets. Vitamin D interplays with PTH to maintain normal serum levels of calcium. Both PTH and calcitriol increase serum calcium levels by activating osteoclastic bone resorption and increasing renal absorption of filtered calcium. Calcitriol also causes increased absorption of calcium from the intestine. Normal serum levels of calcium are 8.8 to 10.3 mg/dL during childhood. An overdose of vitamin D leads to hypercalcemia, hyperphosphatemia, and high calcium/phosphorus product-associated complications. Following the administration of an excess of vitamin D, the vitamin can be found in the circulation for several months, as it is stored in fatty tissues.

Treatment of vitamin D intoxication includes removal of the exogenous source, forced diuresis by adequate hydration and loop diuretics as well as the use of glucocorticoids, which decrease production of $1,25\ (OH)_2$-vitamin D3 and thereby decrease intestinal reabsorption of calcium. In patients with alarmingly high levels or hypercalcemia refractory to conventional therapy, intravenous pamidronate in doses of 0.5 to 1 mg/kg or even lower doses of 0.35 mg/kg are used.

Case Study 14

A previously well 12-year-old boy presented with a 1-month history of polydipsia, polyuria, and lethargy. Over that period, he had been drinking at least 3 L of water daily, reported feeling thirsty, and needed to pass urine approximately every 30 minutes. His parents also reported that he had weight loss over the previous month with reduced appetite secondary to nausea. Of note, he had a long-standing history of drinking approximately 1 L of cow's milk daily. He had no recent acute illnesses or fevers and reported no pain, discomfort, or respiratory distress. He had been treated with azathioprine for 3 years in the past for intractable eczema. His blood glucose level checked by his general practitioner was normal.

Physical examination revealed significant bilateral inguinal lymphadenopathy and a 2-cm palpable liver edge. There were patches of dry skin attributed to previously diagnosed eczema. His cardiovascular, respiratory, neurological, ENT, and musculoskeletal examinations were otherwise unremarkable. There was an evident BCG scar. Vital signs were within normal limits.

Laboratory investigations revealed BUN 43 mg/dL, serum creatinine 1.6 mg/dL, calcium 13.1 mg/dL, ionized calcium 2.3 mg/dL, phosphate 3.4 mg/dL, sodium 139 mmol/L, potassium

3.7 mmol/L, AST 76 U/L, ALT 114 U/L, and lactate dehydrogenase 416 U/L. Serum iPTH levels were suppressed at less than 6 ng/L. Serum 25(OH)-cholecalciferol level was reduced at 38 nmol/L. Urinalysis revealed significant hypercalciuria (calcium/creatinine ratio of 2.91). Full blood count measurements were within normal limits, while blood film revealed only occasional atypical lymphocytes and monocytes. An abdominal ultrasound revealed bilateral hyperechogenic kidneys, which were otherwise unremarkable; and mild hepatosplenomegaly with bulky inguinal lymph nodes bilaterally with speckled hyperechogenicity. A chest radiograph revealed clear lung fields, normal-sized cardiac silhouette with no evidence of a widened mediastinum.

What is the MOST likely diagnosis?

A. Vitamin A intoxication
B. Milk-alkali syndrome
C. Tuberculosis
D. Sarcoidosis

The correct answer is D

Comment: Hypercalcemia results when the entry of calcium into the circulation exceeds its excretion into the urine or deposition into bone. This can occur when there is accelerated bone resorption, excessive gastrointestinal absorption, decreased renal excretion of calcium, or in some disorders, a combination. It is often a clue to an underlying disease process. The differential diagnoses for hypercalcemia in children are wide, which include PHP, FHH, hypercalcemia of malignancy, vitamin D intoxication, chronic granulomatous disorders such as tuberculosis and sarcoidosis, drug-induced hyperkalemia (thiazide diuretics, lithium, theophylline), prolong immobilization, milk-alkali syndrome, and other conditions such as hyperthyroidism, adrenal insufficiency pheochromocytoma.

In our 12-year-old patient with lymphadenopathy and hepatosplenomegaly, the hypercalcemia is likely secondary to malignancy or chronic granulomatous disease. The diagnosis of sarcoidosis was confirmed with the finding of a normal bone marrow biopsy, coupled with a raised serum ACE level and lymph node biopsy showing multiple noncaseating epithelioid cell granulomata.[1,2] Supporting this is the fact that hypercalcemia in our patient was associated with a suppressed serum PTH and PTHrp, increased fractional excretion of calcium, and a high 1,25-dihydroxycholecalciferol level. His presentation with polyuria is attributable to a concentrating defect secondary to hypercalcemia, which in turn led to the increased sensation of thirst.

Symptomatic sarcoidosis is rare in children. In infants and children below the age of 4 years, the most common presentation is with the triad of skin, joint, and eye involvement without the typical pulmonary disease, whereas in older children, involvement of the lungs, lymph nodes, and eyes predominates. In a series of Danish children with sarcoidosis, the most common presenting features were erythema nodosum and iridocyclitis. Other features of sarcoidosis include fatigue, malaise, fever, and weight loss. African American children tend to have a higher incidence of lymph node involvement, hyperglobulinemia, and hypercalcemia. Although the lungs are the most frequently affected organs, the disease can affect any organ system in the body. Up to 30% of patients present with extrapulmonary disease; the most prominent sites involve the skin, eyes, reticuloendothelial system, musculoskeletal system, exocrine glands, heart, kidney, and central nervous system.

Case Study 15

A 6-month-old male infant born by normal vaginal delivery (birth weight, 3.150 kg; length 49 cm) and was found to have hypospadias. The patient suffered decreased appetite, vomiting, constipation, polyuria, and polydipsia during the previous 2 months. Further history taking revealed that the infant's grandmother vitamin D 400,000 IU/week for the last 10 months.

At our appointment, we found hypotonia, irritability, failure to thrive, anterior fontanelle 1.5 × 1 cm, and moderate dehydration. His mother reported that the infant was taking no drugs except prophylaxis with vitamin D (400 IU/day).

Serum chemistry was as follows: calcium 18.67 mg/dL (normal range, 8.4 to 10.2 mg/dL), urea 65 mg/dL (10 to 50 mg/dL), creatinine 0.45 mg/dL, phosphorus 5.7 mg/dL, calcium and phosphorus products 106 mg/dL (normal value < 55 mg), sodium, potassium, chloride, and bicarbonate concentrations were normal. The arterial blood gas, glucose, liver function tests, and complete blood count were also within the normal limits. Urinary electrolyte concentrations were as follows: calcium/creatinine ratio 1.27 mg/mg, uric acid/creatinine 0.45 mg/dL of glomerular filtration rate, beta-2 microglobulin 0.4 mg/L. Serum vitamin D was elevated (160 ng/mL) and serum PTH was suppressed (< 4 pg/mL).

ECG, cardiologic examination, and blood pressure monitoring were normal. Abdominal ultrasound showed bilateral nephrocalcinosis.

Hydration was started with NaCl 0.9% at 7 mL/kg/h to reduce calcemia. After 12 hours, the blood calcium was 15.2 mg/dL. Therefore we added furosemide (1 mg/kg intravenously twice a day) and methylprednisolone (1 mg/kg once a day). After 4 days of therapy, the blood calcium was 13.8 mg/dL and urinary calcium/creatinine ratio was 2.61 mg/mg.

The clinical conditions of the patient improved after 4 days. The serum level of calcium did not decrease after 6 days of therapy with furosemide and methylprednisolone, remaining at 13.8 mg/dL.

What is the MOST likely cause of this patient's hypercalcemia and how would you treat it?

A. Milk-alkali syndrome
B. Tuberculosis
C. Sarcoidosis
D. Vitamin D intoxication

The correct diagnosis is B
Comment: This patient was given 400,000 IU/week of vitamin D for 3 months, giving a total dose of 4,800,000 IU. The elevated serum calcium and vitamin D levels along with hypercalciuria and low PTH level, after excluding other causes of hypercalciuria, supported the diagnosis of vitamin D intoxication.[1-3]

Hydration with saline, use of loop diuretics and corticosteroids followed by pamidronate (1 mg/kg) are the main stay of treatment. Although bisphosphonate is frequently used to treat childhood hypercalcemia due to malignancies, osteogenesis imperfect, and osteoporosis, its use in vitamin D intoxication is very limited. The nitrogen-containing bisphosphonates, including alendronate, ibandronate, pamidronate disodium, risedronate, and zoledronic acid, induce osteoclast apoptosis and are powerful inhibitors of bone resorption. Calcitonin (2 to 4 U/kg bid) given by subcutaneous injection is effective when given early during the course of disease. However, as resistance to the hormone occurs quite rapidly, it is rarely used. Both pamidronate disodium and zoledronic acid can rapidly lower serum and urinary calcium levels in patients with hypercalcemia due to a variety of causes, and the effects can last for weeks.

Case Study 16

A 10-month-old Caucasian female born at term with a noncontributory birth history presented to the emergency department with complaints of generalized swelling and irritability for the past few days. Review of systems revealed loss of motor milestones for the previous 1-month proceeded by an increase in head size a month earlier. The patient was breastfed up to 3 months of age. She was later switched to unpasteurized goat's milk. The mother was supplementing milk with 10 drops of vitamin A with each bottle. Total daily milk intake was between 40 and 50 oz. The mother also added an unknown amount of each: vitamin E drops, blackstrap molasses, flax oil, cod liver oil, and drops of multivitamin preparation.

On physical examination, the patient was afebrile; systolic blood pressure ranged between 110 and 120 mmHg and diastolic was 80 to 90 mmHg (reference: 95th percentile for age, sex, and height was 103/57 mmHg). She was irritable, with a yellowish discoloration of the skin, generalized edema, and enlarged head (48.5 cm; > 95th percentile for age). She also had hepatomegaly with liver palpable 2 cm below the costal margin.

Laboratory tests in the emergency department revealed serum creatinine of 61.8 μmol/L (normal for her age 18 to 35 μmol/L), total calcium of 13.2 mg/dL. Her albumin was 2.0 g/dL, phosphorus was 3.4 mg/dL, PTH was low at less than 0.265 pmol/L (1.30 to 6.80 pmol/L), and alkaline phosphatase was 513 U/L (normal range for her age 150 to 420 U/L). Her liver enzymes were aspartate aminotransferase (AST) of 131 U/L, alanine transaminase (ALT) 37 U/L, total bilirubin 25.65 μmol/L and direct bilirubin 20 μmol/L, prothrombin time (PT) 27.9 seconds and partial thromboplastin time (PTT) 46.2 seconds. Her hemoglobin was 7.8 g/dL, hematocrit 23%, and platelets $137 \times 10^3/\mu L$. Her calcium/creatinine ratio in the urine was 0.29.

Head CT scan done in emergency department showed a step-off of the right medial parietal bone and lateral aspect of right side of the occipital bone about the lambdoid suture, suggestive of linear nonaccidental skull fractures. Subsequently, a skeletal survey showed no fractures but rachitic skeletal changes. Wrists had bilateral symmetric metaphyseal flaring and cupping as well as a majority of ribs had mild flared and cupped metaphyseal appearance at the costochondral margins. Magnetic resonance imaging (MRI) of her brain showed mild ventricular enlargement.

Renal sonogram showed her right kidney to be 8.1 cm and left kidney 8.0 cm (normal size range for the age 5.4 to 7.5 cm). There was also grade II and III bilateral nephrocalcinosis.

Upon admission to the pediatric intensive care unit (PICU), she had good urine output of 4.6 cc/kg/h despite elevated serum creatinine. Her urine volume declined over the next 24 hours and she became significantly hypertensive. Further workup included 25-OH vitamin D and 1,25 dihydroxy vitamin D levels, vitamin A and E levels. She received albumin infusion, which helped reduce edema. She was given amlodipine to treat hypertension. She was started on saline solution at maintenance rate with Lasix 1 mg/kg every 6 hours to manage her elevated calcium levels with no effect after 12 hours of therapy. She was later started on hydrocortisone 10 mg/kg/day to treat hypercalcemia. With also no improvement in hypercalcemia, she was then started on intravenous pamidronate 0.5 mg/kg/dose. During the same day that she received pamidronate, the patient had received blood products, including fresh frozen plasma and packed RBCs. This resulted in fluid overload, and she went into pulmonary edema and respiratory failure and got intubated. She was then started on continuous veno-venous hemofiltration (CVVH). CVVH was done with a blood flow rate of 80 mL/min and replacement fluid contained 4 K/2.5 Ca, which ran at a rate of 250 mL/h, but no dialysate fluid bag was added to the circuit. Her calcium levels normalized within 24 hours on CVVH. Within 48 hours, she was extubated. Her urine output improved and her creatinine normalized. Her hypertension improved once her calcium levels normalized. On hospital day 4, vitamin D levels became available: 25-hydroxy vitamin D level was 22 ng/mL (normal range: 20 to 80 ng/mL) and 1,25-dihydroxyvitamin D levels were 27 pg/mL (normal range: 15 to 75 pg/mL).

What is the MOST likely diagnosis?

    A. Primary hyperparathyroidism
    B. Vitamin A intoxication
    C. Transient hypercalcemia due to *CYP24A1* gene mutation
    D. Granulomatous disease

The correct answer is B

Comment: The patient was a 10-month-old girl who presented with irritability, macrocephaly, loss in milestones, hepatomegaly, anemia, thrombocytopenia, coagulopathy, and severe hypercalcemia of uncertain etiology causing hypertension and renal insufficiency. She underwent an extensive workup to define the etiology of hypercalcemia. She had appropriately low PTH for the degree of hypercalcemia and normal serum phosphorus, which ruled out PHP. Her 25-hydroxyvitamin D levels were normal, ruling out hypervitaminosis D. Her 1,25-dihydroxyvitamin D level was also normal, which was inconsistent with transient hypercalcemia.[1] Transient hypercalcemia is a rare autosomal recessive trait with mutation in the *CYP24A1* gene, the product of which is involved in breakdown of 1,25-dihydroxyvitamin D. Chest x-ray showed no evidence of granulomatous disease (sarcoidosis or tuberculosis). Based on other laboratory and x-ray findings, malignancy-related paraneoplastic syndrome was also a less likely cause of hypercalcemia. FHH was also considered. This condition is inherited as an autosomal dominant trait and results from heterozygous mutations in the *CASR* causing hypocalciuria and hypercalcemia with inappropriately normal PTH levels. The patient had low urine calcium to creatinine ratio for age, but with no family history of hypercalcemia and low PTH, FHH was a less likely diagnosis. Another rare bone disease is hypophosphatasia, which can result in hypercalcemia with metaphyseal dysplasia and severe rachitic changes similar to the findings in our patient. Hypophosphatasia is inherited either in an autosomal dominant or recessive fashion. The latter condition is due to a mutation in the alkaline phosphatase, liver/bone/kidney (*ALPL*) gene, which results in decrease in tissue-nonspecific alkaline phosphatase (TNSALP) in osteocytes and chondrocytes, which impairs bone mineralization leading to rickets. Hypercalcemia is hypothesized to be related to bone resorption in conjunction with impaired bone mineralization. Plasma pyridoxal 5′-phosphate and urinary phosphoethanolamine are elevated in such cases. Our patient had very low serum alkaline phosphatase levels, which ruled out hypophosphatasia.

Within 4 days of admission, vitamin A and E levels became available: vitamin A levels were retinol 1.48 mg/L (0.2 to 0.5 mg/L), retinyl palmitate 2.71 mg/L (0 to 0.1 mg/L); vitamin E level was alpha tocopherol 12 mg/L (3.5 to 8 mg/L). Based on history, clinical, biochemical, and radiological evidence, the child was diagnosed with hypervitaminosis secondary to chronic ingestion of excessive amounts of vitamin A.[2] The mother was supplementing about 10 drops of vitamin A with each bottle of goat milk. The infant received 40 to 50 oz of goat milk daily. This resulted in the ingestion of 20,100 IU/day of vitamin A from a medicinal supplement; the Recommended Daily Allowance for 1 to 3 years is 1000 IU/day. This was in addition to an estimated ingestion of 1936 IU from goat milk per day, which makes the total ingestion 22,000 U daily.

The treatment for vitamin A toxicity is mainly supportive. All sources of vitamin A ingestion must be eliminated from the diet. Intralipids have been used for cardiotoxic lipid-soluble drug intoxications but are of no proven benefit in hypervitaminosis A.

Case Study 17

A 5-year-old boy is evaluated for hypercalcemia. The patient has been asymptomatic. The abnormality was detected on a routine screening laboratory panel. The patient has been followed for 1 year after undergoing a negative evaluation for an occult malignancy. His physical examination remains normal, and his laboratory studies reveal serum calcium 12.5 mg/dL, phosphorous 2.9 mg/dL, PTH 40 pg/mL, and urine calcium 463 mg/24 h.

Which ONE of the following choices would be best for this patient?

A. Continued observation
B. Parathyroidectomy
C. Begin a calcimimetic agent
D. Evaluate family members for genetic defect in the calcium sensing receptor
E. Begin therapy with calcitriol

The correct answer is B

Comment: This patient has PHP and fulfills the criteria for surgical removal of hyperparathyroidism because his 24-hour urinary calcium excretion is greater than 250 mg, and his serum calcium is greater than 1 mg/dL above normal.[1]

Case Study 18

Which ONE of the following statements BEST describes the actions of a high-protein diet (2 g/kg/day) versus a low-protein diet (0.7 g/kg/day) on calcium metabolism?

    A. Intestinal absorption of dietary calcium is 40% higher on a high-protein diet than it is on a low-protein diet

    B. High-protein diet stimulates parathyroid hormone secretion

    C. Hypercalciuria induced by a high-protein diet is unrelated to gastrointestinal calcium absorption

    D. High-protein intake leads to a fall in bone mineral density

    E. Renal tubular defects of high-protein intake on calcium reabsorption are excreted in the proximal tubule.

The correct answer is A

Comment: In the study cited, low dietary protein was associated with secondary hyperparathyroidism because it led to reduce dietary calcium absorption. Recent data also suggest that high dietary protein intake is not associated with a reduction in bone mineral content—in fact, the opposite was found.[1]

Case Study 19

Which ONE of the following statements regarding the use of bisphosphonates in the treatment of the hypercalcemia of malignancy is correct?

    A. A hypercalciuric effect of bisphosphonates contributes to lowering serum calcium.

    B. Pamidronate is the most effective hypocalcemia-inducing bisphosphonate.

    C. Bisphosphonates are as effective after recurrence of hypercalcemia as during the initial treatment.

    D. Bisphosphonates block the hypocalciuric effect of parathyroid hormone-related protein (PTHrp).

    E. When treating hypercalcemia with bisphosphonates, the highest recommended dose should be used initially.

The correct answer is E

Comment: Bisphosphonates do not produce hypercalciuria. Zoledronic acid (bisphosphonate) is 100 times more potent that pamidronate. Bisphosphonates are most effective as an initial treatment for hypercalcemia. PTHrp-induced hypercalciuria is not influenced by bisphosphonates.[1]

Case Study 20

A 7-year-old boy presents in the office, complaining of slowly progressing pain in his upper right chest. The pain began about 2 weeks ago and is described as being similar to a toothache. It is unrelated to exercise or position. It initially responded to nonsteroidal antiinflammatory drugs, but they are no longer effective.

Review of systems reveals that he has noted some urinary urgency and frequency over the last 4 months and has nocturia three times weekly. He has also noted episodes of tingling around his mouth and occasional cramps of his hands and legs in the last several weeks.

Upon examination, vital signs are normal, the chest is clear, and there is tenderness over the fourth rib in the midline. There are no murmurs, and the abdomen is soft and nontender. There is mild hepatosplenomegaly. There is no edema. The neurologic examination is within normal limits. Rectal examination reveals a stony hard-indurated nodule in the left lobe of the prostate gland.

Initial laboratory studies reveal hemoglobin of 11.0 g/dL, white blood counts of 15,600 cells/uL, predominantly leukocytes, BUN 20 mg/dL, creatinine 1.6 mg/dL, sodium 140 mmol/L, chloride 106 mmol/L, potassium 4.0 mmol/L, bicarbonate 25 mmol/L, calcium 6.9 mg/dL, phosphate 3.3 mg/dL, and albumin 3.7 g/dL. Urinalysis is normal.

Which of the following do you expect to find? (Select all that apply)

A. Elevated PTH
B. Low PTH
C. Elevated alkaline phosphatase
D. Low alkaline phosphatase
E. High calcidiol
F. Low calcidiol
G. High calcitriol
H. Low calcitriol

The correct answers are A, C, and E
Comment: The most likely cause of the hypocalcemia is deposition of calcium in osteoblastic metastasis from acute leukemia. Elevated levels of PTH, alkaline phosphatase, and calcitriol characterize this condition.[1]

Case Study 21

Which of the following signs and symptoms are due to the effects of hypercalcemia per se? (Select all that apply)

A. Polyuria
B. Muscle weakness
C. Band keratopathy
D. Shortening of the Q-T interval
E. Constipation
F. Shortness of breath
G. Cognitive dysfunction
H. Supraventricular tachycardia

The correct answers are A, C, D, E, and G
Comment: Chronic hypercalcemia leads to a defect in concentrating ability that may induce polyuria and polydipsia in up to 20% of patients. This is due to down regulation of aquaporin-2 water channels and activation of the normal calcium-sensing receptor in the loop of Henle, which reduces sodium chloride reabsorption in this segment and thereby impairment of the interstitial osmotic gradient.

Hypercalcemia directly shortens the myocardial action potential, which is reflected in a shortened QT interval. Band keratopathy, a reflection of subepithelial calcium phosphate deposits in the cornea, is a very rare finding in patients with hypercalcemia. It extends, as a horizontal band across the cornea in the area that is exposed between the eyelids. Calcium salts probably precipitate in that site because of the higher local pH induced by the evaporation of CO_2. Constipation is the most common gastrointestinal complaint in patients with hypercalcemia. It is likely related to decreased smooth muscle tone. Personality changes and affective disorders have been described at serum calcium concentrations above 12 mg/dL-confusion, organic psychosis, hallucinations, somnolence, and coma is rare until the serum calcium concentration is above 16 mg/dL.[1-10]

Case Study 22

Which of the following factors may be contributing to the renal failure at the initial presentation? (Select all that apply)

    A. Extracellular fluid (ECF) volume contraction
    B. ECF volume expansion
    C. Hypercalcemia-induced renal vasoconstriction
    D. Nephrocalcinosis
    E. Granulomatous glomerulonephritis

The correct answers are A, B, C, and D

Comment: Mild hypercalcemia is only rarely associated with renal insufficiency. Higher elevations in the serum calcium concentration (serum calcium 12 to 15 mg/dL) can lead to a reversible fall in glomerular filtration rate that is mediated by direct renal vasoconstriction and natriuresis-induced volume contraction.[1-10] Long-standing hypercalcemia and hypercalciuria lead to the development of chronic hypercalcemic nephropathy, which may be irreversible and continue to progress despite cure of the underlying condition, such as hyperparathyroidism. Calcification, degeneration, and necrosis of the tubular cells lead to cell sloughing and eventual tubular atrophy as well as interstitial fibrosis and calcification (nephrocalcinosis).

These changes are most prominent in the medulla but can also be seen in the cortex. Interstitial calcium deposition can be detected radiographically. Nephrocalcinosis that can be detected by a plain film of the abdomen is advanced and reflects severe renal parenchymal involvement. Ultrasonography or CT can detect earlier stages of the disease. An interstitial nephritis with granuloma formation is common in sarcoidosis, but the development of clinical disease manifested by renal insufficiency is unusual.

While the patient is receiving therapy, and you are monitoring the serum calcium, it is time to begin ordering diagnostic studies.

Case Study 23

Which of the following would you order first? (Select all that apply)

    A. Parathyroid hormone level
    B. Calcitriol level
    C. Calcidiol level
    D. PTHrp level
    E. Abdominal CT
    F. Abdominal flat plate
    G. Bone marrow examination
    H. Serum electrophoresis

The correct answers are A, B, and F

Comment: The diagnosis of PHP is always high on the first list in a patient presenting with hypercalcemia.

Granulomatous disease is certainly a possibility given the hilar adenopathy and hypercalcemia of several years duration. Measurement of calcitriol is therefore a good idea. An abdominal flat plate to look for nephrocalcinosis is reasonable given the history of renal failure.[1-10]

The PTH level was 2 pg/mL (normal is 10 to 65 pg/mL) and the 1,25(OH)$_2$ D (calcitriol) was 72 ng/mL (normal range is 9 to 47 ng/mL). The abdominal flat plate shows bilateral nephrocalcinosis.

Case Study 24

Which are the most likely diagnoses? (Select all that apply)

A. Primary hyperparathyroidism
B. Malignancy
C. Granulomatous disease
D. Nephrocalcinosis
E. Milk-alkali syndrome
F. UV light toxicity from the tanning salon

The correct answers are C, D, and F
Comment: The elevated calcitriol and low PTH are consistent with granulomatous disease. There is hilar adenopathy on the chest x-ray, which makes the diagnosis of sarcoidosis very likely. It is very unlikely that exposure to a tanning salon alone would lead to elevated calcitriol production that is normally feedback-regulated. However, in a patient with a granulomatous disease where calcitriol production is not feedback-regulated, increased production of 25 (OH) D would aggravate the hypercalcemia.[1-10]

Case Study 25

Which of the following would be appropriate as part of the therapeutic regimen for this patient?

A. Low calcium diet
B. Low oxalate diet
C. Pamidronate
D. Low-dose corticosteroid therapy
E. Avoidance of tanning salon
F. Furosemide administration

The correct answers are A, B, D, and E
Comment: Treatment of the hypercalcemia and hypercalciuria is aimed at reducing intestinal calcium absorption and calcitriol synthesis.

This can be achieved by reducing calcium intake (no more than 400 mg/day), reducing oxalate intake, eliminating dietary vitamin D supplements, avoidance of sun exposure, and low-dose glucocorticoid therapy (10 to 30 mg/day of prednisone). The serum calcium concentration typically begins to fall in 2 days, but the full hypocalcemic response may take 7 to 10 days, depending upon the prednisone dose. Inhibition of calcitriol synthesis by the activated mononuclear cells is thought to play a major role in this response, although inhibition of intestinal absorption and of osteoclast activity also may contribute.

Concurrent restriction of dietary oxalate is required to prevent a marked increase in oxalate absorption and hyperoxaluria. The latter may increase the risk of kidney stone formation, even though urinary calcium excretion is reduced. Oxalate absorption is normally limited by the formation of insoluble calcium oxalate salts in the intestinal lumen. Dietary calcium restriction leads to more free oxalate than can then be absorbed if oxalate intake is unchanged.[1-10]

References

Case Study 1

1. Pecherstorfer M, Schilling T, Blind E. Parathyroid hormone-related protein and life expectancy in hypercalcemic cancer patients. *J Clin Endocrinol Metab*. 1994;78(5):1268–1270.
2. Willis MR. Value of plasma chloride concentration and acid-base status in the differential diagnosis of hyperparathyroidism from other causes of hypercalcaemia. *J ClinPathol*. 1971;24(3):219–227.
3. Patel A, Adeseun G, Goldfarb S. Calcium-alkali syndrome in the modern era. *Nutrients*. 2013;5(12):4880–4893.
4. Patel A, Goldfarb S. Got calcium? Welcome to the calcium-alkali syndrome. *J Am Soc Nephrol*. 2010;21(9):1440–1443.
5. Assadi F. Hypercalcemia: an evidence-based approach to clinical cases. *Iran J Kidney Dis*. 2009;3(2):71–79.

Case Study 2

1. Hosking DJ, Cowley A, Bucknall CA. Rehydration in the treatment of severe hypercalcaemia. *Q J Med*. 1981;50:473–481.
2. Wisneski LA. Salmon calcitonin in the acute management of hypercalcemia. *Calcif Tissue Int*. 1990;46(suppl):S26–S30.
3. Major P, Lortholary A, Hon J, et al. Zoledronic acid is superior to pamidronate in the treatment of hypercalcemia of malignancy: a pooled analysis of two randomized, controlled clinical trials. *J Clin Oncol*. 2001;19:558–567.
4. Assadi F. Hypercalcemia: an evidence-based approach to clinical cases. *Iran J Kidney Dis*. 2009;3(2):71–79.

Case Study 3

1. Berl T. The cAMP system in vasopressin-sensitive nephron segments of the vitamin D-treated rat. *Kidney Int*. 1987;31:1065–1071.
2. Diercks DB, Shumaik GM, Harrigan RA, et al. Electrocardiographic manifestations: electrolyte abnormalities. *J Emerg Med*. 2004;27:153–160.
3. Wilson KS, Alexander S, Chisholm IA. Band keratopathy in hypercalcemia of myeloma. *Can Med Assoc J*. 1982;126:1314–1315.
4. Heath 3rd H. Clinical spectrum of primary hyperparathyroidism: evolution with changes in medical practice and technology. *J Bone Miner Res*. 1991;6(suppl 2):S63–S70, discussion S83–S84.
5. Inzucchi SE. Understanding hypercalcemia. Its metabolic basis, signs, and symptoms. *Postgrad Med*. 2004;115:69–70.
6. Assadi F. Hypercalcemia: an evidence-based approach to clinical cases. *Iran J Kidney Dis*. 2009;3(2):71–79.

Case Study 4

1. Lins LE. Reversible renal failure caused by hypercalcemia. A retrospective study. *Acta Med Scand*. 1978;203:309–314.
2. Caruana RJ, Buckalew Jr VM. The syndrome of distal (type 1) renal tubular acidosis. Clinical and laboratory findings in 58 cases. *Medicine (Baltimore)*. 1988;67:84–99.
3. Assadi F. Hypercalcemia: an evidence-based approach to clinical cases. *Iran J Kidney Dis*. 2009;3(2):71–79.

Case Study 5

1. Insogna KL, Dreyer BE, Mitnick M, et al. Enhanced production rate of 1,25-dihydroxyvitamin D in sarcoidosis. *J Clin Endocrinol Metab*. 1988;66:72–75.
2. Heath 3rd H. Clinical spectrum of primary hyperparathyroidism: evolution with changes in medical practice and technology. *J Bone Miner Res*. 1991;(suppl 2):S63–S70, discussion S83–S84.
3. Assadi F. Hypercalcemia: an evidence-based approach to clinical cases. *Iran J Kidney Dis*. 2009;3(2):71–79.

Case Study 6

1. Insogna KL, Dreyer BE, Mitnick M, et al. Enhanced production rate of 1,25-dihydroxyvitamin D in sarcoidosis. *J Clin Endocrinol Metab.* 1988;66:72–75.
2. Inzucchi SE. Understanding hypercalcemia. Its metabolic basis, signs, and symptoms. *Postgrad Med.* 2004;115:69–70.
3. Assadi F. Hypercalcemia: an evidence-based approach to clinical cases. *Iran J Kidney Dis.* 2009;3(2):71–79.

Case Study 7

1. Montoli A, Colussi G, Minetti L. Hypercalcaemia in Addison's disease: calciotropic hormone profile and bone histology. *J Intern Med.* 1992;232:535–540.
2. Akmal M, Bishop JE, Telfer N, et al. Hypocalcemia and hypercalcemia in patients with rhabdomyolysis with and without acute renal failure. *J Clin Endocrinol Metab.* 1986;63:137–142.
3. Bilezikian JP. Management of acute hypercalcemia. *N Engl J Med.* 1992;326:1196–1203.
4. Kogan BA, Konnak JW, Lau K. Marked hyperoxaluria in sarcoidosis during orthophosphate therapy. *J Urol.* 1982;127:339–340.
5. Assadi F. Hypercalcemia: an evidence-based approach to clinical cases. *Iran J Kidney Dis.* 2009;3(2):71–79.

Case Study 8

1. Inzucchi SE. Understanding hypercalcemia. Its metabolic basis, signs, and symptoms. *Postgrad Med.* 2004;115:69–70.
2. Heath 3rd H. Clinical spectrum of primary hyperparathyroidism: evolution with changes in medical practice and technology. *J Bone Miner Res.* 1991;6(suppl 2):S63–S70, discussion S83–S84.
3. Assadi F. Hypercalcemia: an evidence-based approach to clinical cases. *Iran J Kidney Dis.* 2009;3(2): |71–79. Apr.

Case Study 9

1. Heath 3rd H. Clinical spectrum of primary hyperparathyroidism: evolution with changes in medical practice and technology. *J Bone Miner Res.* 1991;6(suppl 2):S63–S70, discussion S83–S84.
2. Kogan BA, Konnak JW, Lau K. Marked hyperoxaluria in sarcoidosis during orthophosphate therapy. *J Urol.* 1982;127:339–340.
3. Assadi F. Hypercalcemia: an evidence-based approach to clinical cases. *Iran J Kidney Dis.* 2009;3(2):71–79.

Case Study 10

1. Jacobson MA, Gambertoglio JG, Aweeka FT, et al. Foscarnet-induced hypocalcemia and effects of foscarnet on calcium metabolism. *J Clin Endocrinol Metab.* 1991;72:1130–1135.
2. Inzucchi SE. Understanding hypercalcemia. Its metabolic basis, signs, and symptoms. *Postgrad Med.* 2004;115:69–70.
3. Assadi F. Hypercalcemia: an evidence-based approach to clinical cases. *Iran J Kidney Dis.* 2009;3(2):71–79.

Case Study 11

1. Lafferty FW. Differential diagnosis of hypercalcemia. *J Bone Miner Res.* 1991;6(suppl 2):S51–S59.
2. Levi M, Ellis MA, Berl T. Control of renal hemodynamics and glomerular filtration rate in chronic hypercalcemia. Role of prostaglandins, renin-angiotensin system, and calcium. *J Clin Invest.* 1983;71:1624–1632.
3. Shane E, Dinaz I. Hypercalcemia; pathogenesis, clinical manifestations, differential diagnosis, and management. In: Favus MJ, ed. *Primer on the Metabolic Bone Diseases and Disorders of Mineral Metabolism.* 6th ed. Philadelphia: Lippincott Williams & Wilkins; 2006:176–189.
4. Ratcliffe WA, Hutchesson AC, Bundred NJ, et al. Role of assays for parathyroid-hormone-related protein in investigation of hypercalcaemia. *Lancet.* 1992;339:164–167.
5. Assadi F. Hypercalcemia: an evidence-based approach to clinical cases. *Iran J Kidney Dis.* 2009;3(2):71–79.

Case Study 12

1. Iannuzzi MC, Rybicki BA, Teirstein AS. Sarcoidosis. *N Engl J Med.* 2007;357:2153–2165.

2. Gedalia A, Khan TA, Shetty AK, et al. Childhood sarcoidosis: Louisiana experience. *Clin Rheumatol.* 2016;35:1879–1884.
3. Falk S, Kratzsch J, Paschke R, et al. Hypercalcemia as a result of sarcoidosis with normal serum concentrations of vitamin D. *Med Sci Monit.* 2007;13:CS133–CS136.
4. Hilderson I, Van Laecke S, Wauters A, et al. Treatment of renal sarcoidosis: is there a guideline? Overview of the different treatment options. *Nephrol Dial Transplant.* 2014;29:1841–1847.
5. Moudgil A, Przygodzki RM, Kher KK. Successful steroid-sparing treatment of renal limited sarcoidosis with mycophenolate mofetil. *Pediatr Nephrol.* 2006;21:281–285.
6. Villemaire M, Cartier JC, Mathieu N, et al. Renal sarcoid-like granulomatosis during anti-TNF therapy. *Kidney Int.* 2014;86:215.
7. Löffler C, Löffler U, Tuleweit A, et al. Renal sarcoidosis: epidemiological and follow-up data in a cohort of 27 patients. *Sarcoidosis Vasc Diffuse Lung Dis.* 2015;31:306–315.
8. Downie ML, Mulder J, Schneider R, et al. A curious case of growth failure and hypercalcemia: answers. *Pediatr Nephrol.* 2018;33:995–999. https://doi.org/10.1007/s00467-017-3769-2.

Case Study 13

1. Fuleihan G-H. Familial benign hypocalciuric hypercalcemia. *J Bone Miner Res.* 2002;17:51–56.
2. Vanstone MB, Oberfield SE, Shader L, et al. Hypercalcemia in children receiving pharmacologic doses of vitamin D. *Pediatrics.* 2012;129:e1060–e1063.
3. Chatterjee M, Speiser PW. Pamidronate treatment of hypercalcemia caused by vitamin D toxicity. *J Pediatr Endocrinol Metab.* 2007;20:1241–1248.
4. Khanna A. Acquired nephogenic diabetets insipidus. *Semin Nephrol.* 2006;26:244–246.
5. Orbak Z, Doneray H, Keskin F, et al. Vitamin D intoxication and therapy with alendronate (case report and review of literature). *Eur J Pediatr.* 2006;165:583–584.

Case Study 14

1. Iannuzzi MC, Rybicki BA, Teirstein AS. Sarcoidosis. *N Engl J Med.* 2007;357(21):2153–2165.
2. Milman N, Hoffmann AL. Childhood sarcoidosis: long-term follow-up. *Eur Respir J.* 2008;31(3):592–598.

Case Study 15

1. Barrueto Jr F, Wang-Flores HH, Howland MA, et al. Acute vitamin D intoxication in a child. *Pediatrics.* 2005;116:e453–e456.
2. Basso SM, Lumachi F, Nascimben F, et al. Treatment of acute hypercalcemia. *Med Chem.* 2012;8:564–568.
3. Ammenti A, Pelizzoni A, Cecconi M, et al. Nephrocalcinosis in children: a retrospective multi-centre study. *Acta Pediatr.* 2009;98:1628–1631.

Case Study 16

1. Vyas AK, White NH. Case of hypercalcemia secondary to hypervitaminosis A in a 6-year old boy with autism. *Case Rep Endocrinol.* 2011;424712.
2. Doireau V, Macher MA, Brun P, et al. Vitamin A poisoning revealed by hypercalcemia in a child with kidney failure. *Arch Pediatr.* 1996;3:888–890.

Case Study 17

1. Bilezikian JP, Potts Jr JT, Gel-H F, et al. Summary statement from a workshop on asymptomatic primary hyperparathyroidism: a perspective for the 21st century. *J Clin Endocrinol Metab.* 2002;87:5353–5361.

Case Study 18

1. Kerstetter JE, O'Brian KO, Insogna KL. Low protein intake: the impact on calcium and bone homeostasis in humans. *J Nutr.* 2003;133:855S–861.

Case Study 19

1. Berenson JR. Treatment of hypercalcemia of malignancy with bisphosphonates. *Semin Oncol.* 2002;29(6 suppl 21):8–12.

Case Study 20

1. Tommaso CL, Tucci JR. Metabolic studies in a case of hypocalcemia and osteoblablastic metastases. *Arch Intern Med.* 1979;139:238–241.

Case Study 21

1. Berenson JR. Treatment of hypercalcemia of malignancy with bisphosphonates. *Semin Oncol.* 2009;29(6 suppl 21):8–12.
2. Fatemi S, Singer FR, Rude RK. Effect of salmon calcitonin and etidronate on hypercalcemia of malignancy. *Calcif Tissue Int.* 1992;50:107–109.
3. Frick TW, Mithofer K, Fernandez-del Castillo C, et al. Hypercalcemia causes acute pancreatitis by pancreatic secretory block, intracellular zymogen accumulation, and acinar cell injury. *Am J Surg.* 1995;1:167–172.
4. Heath 3rd H. Clinical spectrum of primary hyperparathyroidism. Evolution with changes in medical practice and technology. *J Bone Miner Res.* 1991;6(suppl 2):S63–S70.
5. Lins LE. Reversible renal failure caused by hypercalcemia. A retrospective study. *Acta Med Scand.* 1978;203:309–314.
6. Major P, Lortholary A, Hon J, et al. Zolendronic acid is superior to pamidronate in the treatment of hypercalcemia of malignancy: a pooled analysis of two randomized, controlled clinical trials. *J Clin Oncol.* 2001;19:558–567.
7. Shek CC, Natkunam A, Tsang V, et al. Incidence, causes, and mechanism of hypercalcemia in a hospital population in Hong Kong. *Q J Med.* 1990;77:1277–1285.
8. Suki WN, Yium JJ, Von Minden M, et al. Acute treatment of hypercalcemia with furosemide. *N Engl J Med.* 1970;283:836–840.
9. Wilson KS, Alexander S, Chiaolm IA. Band keratopathy in hypercalcemia of myeloma. *Can Med Ass J.* 1982;126:1314.
10. Winsneski LA. Salmon calcitonin in the acute management of hypercalcemia. *Calcif Tissue Int.* 1990;46:S26–S30.

Case Study 22

1. Berenson JR. Treatment of hypercalcemia of malignancy with bisphosphonates. *Semin Oncol.* 2009;29(6 suppl 21):8–12.
2. Fatemi S, Singer FR, Rude RK. Effect of salmon calcitonin and etidronate on hypercalcemia of malignancy. *Calcif Tissue Int.* 1992;50:107–109.
3. Frick TW, Mithofer K, Fernandez-del Castillo C, et al. Hypercalcemia causes acute pancreatitis by pancreatic secretory block, intracellular zymogen accumulation, and acinar cell injury. *Am J Surg.* 1995;1:167–172.
4. Heath 3rd H. Clinical spectrum of primary hyperparathyroidism. Evolution with changes in medical practice and technology. *J Bone Miner Res.* 1991;6(suppl 2):S63–S70.
5. Lins LE. Reversible renal failure caused by hypercalcemia. A retrospective study. *Acta Med Scand.* 1978;203:309–314.
6. Major P, Lortholary A, Hon J, et al. Zolendronic acid is superior to pamidronate in the treatment of hypercalcemia of malignancy: a pooled analysis of two randomized, controlled clinical trials. *J Clin Oncol.* 2001;19:558–567.
7. Shek CC, Natkunam A, Tsang V, et al. Incidence, causes, and mechanism of hypercalcemia in a hospital population in Hong Kong. *Q J Med.* 1990;77:1277–1285.
8. Suki WN, Yium JJ, Von Minden M, et al. Acute treatment of hypercalcemia with furosemide. *N Engl J Med.* 1970;283:836–840.
9. Wilson KS, Alexander S, Chiaolm IA. Band keratopathy in hypercalcemia of myeloma. *Can Med Ass J.* 1982;126:1314.
10. Winsneski LA. Salmon calcitonin in the acute management of hypercalcemia. *Calcif Tissue Int.* 1990;46:S26–S30.

Case Study 23

1. Berenson JR. Treatment of hypercalcemia of malignancy with bisphosphonates. *Semin Oncol.* 2009;29(6 suppl 21):8–12.

2. Fatemi S, Singer FR, Rude RK. Effect of salmon calcitonin and etidronate on hypercalcemia of malignancy. *Calcif Tissue Int.* 1992;50:107–109.
3. Frick TW, Mithofer K, Fernandez-del Castillo C, et al. Hypercalcemia causes acute pancreatitis by pancreatic secretory block, intracellular zymogen accumulation, and acinar cell injury. *Am J Surg.* 1995;1:167–172.
4. Heath 3rd H. Clinical spectrum of primary hyperparathyroidism. Evolution with changes in medical practice and technology. *J Bone Miner Res.* 1991;6(suppl 2):S63–S70.
5. Lins LE. Reversible renal failure caused by hypercalcemia. A retrospective study. *Acta Med Scand.* 1978;203:309–314.
6. Major P, Lortholary A, Hon J, et al. Zolendronic acid is superior to pamidronate in the treatment of hypercalcemia of malignancy: a pooled analysis of two randomized, controlled clinical trials. *J Clin Oncol.* 2001;19:558–567.
7. Shek CC, Natkunam A, Tsang V, et al. Incidence, causes, and mechanism of hypercalcemia in a hospital population in Hong Kong. *Q J Med.* 1990;77:1277–1285.
8. Suki WN, Yium JJ, Von Minden M, et al. Acute treatment of hypercalcemia with furosemide. *N Engl J Med.* 1970;283:836–840.
9. Wilson KS, Alexander S, Chiaolm IA. Band keratopathy in hypercalcemia of myeloma. *Can Med Ass J.* 1982;126:1314.
10. Winsneski LA. Salmon calcitonin in the acute management of hypercalcemia. *Calcif Tissue Int.* 1990;46:S26–S30.

Case Study 24

1. Berenson JR. Treatment of hypercalcemia of malignancy with bisphosphonates. *Semin Oncol.* 2009;29(6 suppl 21):8–12.
2. Fatemi S, Singer FR, Rude RK. Effect of salmon calcitonin and etidronate on hypercalcemia of malignancy. *Calcif Tissue Int.* 1992;50:107–109.
3. Frick TW, Mithofer K, Fernandez-del Castillo C, et al. Hypercalcemia causes acute pancreatitis by pancreatic secretory block, intracellular zymogen accumulation, and acinar cell injury. *Am J Surg.* 1995;1:167–172.
4. Heath 3rd H. Clinical spectrum of primary hyperparathyroidism. Evolution with changes in medical practice and technology. *J Bone Miner Res.* 1991;6(suppl 2):S63–S70.
5. Lins LE. Reversible renal failure caused by hypercalcemia. A retrospective study. *Acta Med Scand.* 1978;203:309–314.
6. Major P, Lortholary A, Hon J, et al. Zolendronic acid is superior to pamidronate in the treatment of hypercalcemia of malignancy: a pooled analysis of two randomized, controlled clinical trials. *J Clin Oncol.* 2001;19:558–567.
7. Shek CC, Natkunam A, Tsang V, et al. Incidence, causes, and mechanism of hypercalcemia in a hospital population in Hong Kong. *Q J Med.* 1990;77:1277–1285.
8. Suki WN, Yium JJ, Von Minden M, et al. Acute treatment of hypercalcemia with furosemide. *N Engl J Med.* 1970;283:836–840.
9. Wilson KS, Alexander S, Chiaolm IA. Band keratopathy in hypercalcemia of myeloma. *Can Med Ass J.* 1982;126:1314.
10. Winsneski LA. Salmon calcitonin in the acute management of hypercalcemia. *Calcif Tissue Int.* 1990;46:S26–S30.

Case Study 25

1. Berenson JR. Treatment of hypercalcemia of malignancy with bisphosphonates. *Semin Oncol.* 2009;29(6 suppl 21):8–12.
2. Fatemi S, Singer FR, Rude RK. Effect of salmon calcitonin and etidronate on hypercalcemia of malignancy. *Calcif Tissue Int.* 1992;50:107–109.
3. Frick TW, Mithofer K, Fernandez-del Castillo C, et al. Hypercalcemia causes acute pancreatitis by pancreatic secretory block, intracellular zymogen accumulation, and acinar cell injury. *Am J Surg.* 1995;1:167–172.
4. Heath 3rd H. Clinical spectrum of primary hyperparathyroidism. Evolution with changes in medical practice and technology. *J Bone Miner Res.* 1991;6(suppl 2):S63–S70.
5. Lins LE. Reversible renal failure caused by hypercalcemia. A retrospective study. *Acta Med Scand.* 1978;203:309–314.

6. Major P, Lortholary A, Hon J, et al. Zolendronic acid is superior to pamidronate in the treatment of hypercalcemia of malignancy: a pooled analysis of two randomized, controlled clinical trials. *J Clin Oncol.* 2001;19:558–567.
7. Shek CC, Natkunam A, Tsang V, et al. Incidence, causes, and mechanism of hypercalcemia in a hospital population in Hong Kong. *Q J Med.* 1990;77:1277–1285.
8. Suki WN, Yium JJ, Von Minden M, et al. Acute treatment of hypercalcemia with furosemide. *N Engl J Med.* 1970;283:836–840.
9. Wilson KS, Alexander S, Chiaolm IA. Band keratopathy in hypercalcemia of myeloma. *Can Med Ass J.* 1982;126:1314.
10. Winsneski LA. Salmon calcitonin in the acute management of hypercalcemia. *Calcif Tissue Int.* 1990;46:S26–S30.

CHAPTER 9

Hypophosphatemia

Case Study 1

A 30-month-old boy is evaluated for failure to thrive, muscle weakness, bone pain, and difficulty to walk over the last 10 months. The infant was born at term to a 28-year-old gravida 2, para 2 mother via vaginal delivery. The birth weight was 3.1 kg; length, 50 cm; and head circumference, 45 cm. The child's father had rickets as a child, which left severe deformities. He was taking vitamin D and phosphorus supplements. The patient's 6-year-old sister had a history of delayed gross motor milestones and frontal bossing. However, a workup had never been done, nor had the child been treated. A dietary history revealed that the child had been fed a soy-based formula since early infancy because he had been unable to tolerate cow's milk. On examination, he appears as a thin male in no acute distress. Blood pressure is 96/51 mmHg; pulse, 96 beats/min; respiration, 20 breaths/min; temperature, 37°C; weight, 11.3 kg (5th percentile); height, 80 cm (below 3rd percentile); and head circumference, 49 cm (50th percentile). Heart rate is regular and there are no extra sounds or murmurs. The lungs are clear. The abdomen is soft and there are no masses. The extremities are free of rashes or edema. Neurological examination shows moderate proximal-muscle weakness with lower extremity bowing. The rest of physical examination is uneventful. Laboratory studies reveal a hemoglobin level and a leukocyte count within reference ranges and a normal urinalysis. Serum sodium level is 137 mmol/L; potassium, 3.9 mmol/L; chloride, 100 mmol/L; bicarbonate, 28 mmol/L; blood urea nitrogen, 8 mg/dL; creatinine, 0.3 mg/dL; albumin, 4.2 g/dL; calcium, 10.2 mg/dL; phosphate, 1.9 mg/dL; magnesium, 1.7 mg/dL; and alkaline phosphatase, 1829 U/L (reference range, 50 U/L to 330 U/L). A random urine calcium-creatinine ratio is 0.18 (reference range, < 0.22 to 0.26).

Which one of the following is most likely associated with his electrolyte abnormalities? (Select all that apply)

A. Muscle weakness
B. Failure to thrive
C. Bowing of the legs
D. Bone pain
E. Hyperthyroidism

The correct answers are A, B, and D

Comment: Muscle weakness, failure to thrive, radiographic evidence of rickets, and bone pain are classic clinical features of chronic hypophosphatemia. Hypophosphatemia-induced muscle weakness involves skeletal muscle and may cause proximal myopathy, dysphasia, ileus, and even respiratory failure.[1–3]

Case Study 2

Which of the following studies should be done first in attempting to distinguish the diagnosis? (Select all that apply)

A. Fractional excretion of phosphate ($FEPO_4$)
B. Fractional excretion of calcium
C. Arterial blood gases
D. Plasma 25-hydroxyvitamin D level
E. Plasma 1,25-dihydroxyvitamin D level

The correct answer is A

Comment: The first step in the diagnostic approach to hypophosphatemia is to establish whether hypophosphatemia is caused by inadequate dietary phosphate intake, reduced intestinal phosphate absorption, or excessive urinary losses of phosphate and this is done by evaluating the $FEPO_4$.[1,2]

In this patient, the random urine phosphate and creatinine excretion were 60 and 33 mg, respectively, and the $FEPO_4$ was 28.6% (reference range, 10% to 15%).

Case Study 3

Which of the following conditions should now be considered in the differential diagnosis? (Select all that apply)

A. Primary hyperparathyroidism
B. Inadequate dietary intake
C. Malabsorption of intestinal phosphate
D. Ingestion of large quantities of phosphate binding antacids
E. Vitamin D deficiency
F. Fanconi syndrome (FS)
G. X-linked hypophosphatemic rickets
H. Oncogenic osteomalacia
I. Hyperventilation

The correct answers are E, F, G, and H

Comment: The elevated $FEPO_4$ signifies excessive urinary losses of phosphate. Renal phosphate wasting can result from genetic or acquired renal disorders. Acquired renal phosphate wasting syndromes can result from vitamin D deficiency, hyperparathyroidism, oncogenic osteomalacia, and FS. The genetic disorder of renal hypophosphatemic disorders generally manifest in infancy and are usually transmitted as XHR.[1-6] The choice **"A"** is a wrong answer as serum calcium concentration is elevated in patients with primary hyperparathyroidism. Choices **"B, C, and D"** are also incorrect because of the inappropriately high $FEPO_4$. The choice "I" is a wrong answer because hyperventilation lowers serum phosphate level by promoting a shift of phosphate into the cells, leading to respiratory alkalosis and the $FEPO_4$ is appropriately low.

Case Study 4

Additional laboratory studies revealed 25-hydroxyvitamin D was 71.8 ng/mL (reference range, 30 to 100 ng/mL); 1,25-dihydroxyvitamin D, 15 pg/dL (reference range for children, 20 to 70 pg/dL); and intact parathyroid hormone (PTH), 44 pg/mL (4.6 pmol/L; reference range, 10 to 68 pg/mL). There was no aminoaciduria or glucosuria. Radiographic studies revealed florid signs of rickets, including a rachitic rosary and cupping of the ribs, as well as fraying and flaying of the radius, ulna, femur, tibia, and fibula.

What is the most likely diagnosis now? (Select all that apply)

A. Fanconi syndrome

B. X-linked hypophosphatemic rickets

C. Oncogenic osteomalacia

D. Nutritional vitamin D deficiency

The correct answer is B

Comment: The condition appears to be genetic (strong family history of rickets) and the 1,25-dihydroxyvitamin D levels are very low, consistent with this diagnosis. X-linked hypophosphatemic rickets is the most common inherited form of familial hypophosphatemic rickets and is characterized by growth retardation, defective bone mineralization, hypophosphatemia secondary to renal phosphate wasting, and inappropriately low serum concentration of 1,25-dihydroxyvitamin D. Patients with XHR have mutations in PHEX. It has been postulated that PHEX plays a major role in osteoblast cell differentiation and bone mineralization. It also increases renal phosphate reabsorption and promotes conversion of 25-hydroxyvitamin D to 1,25-dihydroxyvitamin D through activation of 1-α-hydroxylase enzymes.[1-3] Choice "A" is incorrect because FS is associated with generalized aminoaciduria and glucosuria. Choices "C and D" are not the correct answers, because of a strong family history of rickets.

Case Study 5

Which one of the following factors is most likely elevated in the plasma? (Select all that apply)

A. Parathyroid hormone-related protein

B. Fibroblast growth factor 23

C. Stanniocalcin-1

D. Calcitonin

The correct answer is B

Comment: Mutation in PHEX is associated with an increase in serum concentration of phosphatonin, including FGF23. The mechanism by which this mutation leads to elevation in FGF23 is unknown. The elevated level of FGF23 inhibits renal and intestinal absorption of phosphate directly by inhibition of sodium-potassium-II cotransporters. It also inhibits activation of 25-hydroxyvitamin D to 1,25-dihydroxyvitamin D through inhibition of 1-α-hydroxylase enzyme directly. Autosomal dominant hypophosphatemic rickets has similar clinical manifestations, with hypophosphatemia, clinical rickets, and inappropriately low levels of 1,25-dihydroxyvitamin D. Genetic studies have identified mutation in FGF23 as the cause of ADHR. The diagnosis of X-linked hypophosphatemic rickets was made based on the available laboratory data.[1,2]

Case Study 6

What should be done next? (Select all that apply)

A. Treat with oral phosphate

B. Treat with oral calcitriol

C. Recommend total parathyroidectomy

D. Order scintigraphy using octreotide labeled with indium-111

The correct answers are A and B

Comment: The goal of therapy is to improve growth, reduce the severity of bone disease, and minimize activity limitations. Phosphate supplements and calcitriol are the mainstays of therapy.

Phosphorus administration lowers the level of ionized calcium in plasma and decreases calcitriol synthesis, leading to secondary hyperparathyroidism. Increased levels of PTH further aggravate urinary phosphate loss. Therefore, calcitriol administration is necessary to increase the intestinal absorption of calcium and phosphorus and to prevent secondary hyperparathyroidism. Therapy with calcitriol is initiated at 15 ng/kg/day to 20 ng/kg/day. The dose is gradually increased over several weeks to 30 ng/kg/day to 60 ng/kg/day. Phosphate salts are given between 0.5 and 4.0 g/day in divided doses every 4 hours. Healing typically starts in 6 to 8 months after the start of therapy. The patient was treated with calcitriol and sodium phosphate, which led to significant improvement in the radiological signs of rickets after 6 months of therapy, and his serum phosphate level returned to normal.[1-4]

Case Study 7

Which of the following acquired clinical disorders has similar clinical and biochemical findings as XHR and ADHR?

A. Primary hyperparathyroidism
B. Tumor-induced (oncogenic) osteomalacia
C. Vitamin D deficiency
D. Cystinosis

The correct answer is B

Comment: Oncogenic osteomalacia is a paraneoplastic syndrome characterized by osteomalacia, hypophosphatemia, renal phosphate wasting, bone pain, and muscle weakness. These patients usually have benign tumors of mesenchymal origin that produce phosphatonins, phosphaturic peptides. Identification of the tumor can involve total body magnetic resonance imaging or scintigraphy using octreotide with indium-111 (since the tumors typically express somatostatin receptors). Patients with this syndrome require a combination of oral phosphate and calcitriol. This is because the use of phosphate alone may lower ionized calcium and lead to secondary hyperparathyroidism. Therapy should continue until the tumor can be identified and removed. Removal of the tumor leads to prompt reversal of the biochemical abnormalities and healing of the bone disease. The vast majority of tumors are benign and do not recur. Prognosis is excellent for complete recovery.[1-3]

Case Study 8

A 22-month-old girl was referred to our clinic upon detection of glycosuria and proteinuria in urine analysis. Her medical history was uneventful except a history of immature teratoma diagnosed on the 20th postnatal day. Physical examination revealed low body weight 9.7 kg and height 76 cm (-1,46 SDS); with normal motor and mental development. A surgical scar tissue was observed on umbilicus. No other pathology was detected. Laboratory investigations showed hypouricemia 1.7 mg/dL (reference: 2 to 5.5 mg/dL) and hypophosphatemia 3.9 mg/dL (reference: 4 to 7 mg/dL). Serum glucose, hepatic and pancreatic enzymes, bilirubin levels, renal functional tests and other electrolytes including sodium, calcium, chloride, potassium, and magnesium were within normal range. The blood gas analyzes were normal (pH: 7.43 mmHg, bicarbonate: 21.9 mmol/L, base excess: 1.0 mmol/L). The total urine analysis revealed + 2 proteinuria, 3 + glycosuria. The urine density was 1015 and pH was 5.5. In spot urine analysis for evaluation of tubular functions were: Fractional sodium excretion (FENa+) was 1%, fractional excretion of potassium (FEK+) 20%, tubular phosphate reabsorption (TPR) 62%, fractional uprate excretion (FEK) 57%, and urine calcium-creatinine ratio 0.15 mg/mg. Urine protein-creatinine ratio was 4 mg/mg. Urine protein electrophoresis was consistent with tubular proteinuria and urine β2 globulin level was high 0.69 μg/L (reference: 0.00 to 0.14). Ophthalmological examination was totally normal.

What is the most likely diagnosis?

A. Galactosemia

B. Tyrosinemia type 1

C. Wilson's disease

D. Ifosfamide-induced Fanconi syndrome

The correct answer is D

Comment: The presence of multiple defects in renal proximal tubular reabsorption, including glycosuria, proteinuria, hypophosphatemia, hyperphosphaturia, hyperuricosuria, and hypouricemia without non-anion gap metabolic acidosis, hypokalemia, and polyuria with episodes of dehydration were suggestive of FS.[1–7]

The differential diagnosis of FS in a young child includes inherited diseases and acquired causes. Cystinosis is the most common disease among inherited etiologies. The others are galactosemia, hereditary fructose intolerance, tyrosinemia, Wilson's disease, Lowe syndrome, Dent's disease, and mitochondrial cytopathies. Acquired causes of FS include the disorders that affect the proximal tubule such as drugs used in chemotherapy, toxins, dysproteinemia, glomerulonephritis, and acute kidney injury.

When examined for inherited diseases, corneal examination and intracellular cystine concentration in white blood cells for cystinosis were normal. Galactosemia was excluded with the lack of vomiting, diarrhea, cataract, and hepatic pathologies. There was not any vomiting, hypoglycemia, or convulsion after the ingestion of fructose, so hereditary fructose intolerance was excluded as well. Hereditary tyrosinemia type I, also known as hepatorenal tyrosinemia, is a tyrosine metabolism defect, affecting the kidneys and peripheral nerves but especially the liver. Hepatomegaly, jaundice, hypoglycemia, or hepatitis was not presented in this patient. Clinical findings of Wilson's disease are usually related to hepatic or central nervous system involvement. The clinical spectrum is variable and rarely presents before the age of 5 years. Hepatic disorders, neuropsychiatric pathologies, or both may predominantly is the initial diagnosis. In our patient, these pathologic findings that suggest Wilson's disease were not present. Lowe and Dent's disease are both X-linked disorders and they are common in males. Congenital glaucoma, cataracts, and mental retardation characterize Lowe syndrome. In Dent's disease, affected males have aminoaciduria, glycosuria, hypercalciuria and nephrocalcinosis, but hemizygous females have only mild aminoaciduria and hypercalciuria. Our patient has a normal mental status and no glaucoma or cataract. It was distinguished from Dent's disease by the absence of hypercalciuria. Mitochondrial cytopathies are a group of diseases with abnormalities in multiple systems including neurologic disorders, pancreatic and hepatic diseases, and cardiomyopathy. No additional systemic involvement suggesting mitochondrial disease was found in our patient's history, physical examination, and laboratory evaluations. Medication is an important cause of acquired FS. A number of chemotherapeutic drugs especially ifosfamide (IFO) and cisplatin are the common causes of FS. Since our patient had a history of immature teratoma, chemotherapy regimen should be questioned. Among chemotherapeutics, IFO is a well-known responsible agent for generalized proximal tubulopathy. When medical records were evaluated, FS was observed after the fourth cycle of neoadjuvant chemotherapy including etoposide (100 mg/m^2 at days 1 to 3), cisplatin (20 mg/m^2 at days 1 to 5), and IFO (1.5 g/m^2 at days 1 to 5) with mesna prophylaxis for six cycles. IFO is known to cause nephrotoxicity. The pathophysiology of IFO toxicity is unclear. It has been reported that chloroacetaldehyde, which is a metabolite of IFO, is responsible for tubular injury in recent studies. Chloroacetaldehyde decreases the antioxidant glutathione (GSH) and adenosine triphosphate (ATP) levels and inhibits the activity of NA$^+$/K$^+$-ATPase pump. The spectrum of tubular dysfunction varies from partial reabsorption defects in amino acids, glucose, sodium, potassium, bicarbonate, and phosphorus to generalized proximal tubulopathy. The common presentation is generalized aminoaciduria with 28%, also 17% present with both phosphaturia and aminoaciduria.

Case Study 9

A 2-year-old child developed hypophosphatemia with serum phosphorous level of 1.6 mg/dL.

Which of the following conditions most likely caused hypophosphatemia in this patient? (Select all that apply)

A. Renal insufficiency
B. Tumor lysis syndrome (TLS)
C. Malnutrition
D. Hypoparathyroidism

The correct answer is C
Comment: Normal serum phosphorus is between 3 and 4.5 mg/dL. Potential causes can include malnutrition and starvation or the use of aluminum hydroxide-based/magnesium-based antacids. Renal insufficiency, hypoparathyroidism, and TLS are causative factors for hyperphosphatemia.[1–4] The patient was started on total parenteral nutrition (TPN).

Case Study 10

What complications can occur with TPN in a malnourished child? (Select all that apply)

A. Hypomagnesemia
B. Hypokalemia
C. Hypophosphatemia
D. Hypoglycemia

The correct answers are A, B, C, and D
Comment: Severely malnourished patients can suffer from shifts in fluids and electrolytes during TPN administration. These shifts can be fatal. During severe malnutrition, the body adjusts its metabolism from carbohydrates to fat and protein for energy. The carbohydrates in the TPN can cause an increase in insulin secretion and cellular uptake in magnesium, potassium, and phosphate.[1–4]

Case Study 11

What are the clinical manifestations of hypophosphatemia? (Select all that may apply)

A. Decreased cardiac output
B. Slow peripheral pulses
C. Weakness
D. Nephrolithiasis
E. Increased clotting

The correct answers are A, B, C, and D
Comment: Clinical manifestations of hypophosphatemia include decreased cardiac contractility, decreased cardiac output, slowed peripheral pulses, shallow respirations, weakness, decreased deep tendon reflexes, decreased bone density, rhabdomyolysis, irritability, confusion, kidney stones, and immune suppression. Increased clotting will not occur as hypophosphatemia decreases platelet aggregation and increases bleeding.[1–4]

Case Study 12

What dietary advice would you give to this patient? (Select all that apply)

    A. Avoid antacids and phosphate binding medications
    B. Decrease calcium-rich foods
    C. Increase calcium-rich foods
    D. Increase phosphorus-rich foods

Comment: Calcium and phosphorus have an inverse relationship. If the phosphorus is low, the calcium is high. The patient will need to increase their phosphorus intake and decrease their calcium intake. It is also important to discontinue antacids and phosphate binder medications as these medications cause phosphorus loss. Increasing calcium-rich foods will further decrease phosphorus levels.[1-4]

Case Study 13

Which of the following electrolyte abnormalities would you expect to see in patients with hypophosphatemia? (Select all that apply)

    A. Hyperkalemia
    B. Hyponatremia
    C. Hypernatremia
    D. Hypercalcemia

The correct answers are A and C
Comment: Phosphorus also has an inverse relationship with calcium and potassium. If the phosphorus is low, the calcium and potassium will be high. Sodium and phosphorus do not have any correlation.

Hypophosphatemia is defined as a serum phosphate level of less than 2.5 mg/dL (0.8 mmol/L). Hypophosphatemia is caused by inadequate intake, decreased intestinal absorption, excessive urinary excretion, or a shift of phosphate from the extracellular to the intracellular compartments. Renal phosphate wasting can result from genetic or acquired renal disorders. Acquired renal phosphate wasting syndromes can result from vitamin D deficiency hyperparathyroidism, oncogenic osteomalacia, and FS. Genetic disorders of renal hypophosphatemic disorders generally manifest in infancy and are usually transmitted as X-linked hypophosphatemic rickets. Symptoms of hypophosphatemia are nonspecific, and most patients are asymptomatic. Severe hypophosphatemia may cause skeletal muscle weakness, myocardial dysfunction, rhabdomyolysis, and altered mental status. The diagnostic approach to hypophosphatemia should begin with the measurement of fractional phosphate excretion; if it is greater than 15% in the presence of hypophosphatemia, the diagnosis of renal phosphorus wasting is confirmed. Renal phosphorus wasting can be divided into three types based upon serum calcium levels: primary hyperparathyroidism (high serum calcium level), secondary hyperparathyroidism (low serum calcium level), and primary renal phosphate wasting (normal serum calcium level). Phosphate supplementations are indicated in patients who are symptomatic or who have a renal tubular defect leading to chronic phosphate wasting. Oral phosphate supplements in combination with calcitriol are the mainstay of treatment. Parenteral phosphate supplementation is generally reserved for patients with life-threatening hypophosphatemia (serum phosphate < 2.0 mg/dL). Intravenous phosphate (0.16 mmol/kg) is administered at a rate of 1 mmol/h to 3 mmol/h until a level of 2 mg/dL is reached.[1-4]

Case Study 14

A 19-year-old girl was diagnosed with hypophosphatemic rickets at the age of 2 years: she presented with growth retardation (worsening since the beginning of walking), bowing of the legs and hypophosphatemia. There was a negative familial history for phosphorus disorders, and a genetic analysis of the main genes involved in hypophosphatemic rickets has not been performed. Therapy was initiated with both phosphate supplementation and alfa-calcidol. Her final adult height was 154 cm and leg deformities were very moderate, without need for surgical correction. There were no dental problems. A mild but stable nephrocalcinosis appeared at the age of 16 years; renal function remained normal during follow-up. However, at the age of 18 years, while she was still receiving phosphate supplements (20 mg/kg/day) and alfa-calcidol (2 μg/day), PTH levels began to rise (i.e., 80 pg/mL, upper normal range of the assay of 65 pg/mL); treatment was continued without modifications and PTH levels continued to increase (PTH: 115 pg/mL). Phosphate supplements and alfa-calcidol were therefore tapered and eventually discontinued. However, clinical symptoms (i.e., muscular and bone pain, asthenia) recurred with serum phosphorus levels of 1.50 mg/dL 3 months after the initial therapeutic withdrawal, leading to the reintroduction of phosphorus (20 mg/kg/day) and alfa-calcidol (1 μg/day), in addition to a native vitamin D supplementation (cholecalciferol, 100,000 units monthly).

What is the most likely cause of hyperparathyroidism and nephrocalcinosis in this patient?

A. Long-term treatment with phosphate supplement and active vitamin D sterol (alfa-calcidol)
B. X-linked hypophosphatemic rickets
C. Primary hyperparathyroidism
D. Vitamin A deficiency

The correct answer is A

Comment: In this case, the patient presented with hypophosphatemia beginning at an early age and investigations revealed evidence for hypophosphatemic ricket. After an initial diagnosis of hypophosphatemic ricket during early childhood based on the association between bone deformities and hypophosphatemia, the patient received long-term treatment with phosphate supplementation and active vitamin D sterol (alfa-calcidol) and as a young adult, the presents with the two main long-term complications secondary to therapies often observed in hypophosphatemic ricket: secondary hyperparathyroidism and nephrocalcinosis.

Hypophosphatemic ricket correspond to a heterogeneous genetic pathology, affecting 1/20,000 children, resulting from mutations in FGF23 or their regulators to induce hypophosphatemia, rickets, dental abnormalities (pulp chambers, dental hypoplasia, dentin abnormalities, and dental abscesses) and bone deformations. Patients present with hypophosphatemia, normal serum calcium, decreased TPR, normal 25 (OH) vitamin D and PTH, and increased alkaline phosphatase levels.

Untreated severe hypophosphatemia can induce hemolysis, rhabdomyolysis, respiratory failure, cardiac dysfunction, and neurological impairment, thus requiring a rapid correction to avoid severe complications.

The recent description of the key role of the FGF23 in the "bone–kidney–parathyroid" axis had led to a better understanding of genetic conditions associated with hypophosphatemia and of the pathophysiology of both phosphate disorders. In hypophosphatemic ricket patients, a careful use of phosphate supplements and active vitamin D sterols should be considered to prevent nephrocalcinosis, secondary hyperparathyroidism, and soft tissue calcifications.[1,2]

Case Study 15

A patient has a phosphate level of 1.0 mg/dL.

Which condition below is not a cause of this phosphate level?

A. Hypoparathyroidism
B. Oncogenic osteomalacia
C. Refeeding syndrome
D. Thermal burns

The correct answer is A[1-5]

Case Study 16

A patient undergoing treatment for rhabdomyolysis with a phosphate level of 6.0 is about to eat their dinner.

What food from his diet would you remove due to its high contents of phosphate?

A. Breaded chicken and French fries
B. Rice and broccoli
C. Macaroni and canned tuna
D. Carrots and peas

The correct answer is A

Case Study 17

A patient's blood tests show they have a critically low PTH.

What effect would this have on phosphate and calcium levels in the blood?

A. Phosphate levels high and calcium levels low
B. Phosphate and calcium levels high
C. Phosphate and calcium levels low
D. Phosphate levels low and calcium levels high

The correct answer is A

Case Study 18

A patient has been undergoing chemotherapy for acute lymphocytic leukemia. The patient has started to exhibit early signs of TLS.

Which of the following findings correlates with TLS?

A. Phosphate level of 6.5
B. Phosphate level of 2.0
C. Phosphate level of 2.9
D. Phosphate level of 4.00

The correct answer is A

Case Study 19

Which patient is likely to present with a phosphate level of 6.0?

A. A patient taking an aluminum hydroxide-based antacid four
B. A patient on TPN therapy
C. A patient who reports drinking a 12 pack of beer daily
D. A patient in end-stage kidney disease

The correct answer is D

Case Study 20

A patient has a phosphate level of 5.6. The doctor orders the patient to take Phoslo.

What education will you provide to this patient regarding this medication?

A. Take the medication with a meal or right after
B. Take the medication before bedtime when phosphate levels are the highest
C. Take the medication with 8 oz of water
D. Take the medication on an empty stomach

The correct answer is A

Case Study 21

A patient is being discharged after being hospitalized with a phosphate level of 1.8.

What type of foods will you encourage the patient to consume in your diet teaching?

A. Organs meats and beef
B. Fresh fruits and vegetables
C. Beans and beets
D. Turnips and cauliflower

The correct answer is A

Case Study 22

A patient is experiencing hypercalcemia and has developed renal calculi.

What is the effect on the phosphate level in hypercalcemia?

A. Phosphate level increases
B. Phosphate level decreases
C. Phosphate level remain the same
D. Phosphate level normalizes

The correct answer is B

Case Study 23

Which of the following would you not expect to see with a phosphate level of 1.2?

A. Positive Trousseau's sign
B. Weakness
C. Confusion
D. Osteomalacia

The correct answer is A[1-4]

Case Study 24

What of the following is not an expected treatment for a phosphate level of 2.2?

A. Administering Phoslo by mouth with meals
B. Administering vitamin-D supplements
C. Encouraging the patient to eat fish, beef, chicken, and organ meats
D. Ensuring patient safety due to risk of bone fracture

The correct answer is A

Comment: Hypophosphatemia is defined as a serum phosphate level of less than 2.5 mg/dL (0.8 mmol/L) in adults. The normal level for serum phosphate in neonates and children is considerably higher, up to 7 mg/dL for infants.

Phosphate is critical for a remarkably wide array of cellular processes. It is one of the major components of the skeleton, providing mineral strength to bone. Phosphate is an integral component of the nucleic acids that comprise DNA and RNA. Phosphate bonds of ATP carry the energy required for all cellular functions. It also functions as a buffer in bone, serum, and urine.

Diet, hormones, and physical factors such as pH regulate serum phosphate concentration. Importantly, because phosphate enters and exits cells under several influences, the serum concentration of phosphate may not reflect true phosphate stores.[1-3] Often, persons with alcoholism who have severely deficient phosphate stores may present for medical treatment with a normal serum phosphate concentration. Only after refeeding will serum phosphate levels decline, often abruptly plummeting to dangerously low levels.

Phosphate is plentiful in the diet. A normal diet provides approximately 1000 to 2000 mg of phosphate, two-thirds of which is absorbed, predominantly in the proximal small intestine. The absorption of phosphate can be increased by increasing vitamin D intake and by ingesting a very low phosphate diet. Under these conditions, the intestine *increases expression of* sodium-coupled phosphate transporters to enhance phosphate uptake.

Regulation of intestinal phosphate transport overall is poorly understood. Although studies had suggested that the majority of small intestine phosphate uptake is accomplished through sodium-independent, unregulated pathways, subsequent investigations have suggested that regulated, sodium-dependent mechanisms may play a greater role in overall intestinal phosphate handling than was previously appreciated.[1-3] Furthermore, intestinal cells may have a role in renal phosphate handling through elaboration of circulating phosphaturic substances in response to sensing a phosphate load. Recent studies have confirmed that the ability of intestinal phosphate transport to influence renal phosphate transport is PTH-dependent; however, the signal to the parathyroid gland remains unknown.

Absorption of phosphate can be blocked by commonly used over-the-counter aluminum, calcium, and magnesium-containing antacids. Mild-to-moderate use of such phosphate binders generally poses no threat to phosphate homeostasis because dietary ingestion greatly exceeds body needs. However, very heavy use of these antacids can cause significant phosphate deficits. Stool losses of phosphate are minor (i.e., 100 to 300 mg/day from sloughed intestinal cells and gastro-intestinal secretions). However, these losses can be increased dramatically in persons with diseases that cause severe diarrhea or intestinal malabsorption.[1-3]

Bone loses approximately 300 mg of phosphate per day, but that is generally balanced by an uptake of 300 mg. Bone metabolism of phosphate is influenced by factors that determine bone formation and destruction, that is, PTH, vitamin D, sex hormones, acid–base balance, and gen-eralized inflammation.

The kidneys to maintain phosphate balance excrete the excess ingested phosphate. The ma-jor site of renal regulation of phosphate excretion is the early proximal renal tubule with some contribution by the distal convoluted tubule. In the proximal tubule, phosphate reabsorption by type 2 sodium phosphate cotransporters is regulated by dietary phosphate, PTH, and vitamin D. High dietary phosphate intake and elevated PTH levels decrease proximal renal tubule phosphate absorption, thus enhancing renal excretion.

Conversely, low dietary phosphate intake, low PTH levels, and high vitamin D levels enhance renal proximal tubule phosphate absorption. To some extent, phosphate regulates its own regulators. High phosphate concentrations in the blood down-regulate the expression of some phosphate trans-porters, decrease vitamin D production, and increase PTH secretion by the parathyroid gland.[1-3]

Distal tubule phosphate handling is less well understood. PTH increases phosphate absorp-tion in the distal tubule, but the mechanisms by which this occurs are unknown. Renal phosphate excretion can also be increased by the administration of loop diuretics.

PTH and vitamin D were previously the only recognized regulators of phosphate metabolism. However, several novel regulators of mineral homeostasis have been identified through studies of serum factors associated with phosphate wasting syndromes such as oncogenic osteomalacia and the hereditary forms of hypophosphatemic rickets, have been discovered.

Medical care for hypophosphatemia is highly dependent on three factors: cause, severity, and duration. Phosphate distribution varies among patients, so no formulas reliably determine the magnitude of the phosphate deficit. The average patient requires 1000 to 2000 mg (32 to 64 mmol) of phosphate per day for 7 to 10 days to replenish the body stores.[1-3]

Oral phosphate supplements, although not curative, are useful for the treatment of the genetic disorders of phosphate wasting and can often normalize phosphate levels and decrease bone pain. Parenteral phosphate supplementation is generally reserved for patients who have life-threatening hypophosphatemia or nonfunctional gastrointestinal syndromes.[1-3]

References

Case Study 1

1. Assadi F. Hypophosphatemia: an evidence-based problem-solving approach to clinical cases. *Iran J Kidney Dis.* 2010;4(3):195–201.
2. Jaureguiberry G, Carpenter TO, Forman S, et al. A novel missense mutation in SLC34A3 that causes he-reditary hypophosphatemic rickets with hypercalciuria in humans identifies threonine 137 as an important determinant of sodium-phosphate cotransport in NaPi-IIc. *Am J Physiol Renal Phsiol.* 2008;295:F371–F379.
3. Planas RF, McBrayer RH, Koen PA. Effects of hypophosphatemia on pulmonary muscle performance. *Adv Exp Med Biol.* 1982;151:283–290.

Case Study 2

1. Schmitt CP, Mehs O. The enigma of hyperparathyroidism in hypophosphatemic rickets. *Pediatr Nephrol.* 2004;19:473–477.
2. Tenenhouse HS, Murer H. Disorders of renal tubular phosphate transport. *J Am Soc Nephrol.* 2003;14:240–248.

Case Study 3

1. Assadi F. Disorders of divalent ion metabolism. In: Assadi F, ed. *Clinical Decisions in Pediatric Nephrology: A Problem-Solving Approach to Clinical Cases.* New York: Springer; 2008:97–123.
2. Schmitt CP, Mehs O. The enigma of hyperparathyroidism in hypophosphatemic rickets. *Pediatr Nephrol.* 2004;19:473–477.
3. Agus ZS, Goldfab S, Sheridan AM. In: Rose BD, ed. *Diagnosis and treatment of hypophosphatemia.* Wellesley: UpToDate; 2009.
4. Jonsson KB, Zahradnik R, Larsson T, et al. Fibroblast growth factor 23 in oncogenic osteomalacia and X-linked hypophosphatemia. *N Engl J Med.* 2003;348:1656–1663.
5. Liu P-Y, Jeng C-Y. Severe hypophosphatemia in a patient with diabetic ketoacidosis and acute respiratory failure. *J Chin Med Assoc.* 2004;67:355–359.
6. Clarke BL, Wynne AG, Wilson DM, et al. Osteomalacia associated with adult Fanconi's syndrome: clinical and diagnostic features. *Clin Endocrinol.* 1995;43:479–490.

Case Study 4

1. Jonsson KB, Zahradnik R, Larsson T, et al. Fibroblast growth factor 23 in oncogenic osteomalacia and x-linked hypophosphatemia. *N Engl J Med.* 2003;348:1656–1663.
2. Tenenhouse HS. X-linked hypophosphataemia: a homologous disorder in humans and mice. *Nephrol Dial Transplant.* 1999;14:333–341.
3. Berndt TJ, Kumar R. Phosphatonins and the regulation of phosphate homeostasis. *Ann Rev Physiol.* 2007;69:341–359.

Case Study 5

1. Jonsson KB, Zahradnik R, Larsson T, et al. Fibroblast growth factor 23 in oncogenic osteomalacia and x-linked hypophosphatemia. *N Engl J Med.* 2003;348:1656–1663.
2. Berndt TJ, Kumar R. Phosphatonins and the regulation of phosphate homeostasis. *Ann Rev Physiol.* 2007;69:341–359.

Case Study 6

1. Siddiqui MF, Bertorini TE. Hypophosphatemia-induced neuropathy: clinical and electrophysiologic findings. *Muscle Nerve.* 1998;21:650–652.
2. Hicks W, Hardy G. Phosphate supplementation for hypophosphataemia and parenteral nutrition. *Curr Opin Clin Nutr Metab Care.* 2001;4:227–233.
3. Nishida Y, Taketani Y, Yamanaka-Okumura H, et al. Acute effect of oral phosphate loading on serum fibroblast growth factor 23 levels in healthy men. *Kidney Int.* 2006;70:2141–2147.
4. Carpenter TO. New perspectives on the biology and treatment of X-linked hypophosphatemic rickets. *Pediatr Clin North Am.* 1997;44:443–466.

Case Study 7

1. Wilkins GE, Granleese S, Hegele RG, et al. Oncogenic osteomalacia: evidence for a humoral phosphaturic factor. *J Clin Endocrinol Metab.* 1995;80:1628–1634.
2. Jan de Beur SM, Streeten EA, Civelek AC, et al. Localization of mesenchymal tumors by somatostatin receptor imaging. *Lancet.* 2002;359:761–763.
3. Perreault MM, Ostrop NJ, Tierney MG. Efficacy and safety of intravenous phosphate replacement in critically ill patient. *Ann Pharmacother.* 1997;31:683–688.

Case Study 8

1. Hall AM, Bass P, Unwin RJ. Drug-induced renal Fanconi syndrome. *QJM.* 2014;107:261–269.
2. Foreman JW. Fanconi syndrome. *Pediatr Clin N Am.* 2019;66:159–167.
3. Yaseen Z, Michoudet C, Baverel G, et al. Mechanisms of the ifosfamide-induced inhibition of endocytosis in the rat proximal kidney tubule. *Arch Toxicol.* 2008;82:607–614.
4. Panezai MA, Owen C, Szerlip HM. Partial Fanconi syndrome induced by ifosfamide. *Proc (Bayl Univ Med Cent).* 2019;32:73–74.
5. Kamran SC, Pendergraft WF, Harmon DC, et al. Ifosfamide-induced Fanconi syndrome and desmopressin-responsive nephrogenic diabetes insipidus. *Am J Med.* 2013;126:7–8.

6. Izzedine H, Launay-Vacher V, Isnard-Bagnis C, et al. Drug-induced Fanconi's syndrome. *Am J Kidney Dis.* 2003;41:292–309.
7. Soyaltın E, Demir BK, Erfidan G, et al. A dilemma of proximal tubule in an infant: hypophosphatemia and hypouricemia without hypokalemia and acidosis: answers. *Pediatr Nephrol.* 2020;35:611–613. https://doi.org/10.1007/s00467-019-04392-7.

Case Study 9

1. Assadi F. Hypophosphatemia: an evidence-based problem-solving approach to clinical cases. *Iran J Kidney Dis.* 2010;4(3):195–201.
2. DiMeglio LA, White KE, Econs MJ. Disorders of phosphate metabolism. *Endocrinol Metab Clin North Am.* 2000;29:591–609.
3. Rubin MF, Narins RG. Hypophosphatemia: pathophysiological and practical aspects of its therapy. *Semin Nephrol.* 1990;10:536–545.
4. Gaasbeek A, Meinders AE. Hypophosphatemia: an update on its etiology and treatment. *Am J Med.* 2005;118:1094–1101.

Case Study 10

1. Assadi F. Hypophosphatemia: an evidence-based problem-solving approach to clinical cases. *Iran J Kidney Dis.* 2010;4(3):195–201.
2. DiMeglio LA, White KE, Econs MJ. Disorders of phosphate metabolism. *Endocrinol Metab Clin North Am.* 2000;29:591–609.
3. Rubin MF, Narins RG. Hypophosphatemia: pathophysiological and practical aspects of its therapy. *Semin Nephrol.* 1990;10:536–545.
4. Gaasbeek A, Meinders AE. Hypophosphatemia: an update on its etiology and treatment. *Am J Med.* 2005;118:1094–1101.

Case Study 11

1. Assadi F. Hypophosphatemia: an evidence-based problem-solving approach to clinical cases. *Iran J Kidney Dis.* 2010;4(3):195–201.
2. DiMeglio LA, White KE, Econs MJ. Disorders of phosphate metabolism. *Endocrinol Metab Clin North Am.* 2000;29:591–609.
3. Rubin MF, Narins RG. Hypophosphatemia: pathophysiological and practical aspects of its therapy. *Semin Nephrol.* 1990;10:536–545.
4. Gaasbeek A, Meinders AE. Hypophosphatemia: an update on its etiology and treatment. *Am J Med.* 2005;118:1094–1101.

Case Study 12

1. Assadi F. Hypophosphatemia: an evidence-based problem-solving approach to clinical cases. *Iran J Kidney Dis.* 2010;4(3):195–201.
2. DiMeglio LA, White KE, Econs MJ. Disorders of phosphate metabolism. *Endocrinol Metab Clin North Am.* 2000;29:591–609.
3. Rubin MF, Narins RG. Hypophosphatemia: pathophysiological and practical aspects of its therapy. *Semin Nephrol.* 1990;10:536–545.
4. Gaasbeek A, Meinders AE. Hypophosphatemia: an update on its etiology and treatment. *Am J Med.* 2005;118:1094–1101.

Case Study 13

1. Assadi F. Hypophosphatemia: an evidence-based problem-solving approach to clinical cases. *Iran J Kidney Dis.* 2010;4(3):195–201.
2. DiMeglio LA, White KE, Econs MJ. Disorders of phosphate metabolism. *Endocrinol Metab Clin North Am.* 2000;29:591–609.
3. Rubin MF, Narins RG. Hypophosphatemia: pathophysiological and practical aspects of its therapy. *Semin Nephrol.* 1990;10:536–545.

4. Gaasbeek A, Meinders AE. Hypophosphatemia: an update on its etiology and treatment. *Am J Med.* 2005;118:1094–1101.

Case Study 14

1. Carpenter TO, Imel EA, Holm IA, et al. A clinician's guide to X-linked hypophosphatemia. *J Bone Miner Res.* 2011;26(7):1381–1388.
2. Razzaque MS. FGF23-mediated regulation of systemic phosphate homeostasis: is Klotho an essential player? *Am J Physiol Renal Physiol.* 2009;296(3):F470–F476.

Case Study 15

1. Razzaque MS. FGF23-mediated regulation of systemic phosphate homeostasis: is Klotho an essential player? *Am J Physiol Renal Physiol.* 2009;296(3):F470–F476.
2. Assadi F. Hypophosphatemia: an evidence-based problem-solving approach to clinical cases. *Iran J Kidney Dis.* 2010;4(3):195–201.
3. DiMeglio LA, White KE, Econs MJ. Disorders of phosphate metabolism. *Endocrinol Metab Clin North Am.* 2000;29:591–609.
4. Rubin MF, Narins RG. Hypophosphatemia: pathophysiological and practical aspects of its therapy. *Semin Nephrol.* 1990;10:536–545.
5. Gaasbeek A, Meinders AE. Hypophosphatemia: an update on its etiology and treatment. *Am J Med.* 2005;118:1094–1101.

Case Study 16

1. Assadi F. Hypophosphatemia: an evidence-based problem-solving approach to clinical cases. *Iran J Kidney Dis.* 2010;4(3):195–201.
2. DiMeglio LA, White KE, Econs MJ. Disorders of phosphate metabolism. *Endocrinol Metab Clin North Am.* 2000;29:591–609.
3. Rubin MF, Narins RG. Hypophosphatemia: pathophysiological and practical aspects of its therapy. *Semin Nephrol.* 1990;10:536–545.
4. Gaasbeek A, Meinders AE. Hypophosphatemia: an update on its etiology and treatment. *Am J Med.* 2005;118:1094–1101.

Case Study 17

1. Assadi F. Hypophosphatemia: an evidence-based problem-solving approach to clinical cases. *Iran J Kidney Dis.* 2010;4(3):195–201.
2. DiMeglio LA, White KE, Econs MJ. Disorders of phosphate metabolism. *Endocrinol Metab Clin North Am.* 2000;29:591–609.
3. Rubin MF, Narins RG. Hypophosphatemia: pathophysiological and practical aspects of its therapy. *Semin Nephrol.* 1990;10:536–545.
4. Gaasbeek A, Meinders AE. Hypophosphatemia: an update on its etiology and treatment. *Am J Med.* 2005;118:1094–1101.

Case Study 18

1. Assadi F. Hypophosphatemia: an evidence-based problem-solving approach to clinical cases. *Iran J Kidney Dis.* 2010;4(3):195–201.
2. DiMeglio LA, White KE, Econs MJ. Disorders of phosphate metabolism. *Endocrinol Metab Clin North Am.* 2000;29:591–609.
3. Rubin MF, Narins RG. Hypophosphatemia: pathophysiological and practical aspects of its therapy. *Semin Nephrol.* 1990;10:536–545.
4. Gaasbeek A, Meinders AE. Hypophosphatemia: an update on its etiology and treatment. *Am J Med.* 2005;118:1094–1101.

Case Study 19

1. Assadi F. Hypophosphatemia: an evidence-based problem-solving approach to clinical cases. *Iran J Kidney Dis.* 2010;4(3):195–201.

2. DiMeglio LA, White KE, Econs MJ. Disorders of phosphate metabolism. *Endocrinol Metab Clin North Am.* 2000;29:591–609.
3. Rubin MF, Narins RG. Hypophosphatemia: pathophysiological and practical aspects of its therapy. *Semin Nephrol.* 1990;10:536–545.
4. Gaasbeek A, Meinders AE. Hypophosphatemia: an update on its etiology and treatment. *Am J Med.* 2005;118:1094–1101.

Case Study 20

1. Assadi F. Hypophosphatemia: an evidence-based problem-solving approach to clinical cases. *Iran J Kidney Dis.* 2010;4(3):195–201.
2. DiMeglio LA, White KE, Econs MJ. Disorders of phosphate metabolism. *Endocrinol Metab Clin North Am.* 2000;29:591–609.
3. Rubin MF, Narins RG. Hypophosphatemia: pathophysiological and practical aspects of its therapy. *Semin Nephrol.* 1990;10:536–545.
4. Gaasbeek A, Meinders AE. Hypophosphatemia: an update on its etiology and treatment. *Am J Med.* 2005;118:1094–1101.

Case Study 21

1. Assadi F. Hypophosphatemia: an evidence-based problem-solving approach to clinical cases. *Iran J Kidney Dis.* 2010;4(3):195–201.
2. DiMeglio LA, White KE, Econs MJ. Disorders of phosphate metabolism. *Endocrinol Metab Clin North Am.* 2000;29:591–609.
3. Rubin MF, Narins RG. Hypophosphatemia: pathophysiological and practical aspects of its therapy. *Semin Nephrol.* 1990;10:536–545.
4. Gaasbeek A, Meinders AE. Hypophosphatemia: an update on its etiology and treatment. *Am J Med.* 2005;118:1094–1101.

Case Study 22

1. Assadi F. Hypophosphatemia: an evidence-based problem-solving approach to clinical cases. *Iran J Kidney Dis.* 2010;4(3):195–201.
2. DiMeglio LA, White KE, Econs MJ. Disorders of phosphate metabolism. *Endocrinol Metab Clin North Am.* 2000;29:591–609.
3. Rubin MF, Narins RG. Hypophosphatemia: pathophysiological and practical aspects of its therapy. *Semin Nephrol.* 1990;10:536–545.
4. Gaasbeek A, Meinders AE. Hypophosphatemia: an update on its etiology and treatment. *Am J Med.* 2005;118:1094–1101.

Case Study 23

1. Assadi F. Hypophosphatemia: an evidence-based problem-solving approach to clinical cases. *Iran J Kidney Dis.* 2010;4(3):195–201.
2. DiMeglio LA, White KE, Econs MJ. Disorders of phosphate metabolism. *Endocrinol Metab Clin North Am.* 2000;29:591–609.
3. Rubin MF, Narins RG. Hypophosphatemia: pathophysiological and practical aspects of its therapy. *Semin Nephrol.* 1990;10:536–545.
4. Gaasbeek A, Meinders AE. Hypophosphatemia: an update on its etiology and treatment. *Am J Med.* 2005;118:1094–1101.

Case Study 24

1. Shaikh A, Berndt T, Kumar R. Regulation of phosphate homeostasis by the phosphatonins and other novel mediators. *Pediatr Nephrol.* 2008;23(8):1203–1210.
2. Thomas L, Bettoni C, Knöpfel T, et al. Acute adaption to oral or intravenous phosphate requires parathyroid hormone. *J Am Soc Nephrol.* 2017;28(3):903–914.
3. Tenenhouse HS, Gauthier C, Martel J, et al. Na$^+$-phosphate cotransport in mouse distal convoluted tubule cells: evidence for Glvr-1 and Ram-1 gene expression. *J Bone Miner Res.* 1998;13(4):590–597.

CHAPTER 10

Hyperphosphatemia

Case Study 1

An 11-year-old girl recently diagnosed with acute myeloid leukemia. After the third chemotherapy course, consisting of cytarabine, mitoxantrone, and intrathecal methotrexate, she was admitted to the hospital because of septic shock during febrile neutropenia. She was treated with meropenem and vancomycin, and blood cultures were positive for *Streptococcus mitis*. Because of persistent fever, the central venous catheter was removed. Nevertheless, the fever persisted and a chest computed tomography (CT) was performed, which revealed multiple abnormalities suggestive of pulmonary aspergillosis, which was confirmed by bronchoalveolar lavage. On day 5 of admission, she was started on amphotericin B, 5 mg/kg in glucose 5%. Because of the persisting neutropenia, granulocyte colony-stimulating factor (G-CSF) was administered. Fever disappeared with neutrophil recovery approximately 5 days after the start of G-CSF and amphotericin B.

Repeated blood tests showed normal renal function (creatinine 0.4 mg/dL, urea 15 mg/dL). Potassium supplementation was started because of hypokalemia. While phosphate concentrations were low at 2 mg/dL on day 5, they rose spontaneously from day 7 and laboratory tests showed progressive hyperphosphatemia, with a maximum of 7 mg/dL.

What is the most likely cause of the hyperphosphatemia observed in this patient?

    A. Hypoparathyroidism
    B. Pseudohyperphosphatemia due to amphoticin B
    C. Vitamin D intoxication
    D. Increased phosphate intake

The correct answer is B

Comment: Serum phosphate concentration is mainly affected by dietary intake and renal excretion of phosphate. Phosphate homeostasis is regulated by the phosphaturic hormones fibroblast growth factor-23 (FGF23) and parathyroid hormone, as well as by growth hormone and vitamin D. Other sources of phosphate include leakage of intracellular phosphate during tumor lysis, rhabdomyolysis, or hemolysis or a transcellular shift of phosphate during diabetic ketoacidosis or lactate acidosis.[1-4]

The differential diagnosis of hyperphosphatemia can be divided into four major groups: (1) increased phosphate intake, (2) transcellular phosphate shift, (3) diminished phosphate excretion, and (4) pseudohyperphosphatemia.[1-4] The patient in this case received no dietary phosphate supplements or phosphate-containing laxatives. The underlying malignancy was in remission and there were no signs of rhabdomyolysis or hemolysis. There was also no transcellular phosphate shift by diabetic ketoacidosis or lactic acidosis.

Laboratory investigations excluded renal insufficiency, and tubular reabsorption of phosphate was normal (87%). Hypoparathyroidism leading to increased tubular reabsorption of phosphate was ruled out. Growth analysis showed no signs of growth hormone excess, although growth hormone concentration was not measured.

Having excluded all in vivo causes, pseudohyperphosphatemia, that is, an artifact during the measurement of phosphate, was considered. This in vitro phenomenon has been reported for immunoglobulins, hyperlipidemia, and hyperbilirubinemia. Although there is an ongoing debate on the clinical relevance of some of these interferences, the influence of elevated levels of paraproteins by Waldenstrom macroglobulinemia and multiple myeloma is well established. Also, sample hemolysis is known to interfere with the laboratory phosphate assay.

In this case, triglyceride and bilirubin concentrations were normal, as were immunoglobulins. Samples from this patient were nonhemolytic. Analysis was therefore extended to medications known to cause pseudohyperphosphatemia, such as heparin and a tissue plasminogen activator. Another drug, which has been linked to interference of the laboratory phosphate assay, is liposomal amphotericin B, an antimycotic antibiotic. In our patient, hyperphosphatemia was first noted 2 days after liposomal amphotericin B had been prescribed for treatment of pulmonary aspergillosis. Therefore, this drug was considered the most probable culprit of the hyperphosphatemia.[1-4]

Case Study 2

You receive a critical laboratory value on a patient with serum phosphorus level of 5.9 mg/dL.

Which of the following conditions MOST likely cussed the elevated serum phosphorus level? (Select all that apply)

A. Renal insufficiency
B. Tumor lysis syndrome
C. Malnutrition
D. Hypoparathyroidism
E. Hyperparathyroidism

The correct answers are A, B, and D
Comment: Normal serum phosphorus is between 3 and 4.5 mg/dL. The patient is experiencing hyperphosphatemia. Potential causes can include renal insufficiency, hypoparathyroidism, and tumor lysis syndrome. Malnutrition and hyperparathyroidism are causes for hypophosphatemia.[1-5]

Case Study 3

A 14-year-old patient with renal insufficiency has recently been diagnosed with hyperphosphatemia.

What foods should the patient avoid to further worsening of high phosphorus levels? (Select all that apply)

A. Collard greens
B. Chicken and beef
C. Broccoli
D. Tofu

The correct answer is B
Comment: Phosphorous is found in bones and is used for activation of vitamins/minerals. In renal insufficiency, the kidneys are unable to excrete phosphorus and it continues to build up in the blood. Fish, nuts, pumpkin, pork, beef, chicken, and squash are all rich in phosphorous.[1-5]

Case Study 4

The physician is reviewing the clinical manifestations for hyperphosphatemia.

What would you expect to find on this patient's clinical findings? (Select all that apply)

A. Bradycardia
B. Hypotension
C. Negative Trousseau sign
D. Shortened ST interval
E. Prolonged QT interval

The correct answers are A, B, and E
Comment: Clinical manifestations you can see with high phosphorous levels are decreased heart rate, hypotension, diminished peripheral pulses, high risk for bleeding, irritable skeletal muscles, hyperactive deep tendon reflexes, prolonged QT intervals, and prolonged ST interval. We will not see negative Trousseau sign, negative Chvostek sign, and shortened ST interval.[1-5]

Case Study 5

Which dietary recommendations would you provide to this patient? (Select all that apply)

A. Avoid laxative and enema medications
B. Increase intake of calcium-rich foods
C. Decease intake of phosphorous-rich foods
D. Avoid phosphate-binding medications

The correct answers are A, B, and C
Comment: Calcium and phosphorus have an inverse relationship. If the phosphorous is high, the calcium is low. The patient will need to decrease their phosphorous intake and increase their calcium intake. It is also important to discontinue laxative and enema medications as these medications cause phosphorous excess. Discontinuing phosphate-binding medications can cause an increase in phosphorus.[1-5]

Case Study 6

Which of the following laboratory abnormalities would you expect to see in patients with hyperphosphatemia? (Select all that apply)

A. Hypokalemia
B. Hyperkalemia
C. Hypercalcemia
D. Hypocalcemia

The correct answers are A and D
Comment: Phosphorous also has an inverse relationship with calcium and potassium. If the phosphorous is high, the calcium and potassium will be low. The normal plasma inorganic phosphate (Pi) concentration in an adult is 2.5 to 4.5 mg/dL, and men have a slightly higher concentration than women. In children, the normal range is 4 to 7 mg/dL. A plasma phosphate level higher than 4.5 mg/dL is hyperphosphatemia. Phosphate plays an essential role in many

biological functions such as the formation of adenosine triphosphate (ATP), cyclic adenosine monophosphate (cAMP), phosphorylation of proteins, etc. Phosphate is also present in nucleic acids and acts as an important intracellular buffer.[1-5]

Normal adult dietary phosphate intake is around 1000 mg/day. Ninety percent of this is absorbed primarily in the jejunum. In the small intestine, phosphate is absorbed both actively and by passive paracellular diffusion. Active absorption is through sodium-dependent phosphate cotransporter type IIb (NPT2b).[1-5]

Kidneys excrete 90% of the daily phosphate load while the gastrointestinal tract excretes the remainder. As phosphorus is not significantly bound to albumin, most of it gets filtered at the glomerulus. Therefore, the number of functional nephrons plays a significant role in phosphorus homeostasis; 75% of filtered phosphorus is reabsorbed in the proximal tubule, approximately 10% in the distal tubule, and 15% is lost in the urine. In the luminal side of the proximal tubule, the primary phosphorus transporter is the type II Na/Pi cotransporter (NPT2a). The activity of this transporter is increased by low serum phosphorus and 1,25(OH) 2 vitamin D, increasing reabsorption of phosphorus. Renal tubular phosphorus reabsorption also increases by volume depletion, chronic hypocalcemia, metabolic alkalosis, insulin, estrogen, thyroid hormone, and growth hormone. Tubular reabsorption of phosphorus decreases by parathyroid hormone (PTH), phosphatonins, acidosis, hyperphosphatemia, chronic hypercalcemia, and volume expansion.[1-5]

Phosphorus is transported out of the renal cell by a phosphate-anion exchanger located in the basolateral membrane. Phosphate homeostasis is under direct hormonal influence of calcitriol, PTH, and phosphatonins, including fibroblast growth factor 23 (FGF-23). Receptors for vitamin D, FGF-23, PTH, and calcium-sensing receptor (CaSR) also play an important role in phosphate homeostasis. Serum phosphate level is maintained through a complex interaction between intestinal phosphate absorption, renal phosphate handling, and the transcellular movement of phosphate that occurs between intracellular fluid and bone storage pool. A transient shift of phosphate into the cells is also stimulated by insulin and respiratory alkalosis.[1-5]

PTH is an important hormone that controls calcium and phosphate concentration through stimulation of renal tubular calcium reabsorption and bone resorption. PTH also stimulates the conversion of 25-hydroxy vitamin D to 1,25 dihydroxy vitamin D in renal tubular cells, which promotes intestinal calcium absorption as well as bone turnover. Any changes in ionized calcium concentration gets sensed by CaSR on the surface of parathyroid cells, Increase in calcium activates these receptors, which inhibit parathyroid hormone secretion and decreases renal tubular reabsorption of calcium through second messengers.[1-5]

Hypocalcemia, induced by increased phosphate levels, can also produce these effects. However, changes in phosphate concentration should be significant to produce substantial changes in serum calcium. Hyperphosphatemia can also directly stimulate parathyroid hormone synthesis as well as parathyroid cellular proliferation. Several drugs, such as penicillin, corticosteroids, some diuretics, furosemide, and thiazides, can induce hyperphosphatemia as an adverse reaction.[1-5]

1,25 dihydroxycholecalciferol (DHCC) is the activated form of vitamin D. It increases intestinal phosphate absorption by enhancing the expression of NPT2b transporter and stimulates renal phosphate absorption by increasing expression of NPT2a and NPT2c in the proximal tubule. 1,25 DHCC also enhances FGF23 production. The 1,25(OH) 2D also suppresses the synthesis of PTH and enhances FGF23 production.[1-5]

FGF23 is a phosphatonin that is produced primarily by osteocytes and, to a lesser extent, by osteoblasts. It is a hormone that consists of 251 amino acid residues, including a signal peptide comprising 24 amino acids.

It inhibits renal tubular reabsorption of phosphate. FGF23 exerts its effects by binding to the FGFR1-Klotho complex. Alpha Klotho serves as a coreceptor. FGF23 suppresses NPT2a and NPT2c expression at the proximal renal tubules, thereby inhibiting renal phosphate reabsorption. FGF23 also reduces the circulatory level of 1,25(OH) 2D by decreasing the expression of 1-alpha-hydroxylase and increasing the expression of 24-hydroxylase.

Renal failure is the most common cause of hyperphosphatemia. A glomerular filtration rate of less than 30 mL/min significantly reduces the filtration of Pi, increasing its serum level.

Other less common causes include a high intake of phosphorus or increased renal reabsorption. High intake of phosphate can result due to excessive use of phosphate-containing laxatives or enemas, and vitamin D intoxication. Vitamin D increases intestinal phosphate absorption.[1-5]

Hypoparathyroidism, acromegaly, and thyrotoxicosis enhance renal phosphate reabsorption resulting in hyperphosphatemia.

Hyperphosphatemia can also be due to genetic causes. Several genetic deficiencies can lead to hypoparathyroidism, pseudohypoparathyroidism, and decreased FGF-23 activity.

Pseudohyperphosphatemia is a laboratory artifact sometimes seen in patients with hyperglobulinemia, hyperlipidemia, and hyperbilirubinemia. This artifact is due to interference in phosphate assay.[1-5]

Case Study 7

Patients with hyperphosphatemia may present with which symptoms?

A. Muscle cramps, tetany, and periorbital numbness
B. Hyperhidrosis
C. Migraine, persistent dizziness
D. Pallor, skin discoloration

The correct answer is A

Comment: Most patients with hyperphosphatemia are asymptomatic. However, some may experience hypocalcemic symptoms, including muscle cramps, tetany, and perioral numbness or tingling. Other possible symptoms include bone and joint pain, pruritus, and rash. More often, patients report symptoms related to the underlying cause of the hyperphosphatemia.[1-8]

Case Study 8

Which might be suggestive of renal failure, hypoparathyroidism, and pseudohypoparathyroidism as a cause of hyperphosphatemia?

A. Relatively low levels of intact parathyroid hormone (PTH)
B. High serum calcium and phosphate levels
C. Low levels of PTH and vitamin D
D. Low serum calcium levels with high phosphate levels

The correct answer is D

Comment: Low serum calcium levels along with high phosphate levels are observed with renal failure, hypoparathyroidism, and pseudohypoparathyroidism. Blood urea nitrogen (BUN) and creatinine values can also help to determine whether renal failure is the cause of hyperphosphatemia.

Relatively low levels of intact PTH along with normal renal function can be found in patients with primary or acquired hypoparathyroidism. High serum calcium and increased phosphate levels are observed with vitamin D intoxication and milk-alkali syndrome. Low levels of PTH and vitamin D are seen in milk-alkali syndrome.[1-8]

Case Study 9

How often should serum levels of phosphate and calcium be assessed in patients with chronic kidney disease (CKD)?

A. Every 6 to 12 months in patients with stage 3 CKD
B. Every 1 to 2 months among patients with stage 4 CKD
C. Every 3 to 6 months in all patients with CKD, regardless of stage
D. Every 1 to 3 months in patients with stage 3 CKD

The correct answer is A

Comment: In patients with CKD, the development of metabolic bone disease involves a complex interaction of phosphate, calcium, and parathyroid hormone (PTH). As such, serial assessments of all three parameters are recommended in patients with CKD stage G3a-G5D to guide treatment. According to the Kidney Disease: Improving Global Outcomes (KDIGO) guidelines, reasonable monitoring intervals are as follows[1-8]:

- CKD G3a-G3b—Serum phosphate and calcium, every 6 to 12 months; PTH, based on baseline level and CKD progression
- CKD G4—Serum phosphate and calcium, every 3 to 6 months; PTH, every 6 to 12 months
- CKD G5, including G5D—Serum phosphate and calcium, every 1 to 3 months; PTH, every 3 to 6 months

Case Study 10

When should phosphate-lowering therapies be initiated in patients with chronic kidney disease (CKD)?

A. In all circumstances, unless contraindicated
B. Upon initiation of dialysis
C. Only in patients with progressive or persistent hyperphosphatemia
D. To those with glomerular filtration rate (GFR) less than 8 to $10 \, \text{mL/min/1.73} \, \text{m}^2$

The correct answer is C

Comment: In earlier releases of the Kidney Disease: Improving Global Outcomes (KDIGO) guidelines, clinicians were advised to maintain phosphate in the normal range in patients with CKD. However, while acknowledging that preventing, rather than treating, hyperphosphatemia may be beneficial in patients with advanced CKD, the working group believes more data are needed to ascertain the risk/benefit ratio. Thus, current recommendations suggest phosphate-lowering therapies be administered to patients with progressive or persistent hyperphosphatemia only.[1-8]

Case Study 11

What role do dietary interventions play in the management of phosphate levels in patients with chronic kidney disease (CKD)?

A. Dietary phosphate restriction is no longer recommended
B. Dietary phosphate intake should be limited in all patients with advanced CKD (stages 3 to 5)
C. Dietary phosphate restriction should only be used in conjunction with phosphate-lowering therapies
D. Dietary phosphate intake should be limited in all patients with CKD regardless of stage

The correct answer is B

Comments: Restricting dietary phosphate is an important practice for patients with advanced CKD and it is one of the strategies for correcting hyperphosphatemia. However, it is a complex and challenging task, and diet alone is often insufficient and unreliable for keeping phosphate concentrations within the recommended range. Consequently, many patients are advised to restrict dietary phosphate intake in addition to adequate dialysis and phosphate-lowering therapies.[1-8]

Renal failure is the most common cause of hyperphosphatemia. A glomerular filtration rate of less than 30 mL/min significantly reduces the filtration of inorganic phosphate, increasing its serum level.

Other less common causes include a high intake of phosphorus or increased renal reabsorption. High intake of phosphate can result due to excessive use of phosphate-containing laxatives or enemas, and vitamin D intoxication. Vitamin D increases intestinal phosphate absorption.

Hypoparathyroidism, acromegaly, and thyrotoxicosis enhance renal phosphate reabsorption resulting in hyperphosphatemia. Hyperphosphatemia can also be due to genetic causes. Several genetic deficiencies can lead to hypoparathyroidism, pseudohypoparathyroidism, and decreased fibroblast growth factor 23 (FGF-23) activity.[1-8]

Pseudohyperphosphatemia is a laboratory artifact sometimes seen in patients with hyperglobulinemia, hyperlipidemia, and hyperbilirubinemia. This artifact is due to interference in phosphate assay.

An acute increase in phosphate load can be due to exogenous or endogenous causes. Phosphate being the major intracellular anion, massive tissue breakdown due to any cause can lead to the release of intracellular phosphate into the extracellular fluid. Massive tissue breakdown can result from rhabdomyolysis, tumor lysis syndrome, or severe hemolysis.

Approximately, kidneys excrete 90% of daily phosphate load; a decrease in renal function causes decreased secretion and increased retention of phosphate. High serum phosphate levels are seen only in the late stages of chronic kidney disease. Activation of compensatory mechanisms, including an increase in FGF23 and parathyroid hormone (PTH) secretion, prevent an increase in serum phosphate during the early stages of CKD. Both FGF 23 and PTH increase fractional excretion of phosphate per functioning nephron, compensating for the progressive loss of functioning nephron mass. As CKD progresses, these mechanisms are unable to overcome the input of phosphate from dietary intake, leading to hyperphosphatemia.[1-8]

Renal failure also results in reduced synthesis of calcitriol and secondary hyperparathyroidism, causing increased osteoclastic bone reabsorption and release of calcium and phosphate into the circulation. Metabolic acidosis in renal failure can also contribute to hyperphosphatemia by the cellular shift of phosphate from cells. Lactic acidosis and diabetic ketoacidosis can rarely cause massive cellular shifts of phosphate out of the cells.[1-8]

Pseudohypoparathyroidism (PHP) is a rare condition characterized by a resistance to PTH at its receptor. Its manifestations include low serum calcium, high serum phosphate, and inappropriately high PTH levels. PTH resistance can result from impaired cyclic adenosine monophosphate (cAMP) generation, accelerated cAMP degradation, or impaired cAMP-dependent protein kinase activation. Impaired production of cAMP and the defects in the Gsa protein, which couples PTH1 receptor to adenylyl cyclase, are most common. As this signal transduction pathway is used by many G-protein–coupled receptors (GPCRs), reduced responsiveness to numerous other hormones, including thyroid-stimulating hormone (TSH), is also seen.[1-8]

Hypoparathyroidism is also a rare disease that results in hypocalcemia. The most common cause is an injury to or removal of the parathyroid gland during anterior neck surgery. Symptoms include paresthesias, muscle cramps, seizures, and laryngospasm. It can also result from mutations in the autoimmune regulator (AIRE) gene resulting in hypoparathyroidism, mucocutaneous candidiasis, adrenal insufficiency, and malabsorption. AIRE plays a role in shaping central immunological tolerance by building the thymic microarchitecture, facilitating the negative selection of T cells in the thymus, and inducing a specific subset of regulatory T cells. The mutation in this gene leads to a form of hypoparathyroidism called autoimmune polyglandular failure type 1 (APS1), also called autoimmune polyendocrinopathy candidiasis ectodermal dystrophy (APECED). In this disease, hypoparathyroidism is usually the first of multiple autoimmune endocrine disorders to appear.[1-8]

Albright hereditary osteodystrophy (AHO) findings include short stature, shortened fourth metacarpals and other bones of the hands and feet, rounded face, obesity, dental hypoplasia, and soft-tissue calcifications/ossifications and cognitive impairment. Patients with pseudohypoparathyroidism have AHO and PTH resistance resulting in hypocalcemia and hyperphosphatemia. Patients with pseudo-pseudohypoparathyroidism (pseudo PHP) have an AHO phenotype but no impairment in mineral metabolism, that is, normal calcium and phosphate levels.[1-8]

The Kidney Disease: Improving Global Outcomes (KDIGO) guidelines for the management of hyperphosphatemia suggest that, in dialysis patients, phosphate levels require lowering toward the normal range; however, there is no given specific target level. In chronic kidney disease patients not receiving dialysis, serum phosphate levels require maintenance in the normal range (i.e., under 4.5 mg/dL [1.45 mmol/L]). There are several strategies to control phosphate levels.[1-8]

If renal function is good, renal phosphate excretion can increase through extracellular volume expansion by saline infusion and diuretics. Dietary restriction of phosphate is effective both in predialysis and in dialysis patients. KDIGO recommends a daily phosphate intake of 800 to 1000 mg/dL with a daily protein intake of 1.2 g/kg body weight. Also, it is reasonable to consider phosphate sources (e.g., animal, vegetable, additives) in making dietary recommendations. Severe protein restriction can cause malnutrition and, eventually, poorer outcomes. If renal function is impaired, it is an indication for hemodialysis.[1-8]

In patients with persistently or progressively elevated phosphate despite dietary phosphate restriction, phosphate binders are the agent of choice. These are also used, concurrently with dietary restriction, when phosphate levels at presentation are very high (> 6 mg/dL).

Phosphate binders reduce the absorption of dietary phosphate in the gastrointestinal tract, by exchanging the anion phosphate with an active cation (carbonate, acetate, oxyhydroxide, and citrate) to form a nonabsorbable compound that gets excreted in the feces. Aluminum-based agents are amongst the most effective and best tolerated. But doubts regarding their potential to cause aluminum toxicity, presenting with encephalopathy, osteomalacia, microcytic anemia, and premature death, have discouraged their prolonged use. Calcium-based binders (e.g., calcium carbonate and calcium acetate) are effective and do not have adverse effects associated with aluminum-based agents. However, they can lead to a positive calcium balance, which can aggravate the development of ectopic calcification in the media and intima of arterial vessels, a major contributing factor for the excess cardiovascular mortality observed in CKD patients. Magnesium carbonate effectively reduces serum phosphate levels and shows good gastrointestinal tolerance. It also reduces vascular calcification by interfering with hydroxyapatite formation.[1-8]

Sevelamer is a cross-linked polymer that exchanges phosphate with hydrochloride (HCl) or carbonate in the gastrointestinal tract. The phosphate-laden polymer gets excreted in the feces. Both sevelamer HCl and sevelamer carbonate are options. Besides controlling hyperphosphatemia, sevelamer also improves endothelial function, binds bile salts, resulting in a significant reduction in serum total cholesterol and low-density lipoprotein cholesterol. However, this action may interfere with the absorption of fat and fat-soluble vitamins.[1-8]

Lanthanum carbonate is a chewable, calcium-free phosphate binder, which uses metal lanthanum for phosphate chelation. Lanthanum carbonate binds phosphate to form the nonabsorbable compound lanthanum phosphate.

Ferric citrate exchanges citrate with phosphate in the gastrointestinal tract to form ferric phosphate, which is insoluble and excreted in the feces. An additional advantage of ferric citrate is that it increases serum ferritin, reducing the need for intravenous iron and erythropoietin stimulating agents in chronic kidney disease.[1-8]

Sucroferric oxyhydroxide is a chewable, iron-based phosphate binder. A lower dose helps in better compliance. As iron gets excreted as part of the phosphate complex, it does not cause iron overload.

Nicotinic acid and nicotinamide are drugs used in lowering sodium-dependent intestinal phosphate absorption via a reduction in NaPi-IIb expression. The degree of reduction is modest. Adverse effects included flushing, nausea, diarrhea, thrombocytopenia, and accumulation of potentially toxic metabolites.

Tenapanor inhibits sodium/hydrogen ion-exchanger isoform 3 (NHE3), which plays a role in secondary active phosphate absorption. It thus reduces intestinal sodium and phosphate absorption.[1-8]

Both peritoneal and hemodialysis remove phosphate, but the amount of phosphate absorbed from a normal diet is for more than that removed by any of these dialysis methods. Recommendations are for more intensive dialysis to improve phosphate removal.

For better control of hyperphosphatemia, control of secondary hyperparathyroidism is essential, using vitamin D metabolites and the calcium-sensing receptor agonists. Calcitriol or synthetic vitamin D analogs should not be given unless the serum phosphate concentration is less than 5.5 mg/dL and the serum calcium is less than 9.5 mg/dL, as these agents can increase the serum calcium and phosphate, leading to metastatic and vascular calcification in patients with hyperphosphatemia before treatment.[1-8]

For all dialysis patients, the target serum levels of phosphate should be between 3.5 and 5.5 mg/dL (1.13 and 1.78 mmol/L). Serum levels of corrected total calcium should be maintained lower than 9.5 mg/dL (< 2.37 mmol/L). The values of the parathyroid hormone (PTH) should remain less than two to nine times the upper limit for the PTH assay.[1-8]

References

Case Study 1

1. Lane JW, Rehak NN, Hortin GL, et al. Pseudohyperphosphatemia associated with high-dose liposomal amphotericin B therapy. *Clin Chim Acta.* 2008;387:145–149.
2. Larner AJ. Pseudohyperphosphatemia. *Clin Biochem.* 1995;28:391–393.
3. Liamis G, Liberopoulos E, Barkas F, et al. Spurious electrolyte disorders: a diagnostic challenge for clinicians. *Am J Nephrol.* 2013;38:50–57.
4. Albersen M, Bökenkamp A, Schotman H, et al. Hyperphosphatemia in an 11-year-old girl with acute myeloid leukemia: answers. *Pediatr Nephrol.* 2019;34:627–629. https://doi.org/10.1007/s00467-018-4101-5.

Case Study 2

1. Broman M, Wilsson AMJ, Hansson F, et al. Analysis of hypo- and hyperphosphatemia in an intensive care unit cohort. *Anesth Analg.* 2017;124(6):1897–1905.
2. Martin KJ, González EA. Prevention and control of phosphate retention/hyperphosphatemia in CKD-MBD: what is normal, when to start, and how to treat? *Clin J Am Soc Nephrol.* 2011;6(2):440–446.
3. Leaf DE, Wolf M. A physiologic-based approach to the evaluation of a patient with hyperphosphatemia. *Am J Kidney Dis.* 2013;61(2):330–336.
4. Knoderer CA, Knoderer HM. Hyperphosphatemia in pediatric oncology patients receiving liposomal amphotericin B. *J Pediatr Pharmacol Ther.* 2011;16(2):87–91.
5. Leung J, Crook M. Disorders of phosphate metabolism. *J Clin Pathol.* 2019;72(11):741–747.

Case Study 3

1. Broman M, Wilsson AMJ, Hansson F, Klarin B. Analysis of hypo- and hyperphosphatemia in an intensive care unit cohort. *Anesth Analg.* 2017;124(6):1897–1905.
2. Martin KJ, González EA. Prevention and control of phosphate retention/hyperphosphatemia in CKD-MBD: what is normal, when to start, and how to treat? *Clin J Am Soc Nephrol.* 2011;6(2):440–446.
3. Leaf DE, Wolf M. A physiologic-based approach to the evaluation of a patient with hyperphosphatemia. *Am J Kidney Dis.* 2013;61(2):330–336.

4. Knoderer CA, Knoderer HM. Hyperphosphatemia in pediatric oncology patients receiving liposomal amphotericin B. *J Pediatr Pharmacol Ther.* 2011;16(2):87–91.
5. Leung J, Crook M. Disorders of phosphate metabolism. *J Clin Pathol.* 2019;72(11):741–747.

Case Study 4

1. Broman M, Wilsson AMJ, Hansson F, et al. Analysis of hypo- and hyperphosphatemia in an intensive care unit cohort. *Anesth Analg.* 2017;124(6):1897–1905.
2. Martin KJ, González EA. Prevention and control of phosphate retention/hyperphosphatemia in CKD-MBD: what is normal, when to start, and how to treat? *Clin J Am Soc Nephrol.* 2011;6(2):440–446.
3. Leaf DE, Wolf M. A physiologic-based approach to the evaluation of a patient with hyperphosphatemia. *Am J Kidney Dis.* 2013;61(2):330–336.
4. Knoderer CA, Knoderer HM. Hyperphosphatemia in pediatric oncology patients receiving liposomal amphotericin B. *J Pediatr Pharmacol Ther.* 2011;16(2):87–91.
5. Leung J, Crook M. Disorders of phosphate metabolism. *J Clin Pathol.* 2019;72(11):741–747.

Case Study 5

1. Broman M, Wilsson AMJ, Hansson F, et al. Analysis of hypo- and hyperphosphatemia in an intensive care unit cohort. *Anesth Analg.* 2017;124(6):1897–1905.
2. Martin KJ, González EA. Prevention and control of phosphate retention/hyperphosphatemia in CKD-MBD: what is normal, when to start, and how to treat? *Clin J Am Soc Nephrol.* 2011;6(2):440–446.
3. Leaf DE, Wolf M. A physiologic-based approach to the evaluation of a patient with hyperphosphatemia. *Am J Kidney Dis.* 2013;61(2):330–336.
4. Knoderer CA, Knoderer HM. Hyperphosphatemia in pediatric oncology patients receiving liposomal amphotericin B. *J Pediatr Pharmacol Ther.* 2011;16(2):87–91.
5. Leung J, Crook M. Disorders of phosphate metabolism. *J Clin Pathol.* 2019;72(11):741–747.

Case Study 6

1. Broman M, Wilson AMJ, Hansson F, et al. Analysis of hypo- and hyperphosphatemia in an intensive care unit cohort. *Anesth Analg.* 2017;124(6):1897–1905.
2. Martin KJ, González EA. Prevention and control of phosphate retention/hyperphosphatemia in CKD-MBD: what is normal, when to start, and how to treat? *Clin J Am Soc Nephrol.* 2011;6(2). 440–336.
3. Leaf DE, Wolf M. A physiologic-based approach to the evaluation of a patient with hyperphosphatemia. *Am J Kidney Dis.* 2013;61(2):330–336.
4. Knoderer CA, Knoderer HM. Hyperphosphatemia in pediatric oncology patients receiving liposomal amphotericin B. *J Pediatr Pharmacol Ther.* 2011;16(2):87–91.
5. Leung J, Crook M. Disorders of phosphate metabolism. *J Clin Pathol.* 2019;72(11):741–747.

Case Study 7

1. Martin KJ, González EA. Prevention and control of phosphate retention/hyperphosphatemia in CKD-MBD: what is normal, when to start, and how to treat? *Clin J Am Soc Nephrol.* 201;6(2):440–446.
2. Fathi I, Sakr M. Review of tumoral calcinosis: a rare clinico-pathological entity. *World J Clin Cases.* 2014;16;2(9):409–414.
3. Linglart A, Levine MA, Jüppner H. Pseudohypoparathyroidism. *Endocrinol Metab Clin North Am.* 2018;47(4):865–888.
4. Bruserud Ø, Oftedal BE, Wolff AB, et al. AIRE-mutations and autoimmune disease. *Curr Opin Immunol.* 2016;43:8–15.
5. Gafni RI, Collins MT. Hypoparathyroidism. *N Engl J Med.* 2019;380(18):1738–1747.
6. Beto J, Bhatt N, Gerbeling T, et al. Overview of the 2017 KDIGO CKD-MBD update: practice implications for adult hemodialysis patients. *J Ren Nutr.* 2019;29(1):2–15.
7. Barreto FC, Barreto DV, Massy ZA, et al. Strategies for phosphate control in patients with CKD. *Kidney Int Rep.* 2019;4(8):1043–1056.
8. Monge M, Shahapuni I, Oprisiu R, et al. Reappraisal of 2003 NKF-K/DOQI guidelines for management of hyperparathyroidism in chronic kidney disease patients. *Nat Clin Pract Nephrol.* 2006;2(6):326–336.

Case Study 8

1. Martin KJ, González EA. Prevention and control of phosphate retention/hyperphosphatemia in CKD-MBD: what is normal, when to start, and how to treat? *Clin J Am Soc Nephrol.* 201;6(2):440–446.
2. Fathi I, Sakr M. Review of tumoral calcinosis: a rare clinico-pathological entity. *World J Clin Cases.* 2014;16;2(9):409–414.
3. Linglart A, Levine MA, Jüppner H. Pseudohypoparathyroidism. *Endocrinol Metab Clin North Am.* 2018;47(4):865–888.
4. Bruserud Ø, Oftedal BE, Wolff AB, et al. AIRE-mutations and autoimmune disease. *Curr Opin Immunol.* 2016;43:8–15.
5. Gafni RI, Collins MT. Hypoparathyroidism. *N Engl J Med.* 2019;380(18):1738–1747.
6. Beto J, Bhatt N, Gerbeling T, et al. Overview of the 2017 KDIGO CKD-MBD update: practice implications for adult hemodialysis patients. *J Ren Nutr.* 2019;29(1):2–15.
7. Barreto FC, Barreto DV, Massy ZA, et al. Strategies for phosphate control in patients with CKD. *Kidney Int Rep.* 2019;4(8):1043–1056.
8. Monge M, Shahapuni I, Oprisiu R, et al. Reappraisal of 2003 NKF-K/DOQI guidelines for management of hyperparathyroidism in chronic kidney disease patients. *Nat Clin Pract Nephrol.* 2006;2(6):326–336.

Case Study 9

1. Martin KJ, González EA. Prevention and control of phosphate retention/hyperphosphatemia in CKD-MBD: what is normal, when to start, and how to treat? *Clin J Am Soc Nephrol.* 201;6(2):440–446.
2. Fathi I, Sakr M. Review of tumoral calcinosis: a rare clinico-pathological entity. *World J Clin Cases.* 2014;16;2(9):409–414.
3. Linglart A, Levine MA, Jüppner H. Pseudohypoparathyroidism. *Endocrinol Metab Clin North Am.* 2018;47(4):865–888.
4. Bruserud Ø, Oftedal BE, Wolff AB, et al. AIRE-mutations and autoimmune disease. *Curr Opin Immunol.* 2016;43:8–15.
5. Gafni RI, Collins MT. Hypoparathyroidism. *N Engl J Med.* 2019;380(18):1738–1747.
6. Beto J, Bhatt N, Gerbeling T, et al. Overview of the 2017 KDIGO CKD-MBD update: practice implications for adult hemodialysis patients. *J Ren Nutr.* 2019;29(1):2–15.
7. Barreto FC, Barreto DV, Massy ZA, et al. Strategies for phosphate control in patients with CKD. *Kidney Int Rep.* 2019;4(8):1043–1056.
8. Monge M, Shahapuni I, Oprisiu R, et al. Reappraisal of 2003 NKF-K/DOQI guidelines for management of hyperparathyroidism in chronic kidney disease patients. *Nat Clin Pract Nephrol.* 2006;2(6):326–336.

Case Study 10

1. Martin KJ, González EA. Prevention and control of phosphate retention/hyperphosphatemia in CKD-MBD: what is normal, when to start, and how to treat? *Clin J Am Soc Nephrol.* 201;6(2):440–446.
2. Fathi I, Sakr M. Review of tumoral calcinosis: a rare clinico-pathological entity. *World J Clin Cases.* 2014;16;2(9):409–414.
3. Linglart A, Levine MA, Jüppner H. Pseudohypoparathyroidism. *Endocrinol Metab Clin North Am.* 2018;47(4):865–888.
4. Bruserud Ø, Oftedal BE, Wolff AB, et al. AIRE-mutations and autoimmune disease. *Curr Opin Immunol.* 2016;43:8–15.
5. Gafni RI, Collins MT. Hypoparathyroidism. *N Engl J Med.* 2019;380(18):1738–1747.
6. Beto J, Bhatt N, Gerbeling T, et al. Overview of the 2017 KDIGO CKD-MBD update: practice implications for adult hemodialysis patients. *J Ren Nutr.* 2019;29(1):2–15.
7. Barreto FC, Barreto DV, Massy ZA, et al. Strategies for phosphate control in patients with CKD. *Kidney Int Rep.* 2019;4(8):1043–1056.
8. Monge M, Shahapuni I, Oprisiu R, et al. Reappraisal of 2003 NKF-K/DOQI guidelines for management of hyperparathyroidism in chronic kidney disease patients. *Nat Clin Pract Nephrol.* 2006;2(6):326–336.

Case Study 11

1. Martin KJ, González EA. Prevention and control of phosphate retention/hyperphosphatemia in CKD-MBD: what is normal, when to start, and how to treat? *Clin J Am Soc Nephrol.* 201;6(2):440–446.

2. Fathi I, Sakr M. Review of tumoral calcinosis: a rare clinico-pathological entity. *World J Clin Cases*. 2014;16;2(9):409–414.
3. Linglart A, Levine MA, Jüppner H. Pseudohypoparathyroidism. *Endocrinol Metab Clin North Am*. 2018;47(4):865–888.
4. Bruserud Ø, Oftedal BE, Wolff AB, et al. AIRE-mutations and autoimmune disease. *Curr Opin Immunol*. 2016;43:8–15.
5. Gafni RI, Collins MT. Hypoparathyroidism. *N Engl J Med*. 2019;380(18):1738–1747.
6. Beto J, Bhatt N, Gerbeling T, et al. Overview of the 2017 KDIGO CKD-MBD update: practice implications for adult hemodialysis patients. *J Ren Nutr*. 2019;29(1):2–15.
7. Barreto FC, Barreto DV, Massy ZA, et al. Strategies for phosphate control in patients with CKD. *Kidney Int Rep*. 2019;4(8):1043–1056.
8. Monge M, Shahapuni I, Oprisiu R, et al. Reappraisal of 2003 NKF-K/DOQI guidelines for management of hyperparathyroidism in chronic kidney disease patients. *Nat Clin Pract Nephrol*. 2006;2(6):326–336.

CHAPTER 11

Hypomagnesemia

Case Study 1

You are asked to evaluate a family with a high incidence of hypercalciuria and nephrolithiasis, and you find that two children born to a sibling with hypercalciuria and nephrolithiasis died in early childhood of kidney failure and had nephrocalcinosis. An extensive work-up reveals that the family members affected with hypercalciuria also demonstrated hypermagnesuria.

Which one of the following is the most likely basis for this disorder?

A. Isolated recessive hypomagnesemia
B. Familial hypomagnesemia secondary to mutations in paracellin-1 gene
C. Familial defect in calcium-sensing receptor
D. Hypomagnesemia with secondary hypercalciuria associated with a defect in tubular transport of phosphate
E. Impaired proximal tubular oxalate transporter

The correct answer is B

Comment: Isolated recessive hypomagnesemia is not associated with hypercalciuria, and defects in the calcium-sensing receptor are not associated with nephrolithiasis or kidney failure in this fashion. Defects in the tubular reabsorption of phosphate are associated with hypocalcemia. An abnormality in oxalate transport would not produce hypercalciuria. The combination of hypomagnesemia, hypercalciuria, nephrocalcinosis, and kidney failure suggests the presence of familiar hypomagnesemia due to paracellin-1 gene mutation, a tight-junction protein-mediating paracellular transport.[1-8]

Case Study 2

A 16-year-old girl complained of easy fatigability and generalized muscle weakness. She denied vomiting or the use of any medications. Physical examination revealed a thin anxious girl with a normal blood pressure. Her examination was otherwise unremarkable. Her serum sodium was 141 mmol/L; potassium, 2.1 mmol/L; chloride, 85 mmol/L; bicarbonate, 45 mmol/L; calcium, 9.5 mg/dL (reference: 8.5 to 10.3 mg/dL); phosphate, 3.2 mg/dL (reference: 2.8 to 4.5 mg/dL); magnesium, 1.2 mg/dL (reference: 1.8 to 2.3 mg/dL); and albumin, 4.6 g/dL (reference: 3.5 to 5.0 g/dL).

Which of the following statements is true? (Select all that may apply)

A. Hypokalemia can alter the renal handling of magnesium and cause hypomagnesemia
B. Hypomagnesemia can alter the renal handling of potassium and cause hypokalemia
C. Both statements are true
D. Neither statement is true

The correct answer is B

Comment: Magnesium is required for adequate renal health handling of potassium. Hypomagnesemia can cause hypokalemia because of the increased urinary loss of potassium, likely by opening potassium channels in the thick ascending loop of Henle. This may become apparent when hypokalemia persists despite potassium supplementation.[1-4]

Case Study 3

Which of the following studies would be the best initial laboratory to determine the cause of the hypomagnesemia in this patient? (Select all that apply)

    A. Urine diuretic screen
    B. Plasma renin and aldosterone levels
    C. Plasma cortisol level
    D. Twenty-four-hour urine for potassium and aldosterone levels
    E. Twenty-four-hour urine for magnesium, calcium, chloride, and creatinine levels

The correct answers are A and E

Comment: The findings of hypokalemia, metabolic alkalosis, and a normal blood pressure suggest the diagnosis of secondary hyperaldosteronism, vomiting, diuretic abuse, Bartter syndrome, or Gitelman syndrome. Measurement of urinary chloride, calcium, and magnesium is useful in the differentiation between these disorders. The urinary chloride concentration is typically less than 15 mmol/L in hypovolemia due to surreptitious vomiting. In contrast, a urinary chloride greater than 15 mmol/L suggests diuretic abuse, Bartter syndrome, or Gitelman syndrome. Measurement of the urine calcium will help to distinguish between Bartter syndrome and Gitelman syndrome. Screening urine for diuretics is indicated if surreptitious ingestion is suspected. Measurement of the urinary magnesium will help to distinguish between gastrointestinal (GI) and renal losses as the major contributor.[1-3]

Case Study 4

The fractional excretion of magnesium was 6.5%, the urine chloride was 56 mEq/L, and the urine calcium-creatinine ratio was 3.2 (reference range: < 0.22).

What is the most likely diagnosis now? (Select all that apply)

    A. Bartter syndrome
    B. Primary hyperaldosteronism
    C. Loop diuretic abuse
    D. Apparent mineralocorticoid excess
    E. Liddle syndrome
    F. Gitelman syndrome

The correct answers are A and C

Comment: Bartter syndrome can cause hypokalemia, metabolic alkalosis, and renal magnesium wasting, and hypomagnesemia without hypertension in a manner similar to that of loop diuretics.

Bartter syndrome is caused by mutations in a furosemide-sensitive ion transport mechanism in the loop of Henle and is associated with hypercalciuria.[1,2]

Case Study 5

Which study would you like now to differentiate between Bartter syndrome and diuretic abuse?

    A. Plasma renin activity and plasma aldosterone level
    B. Twenty-four-hour urine for calcium, magnesium, and creatinine
    C. Twenty-four-hour urine for sodium, potassium, and creatinine
    D. Urine diuretic screen

The correct answer is D
Comment: A diuretic screen is the only way to rule out diuretic abuse. The diuretic screen was negative.[1,2]

Case Study 6

Suppose the laboratory staff call to tell you that the urinary calcium–creatinine ratio was misreported and the correct value is 0.20, not 3.2.

What is the most likely diagnosis now?

    A. Gitelman syndrome
    B. Bartter syndrome
    C. Primary hyperparathyroidism
    D. Isolated recessive renal magnesium wasting

The correct answer is A
Comment: Gitelman syndrome is the only condition among the above, which is associated with hypocalciuria. Gitelman syndrome is a variant of Bartter syndrome, characterized by hypokalemia, metabolic alkalosis, hypomagnesemia, renal magnesium wasting, and normal blood pressure. Gitelman syndrome is caused by loss-of-function mutations in a thiazide-sensitive ion transport mechanism in the distal nephron and is associated with hypocalciuria. Bartter syndrome and primary hyperparathyroidism are associated with hypercalciuria. Isolated recessive magnesium wasting is characterized by renal magnesium wasting in the absence of hypocalcemia or hypercalciuria.[1-4]

Case Study 7

Which of the following would be most beneficial therapeutic effects in a patient with Gitelman syndrome? (Select all that apply)

    A. Thiazide diuretics
    B. Potassium-sparing diuretics
    C. Low-salt diet
    D. Oral magnesium and potassium supplementation
    E. Loop diuretic

The correct answers are B and D
Comment: Magnesium supplements are typically necessary to increase the serum magnesium and the serum potassium concentrations. Amiloride can be very useful in this condition, because it may help to enhance distal tubular reabsorption of magnesium, as well as inhibit potassium secretion. She was treated with magnesium and potassium supplementation and amiloride. Serum

potassium level improved to 3.2 mEq/L and serum magnesium level rose to 2.2 mg/dL. Six months later, she was brought to the emergency department because of shock due to internal bleeding as a result of automobile accident. She received 7 units of blood transfusion and underwent repair of hepatic laceration. She was oliguric post operation for 4 days. The laboratory data revealed a hemoglobin of 12.6 g/dL; blood urea nitrogen (BUN), 55 mg/dL; serum creatinine, 3.9 mg/dL; serum sodium, 137 mmol/L; serum chloride, 95 mmol/L; serum potassium, 4.9 mmol/L; serum bicarbonate, 20 mmol/L; serum calcium, 5.5 mg/dL; serum phosphate, 5.5 mg/dL; and serum albumin, 3.9 g/dL. Urinalysis showed trace protein, negative for blood and glucose. The electrocardiography showed significant prolongation of the QT interval.[1–4]

Case Study 8

What should be done next to define the likely cause of the hypocalcemia?

    A. Draw blood for a parathyroid hormone (PTH) assay
    B. Give intravenous magnesium
    C. Draw blood for a plasma magnesium level
    D. Draw blood for a calcidiol level
    E. Draw blood for a calcitriol level

The correct answer is C

Comment: Hypermagnesemia can suppress parathyroid hormone level and can cause hypocalcemia. Checking the plasma magnesium level to look for hypermagnesemia as the cause of hypocalcemia is the best choice in this situation. The plasma magnesium level was 5.8 mg/dL. The physician in the emergency department rechecked her medications and realized that no one had discontinued the supplemental magnesium that she was receiving for Gitelman syndrome. Thus, hypermagnesemia and subsequent hypocalcemia may have ensued when she developed acute kidney failure. Hemodialysis was instituted and the magnesium supplements were discontinued. Hypermagnesemia resolved and hemodialysis was discontinued after two treatments. Serum creatinine level slowly returned to normal level over 7 days. She was subsequently returned on magnesium supplements.[1,2]

Case Study 9

You are asked to see a 19-year-old woman complaining of cramps and tightening in her throat. Past medical history is significant for mild hypertension for which she is being treated with hydrochlorothiazide, 12.5 mg/day. She had a total thyroidectomy for a large toxic, multinodular goiter 6 months earlier and is maintained on 1-thyroxine, 100 μg/day. Bone densitometry was consistent with osteoporosis, and she was started on alendronate, 10 mg/day. Five days prior to admission, she began to note intermittent severe cramps in her hands and feet. On the day of admission, she noted some tightening in her throat and came to the emergency room. She denies the use of any other medications or over-the counter supplements. On examination, her blood pressure is 140/86 mmHg; pulse, 86 beats/min; respiration, 12 breaths/min; temperature, 37°C; weight, 52.5 kg; and height, 159 cm. The rest of the physical examination revealed no abnormal sign. Laboratory studies revealed a hemoglobin of 13.0 g/L; leukocyte count, 5.1×10^9/L; sodium, 138 mmol/L; potassium, 4.1 mmol/L; chloride, 100 mmol/L; bicarbonate, 27 mmol/L; blood urea nitrogen, 6 mg/dL; creatinine, 0.7 mg/dL; calcium, 7.3 mg/dL (reference range: 8.5 to 10.3 mg/dL); phosphate, 6.3 mg/dL (reference range: 2.8 to 4.5 mg/dL); magnesium, 1.5 mg/dL (reference range: 1.8 to 2.3 mg/dL); and albumin, 4.2 g/dL (reference range: 3.5 to 5.0 g/dL). Urinalysis showed trace protein, and it was negative for glucose and blood. Her electrocardiography showed prolonged QT intervals.

What would you do at this point? (Select all that apply)

A. Draw parathyroid hormone level
B. Draw serum magnesium level
C. Draw calcitriol level
D. Draw calcidiol level
E. Give intravenous magnesium

The correct answers are A, B, and E
Comment: The combination of hypocalcemia and hypomagnesemia in the absence of kidney failure certainly suggests the presence of hypoparathyroidism. Hypomagnesemia can cause suppression of parathyroid hormone secretion and/or resistance to parathyroid hormone and produce acute hypocalcemia. It is appropriate to consider this and draw a serum magnesium level. In the absence of renal insufficiency, magnesium infusion is safe and reasonable while waiting for the results to come back from the laboratory. She remained symptomatic despite the intravenous magnesium administration. However, she responded to intravenous calcium and experienced relief of her acute symptoms. Her laboratory studies, which were obtained in the emergency department, returned as follows: PTH 15 ng/mL and serum magnesium 2.0 mg/dL.[1-3]

Case Study 10

What is the primary diagnosis?

A. Hypoparathyroidism
B. Alendronate toxicity
C. Vitamin D deficiency
D. Hypomagnesemia
E. Pseudohypoparathyroidism

The correct answer is A
Comment: She has hypocalcemia and a parathyroid hormone value that is inappropriately in the low-normal range, consistent with hyperparathyroidism. She likely had subclinical hypoparathyroidism that was undiagnosed and that now has been masked by alendronate therapy.[1-3]

Case Study 11

A 16-year-old girl presented for evaluation of severe hypomagnesemia of more than 10 years' duration (average serum magnesium concentration, 1.1; range, 0.5 to 2.8 mg/dL). She has a history of psychiatric disorders, including major depression, attention-deficit/hyperactivity disorder, anorexia nervosa, and past laxative abuse. Hypokalemia has rarely accompanied the hypomagnesemia (average serum potassium concentration, 4.0 (range, 3.4 to 4.8 mmol/L). There is no family history of renal or electrolyte disorders. She does not use tobacco, alcohol, or illicit substances. Based on psychiatric history, hypomagnesemia had previously been attributed to suspected surreptitious diuretic use. She denies vomiting, diuretic or laxative abuse, recent weight change, or diarrhea despite high-dose oral magnesium supplementation. Her concerns were diffuse myalgia and paresthesias of the upper extremities, upper back, neck, and thighs.

Relevant medications included intravenous magnesium sulfate infusions twice weekly and oral magnesium oxide, 4800 mg total daily dose. Examination revealed heart rate of 100 beats/min, blood pressure of 102/66 mmHg, body mass index of 23.4 kg/m², and afebrile temperature. She had diffuse tenderness to neck and upper-back palpation. Chvostek sign was negative.

Serum chemistry revealed sodium 136 mmol/L, potassium 4.3 mmol/L, chloride 98 mmol/L, bicarbonate 31 mmol/L, BUN 31 mg/dL, creatinine 1.1 mg/dL, magnesium 1.0 mg/dL, calcium 9.1 mg/dL, phosphorous 3.5 mg/dL, albumin 4.1 g/dL, parathyroid hormone (PTH) 31 pg/dL, and 25-hydroxyvitamin D 30 ng/mL. A 24-hour urine collection showed hypermagnesuria (magnesium excretion, 50 mg) and likely hypocalciuria (calcium excretion, 59 mg). Fractional excretion of magnesium was 10.6%. Renal ultrasound revealed a 1.2-cm simple left upper pole cyst.

What is the most likely cause of hypomagnesemia in this patient?

A. Hypomagnesemia related to Bartter syndrome
B. Hypomagnesemia related to Gitelman syndrome
C. Isolated dominant hypomagnesemia
D. Autosomal dominant tubulointerstitial kidney disease (ADTKD)

The correct answers are A, B, C, and D

Comment: Hypomagnesemia is broadly classified by either excessive gastrointestinal or renal losses. Gastrointestinal causes include those caused by short bowel and gastric bypass surgeries, malabsorption syndromes, and medications such as laxatives and proton pump inhibitors. Renal causes consist of processes that increase filtration or interfere with the reabsorption of magnesium along the nephron. These include an array of medications, most notably thiazide and loop diuretics, as well as aminoglycosides, amphotericin, pentamidine, cisplatin, calcineurin inhibitors, and antibodies targeting epidermal growth factors. Genetic causes of renal magnesium losses include Bartter and Gitelman syndromes.[1,2]

Case Study 12

What is the likely mechanism of hypomagnesemia in this patient?

A. Isolated dominant hypomagnesemia
B. Autosomal dominant tubulointerstitial kidney disease (ADTKD)
C. Gitelman syndrome
D. Bartter syndrome

The correct answers are A and B
Comment: The patient denied laxative abuse or diarrhea and was not taking medications that interfere with gastrointestinal magnesium absorption, such as a proton pump inhibitor. A renal magnesium wasting disorder was therefore considered and supported by elevated fractional excretion of magnesium (10.6%) despite a low serum magnesium concentration. The diuretic screen was negative. A genetic disorder was suspected. Classic Gitelman syndrome seemed less likely as the cause in the absence of hypokalemia, but a variant was considered.[1,2]

Case Study 13

What diagnostic studies would you now order?

A. Genetic testing
B. Twenty-four-hour urine collection for potassium
C. Twenty-four-hour urine collection for magnesium
D. Malabsorption syndrome

The correct answer is A
Genetic testing revealed a heterozygous hepatocyte nuclear factor 1β(HNF1B) whole-gene deletion located on chromosome 17q12, which encodes a transcription factor involved in multisystem

organogenesis. The variant is inherited in an autosomal dominant tubulointerstitial kidney disease (ADTKD) or de novo pattern. It manifests with a wide array of phenotypes, including hypomagnesemia, and is frequently associated with maturity-onset diabetes type 5. In one cohort, there was a 62% prevalence of hypomagnesemia associated with *HNF1B* mutations. Although not well understood, the encoded protein is thought to affect distal tubule magnesium handling. Although this patient's presentation is atypical given the lack of notable organ system developmental abnormalities, it is intriguing to consider her psychiatric disease as a potential component of the phenotype, given reported associations. The finding did not alter treatment. However, confirming a diagnosis accorded the patient's clinical and emotional validation, prevented further specialist referral and repetitive workup, and ultimately strengthened the patient-clinician relationship by promoting trust.[1-5]

Case Study 14

A 1-month-old male infant was admitted to the hospital with a history of recurrent convulsive seizures of 2 weeks duration. He was born at term (40-week gestation) at a normal birth weight of 2.76 kg following an uneventful pregnancy. He was the first child of healthy parents; there was no history of consanguinity. The infant was well until the 14th day of life when he developed convulsive seizures. On admission, the physicians observed tetanic manifestations, such as carpopedal spasms and convulsive seizures. The patient's serum calcium level was 5.0 mg/dL (normal range 8.0 to 10.5 mg/dL), and the inorganic phosphate level was 6.2 mg/dL (normal range 2.5 to 4.5 mg/dL). Calcium gluconate and parathyroid hormone (PTH) were administered intramuscularly in high doses, but the tetanic convulsions did not resolve. At that time, the serum magnesium level was measured and found to be extremely low at 0.16 mmol/L (normal range 1.44 to 1.81 mmol/L). The urinary excretion of magnesium was also low at 0.13 mEq/day (normal 0.31 mEq/L).

Parenteral magnesium therapy (8 mmol/day) was started. After a few days, the serum concentrations of magnesium and calcium increased to nearly normal levels, and the tetanic manifestations disappeared completely. Oral magnesium therapy (magnesium chloride 1 mmol/kg/day) has been continued without any further tetanic manifestations. The magnesium supplement was discontinued on two occasions, and the tetanic convulsions reappeared promptly.

The fractional excretion of magnesium for this patient was 2.7% despite a very low level of serum magnesium (normal range 2.1% to 14.3% in normagnesemic individuals but is close to 0 if there is permanent depletion of magnesium), indicating the presence of a renal magnesium leak. The intestinal absorption of magnesium [(Mg in stool/Mg intake) × 100 (%)] was lower (19.6%) than the amount of absorption observed in people with normal levels of magnesium (50.2%). The serum calcium and magnesium levels of the parents were within normal limits.

What is the most likely cause of hypomagnesemia in this child?

    A. Hypomagnesemia related to Bartter syndrome
    B. Hypomagnesemia related to Gitelman syndrome
    C. Hypomagnesemia related to tubulointerstitial disease
    D. Hypomagnesemia with secondary hypocalcemia (HSH) due to *TRPM6* mutation

The correct answer is D

Comment: HSH, also known as primary infantile hypomagnesemia or hypomagnesemic tetany, is a rare autosomal recessive disease characterized by profound hypomagnesemia associated with hypocalcemia. The basic abnormality in the condition is defective intestinal absorption of magnesium, usually associated with a tendency toward renal magnesium wasting. This condition usually presents during the newborn period. In affected individuals, hypocalcemia is caused by an impaired response to parathyroid hormone (PTH). Patients with HSH usually present during the first few months of life with symptoms of hypocalcemia including recurrent seizures and other symptoms of increased neuromuscular excitability (cramps, tetany) that fail to respond to Ca therapy. This condition usually requires life-long, high-dose Mg supplementation, which corrects both the hypocalcemia and the hypomagnesemia. The diagnosis of HSH can be challenging for pediatricians because the condition is rare, the symptoms are nonspecific, and it is associated with more common metabolic diseases, including hypocalcemia. As a result, late diagnoses or misdiagnoses have been reported in some patients. If an early diagnosis cannot be made or the treatment is not initiated immediately, any convulsions may be fatal or may result in chronic, irreversible neurological complications. Some patients develop moderate mental retardation and a failure to thrive, associated with pronounced diarrhea.

Hypomagnesemia in infancy can also be secondary to malabsorption, persistent diarrhea, or short-bowel syndrome. However, in these situations, the hereditary magnesium-losing disorders (Gitelman syndrome, isolated recessive hypomagnesemia, autosomal dominant hypocalcemia, autosomal dominant hypoparathyroidism, familial hypocalciuric hypercalcemia, and familial hypomagnesemia with hypercalciuria/nephrocalcinosis) should also be considered as potential diagnoses.

The treatment of HSH is administration of magnesium. At diagnosis, parenteral administration is preferred, whereas maintenance therapy consists of high doses orally. Some patients may need parenteral courses, particularly during hypomagnesemia outbreaks. Monthly IV infusions of magnesium may also be useful in some patients. In our patient, there were only occasional asymptomatic periods of mildly lowered magnesium levels during treatment with magnesium orally and occasional IV administration. Some patients present with significant diarrhea, which may be related to chronic magnesium supplementation orally and may be a major cause of the abandonment of therapy.[1,2]

Case Study 15

A 4-week-old female infant was admitted for evaluation of seizure disorder in the last 24 hours. The parents noted rhythmic limb movements associated with eyes deviated to the right, lasting for a few minutes without skin color change or fever. The infant appeared awake and alert among the episodes. She was born following an uneventful full-term pregnancy by spontaneous delivery. The birth weight was 3100 g. The infant presented a normal psychomotor development, was formula-fed, and did not receive any medication. There was no family history of febrile seizures, epilepsy, neurological disease, or early childhood death. On admission, axillary temperature was 36.5°C, heart rate 153 beats/min, oxygen saturation 99% while she was breathing ambient air, blood pressure 90/62 mmHg, body weight 4100 g. General conditions and results of neurologic examination were unremarkable. Twenty minutes after the admission, the baby experienced three new episodes of seizures characterized by mouth opening, staring with eyes deviated to the right and jerking of the right arm, followed by tonic extension of the left arm, jerking of the right leg, and vocalization. Each seizure lasted for approximately 2 minutes. Electroencephalography (EEG) showed a discharge of alpha rhythmic waves mixed with spikes starting from the left central region, then spreading to the left frontal, temporal, and right central regions. Routine blood tests revealed the following: sodium 134 mmol/L, potassium 5.5 mmol/L, chloride 97 mmol/L, calcium 6.8 mg/dL, phosphorus 9.4 mg/dL, magnesium 0.74 mg/dL, and glucose 86 mg/dL. Liver and kidney functions were normal. Intravenous phenobarbital (10 mg/kg) was administered, followed by 5 mg/kg for 5 days and no further seizure was observed. Oral magnesium sulfate (10% at 2 mL four times a day) was also provided. Five days after admission, blood exams revealed calcium level of 8.6 mg/dL, phosphorus of 6.5 mg/dL, and magnesium of 1.90 mg/dL. A second EEG showed normal cerebral activity. The patient was discharged in good condition without any evidence of neurological sequelae. Magnesium supplementation was prescribed for the following 2 months. In the subsequent 6 months, the patient was doing well and blood magnesium and calcium levels were within normal values.

What is the most likely cause of hypomagnesemia in this infant? (Select all that apply)

A. Prematurity
B. Immature renal tubular function
C. Maternal diabetes
D. Genetic disorders

The correct answer is B
Comment: The main causes for hypomagnesemia in newborns are maternal diabetes, prematurity, hypercalcemia, diuretics, rapid extracellular volume expansion, immature tubular function, and genetic disorders. In our patient, hypomagnesemia was likely due to a transient immature tubular function, considering that no risk factor for magnesium deficiency was present and that blood magnesium levels were normal during the following 6 months without any supplementation.[1-3]

Case Study 16

A 17-year-old female complaining of cramps and tightening in her throat. Past medical history is significant for mild hypertension for which she is being treated with hydrochlorothiazide, 12.5 mg/day.

She had a total thyroidectomy for a large toxic, multinodular goiter 2 years ago and is maintained on 1-thyroxine 100 g/day. Bone densitometry was consistent with osteoporosis and she was started on alendronate 10 mg/day. Several days later, she began to note intermittent severe cramps in her hands and feet. Today, she noted some tightening in her throat and came to the emergency room. She denies the use of any other medications or over-the counter supplements. She avoids all dairy products.

Upon examination, her BP is 140/86 mmHg, pulse 86 beats/min, respirations 12 breaths/min, and temperature 37°C, weight 62.5 kg, and height 159 cm. The rest of the physical examination was normal. Laboratory studies revealed hemoglobin 13.0 g/L, white blood count 5100 cells/μL, sodium 138 mmol/L, potassium 4.1 mmol/L, chloride 100 mmol/L, bicarbonate 27 mmol/L, BUN 6 mg/dL, creatinine 0.7 mg/dL, calcium 7.7 mg/dL, phosphate 6.3 mg/dL, magnesium 1.9 mg/dL, and albumin 4.2 g/dL. Urinalysis showed trace protein, negative for glucose and blood. Her EKG showed prolonged QT intervals.

What would you do at this point? (Select all that apply)

A. Draw PTH level
B. Draw serum magnesium level
C. Draw calcitriol level
D. Draw calcidiol level
E. Give intravenous magnesium

The correct answers are A, B, and E
Comment: The combination of hypocalcemia and hypophosphatemia in the absence of renal failure certainly suggests the presence of hypoparathyroidism. Hypomagnesemia (usually due to diarrhea) can cause suppression of PTH secretion and/or resistance to PTH, and produce acute hypocalcemia.

It is appropriate to consider this and draw a serum magnesium level. In the absence of renal insufficiency, magnesium infusion is safe and reasonable while waiting for the results to come back from the laboratory.

Her symptoms did not abate and her serum calcium was unchanged following administration of magnesium. She was given intravenous calcium and experienced relief of her acute symptoms. She was maintained on intravenous calcium for several days until her laboratory studies, which were obtained in the ER, returned as follows: PTH 15 ng/mL, serum magnesium 2.0 mg/dL.[1,2]

Case Study 17

What is the primary diagnosis?

    A. Hypoparathyroidism
    B. Alendronate toxicity
    C. Vitamin D deficiency
    D. Hypomagnesemia
    E. Pseudohypoparathyroidism

The correct answer is A
Comment: She has hypocalcemia and a PTH value that is inappropriately in the low-normal range consistent with hypoparathyroidism. Permanent hypothyroidism occurs in 2% to 10% of cases after thyroid surgery. She likely had subclinical hypoparathyroidism that was undiagnosed and that now has been masked by alendronate therapy.[1,2]

Case Study 18

A 12-year-old male presents to the ER with acute abdominal pain. He noted the onset of steady right upper quadrant pain yesterday. The pain radiates in a band-like fashion to the back and is relieved somewhat by bending forward. He has also experienced nausea and vomiting for the last 10 hours. He has had multiple hospitalizations in the past with similar presentation. Review of symptoms reveal that he has been having loose, greasy, foul-smelling stools that are difficult to flush for the last month. Current medications include Dilantin and phenobarbital for a history of generalized seizures over the last several years. Upon examination, he appears restless and is in significant pain. Vital signs reveal a temperature of 39°C, BP of 103/65 mmHg, a pulse of 110 beats/min, and a respiratory rate of 25 breaths/min with shallow respirations. The chest is clear. There is epigastric distention and tenderness with guarding. The liver and spleen are not palpable. There is no edema. The neurological examination is intact.

Which of the following may be contributing to the hypocalcemia? (Select all that apply)

    A. Hypophosphatemia
    B. Hyperphosphatemia
    C. Hypomagnesemia
    D. Hypermagnesemia
    E. Low calcidol
    F. Extravascular deposition of calcium

The correct answers are C, E, and F
Comment: Vitamin D deficiency, hypomagnesemia, and precipitation of calcium soaps in the abdominal cavity all may play a role in patients with chronic pancreatitis.[1]

Case Study 19

Which of the following may be contributing to the low levels of calcidiol in this patient? (Select all that apply)

A. Renal failure
B. Malabsorption
C. Dietary deficiency of vitamin D
D. Dilantin
E. Liver disease

The correct answers are B, C, D, and E

Comment: Liver disease (loss of 80% to 90% of functioning tissue) can be associated with reduced hydroxylation of vitamin D to calcidiol. Penobarbital and Dilantin increase the activity of the p450 mitochondrial system, which can metabolize calcidiol into inactive metabolites. Dilantin may also interfere with the absorption of vitamin D. Dietary vitamin D deficiency and/or malabsorption associated with chronic pancreatitis is typically a feature in alcoholic patients.[1]

Case Study 20

A 19-year-old, HIV-positive male noted the onset of blurring vision several weeks ago. Indirect ophthalmoscopy revealed white, fluffy retinal lesions, located close to retinal vessels and associated with hemorrhage. Cytomegalovirus (CMV) retinitis was diagnosed and he was begun on intravenous therapy with foscarnet, 120 mg/kg IV, twice daily. This was to be continued for 2 weeks to be followed by maintenance therapy with intravenous 90 mg/kg, once daily. He complained of several episodes of numbness and tingling, particularly around his mouth, with the first several treatments. This morning he experienced a generalized seizure immediately following completion of his treatment.

Laboratory studies included a hemoglobin 10.0 g/dL, white blood count 4600 cells/μL, BUN 8 mg/dL, creatinine 1.0 mg/dL, sodium 140 mmol/L, potassium 4.0 mmol/L, chloride 108 mmol/L, bicarbonate, 25 mmol/L, calcium 9.9 mg/dL, phosphate 3.5 mg/dL, magnesium 1.9 mg/dL, and albumin 3.7 g/dL.

His clinicians are concerned and confused. His symptoms sound like hypocalcemia but his serum calcium concentration and serum albumin concentration are normal.

What would you recommend be done next? (Select all that apply)

A. Measure a PTH level
B. Reduce the foscarnet dose and measure the serum-ionized calcium at the end of the net infusion
C. Measure a calcidol level
D. Measure serum ionized magnesium level
E. Order a head CT scan
F. Check a blood gas during the infusion

The correct answers are B, E, and F

Comment: Foscarnet (trisodium phosphonoformate) has been shown to chelate serum calcium. The plasma-ionized calcium (but not total) typically falls by a mean value of 0.17 mmol/L with a 90 mg/kg dose, and by 0.29 mmol/L with a 120 mg/kg dose. These changes are clinically significant and can be associated with paresthesias and seizures. Acute respiratory alkalosis associated with hyperventilation due to pain or anxiety can also reduce the ionized calcium concentration.[1]

Case Study 21

The patient is a 14-year-old female who presents with a 7-month history of aching in her bones affecting her arms and legs. More recently, she has noted the onset of muscle weakness such that her gait has become cautious and she uses her arms to rise from a sitting position. She has no significant past medical history and she does not smoke or drink alcohol. She denies the use of any medications. Her most recent office visit was 6 months ago, at which time there were no abnormal physical or laboratory findings. Upon examination, she appears as a thin female in no acute distress. BP is 126/78 mmHg, pulse 76 beats/min, respirations 12 breaths/min, and temperature 37°C, weight 55.0 kg, and height 160 cm. The rest of the physical exam is normal.

Laboratory studies showed normal hemoglobin, white cell count, and urinalysis. Serum sodium is 140 mmol/L, potassium 3.9 mmol/L, chloride 101 mmol/L, bicarbonate, 28 mmol/L, BUN 8 mg/dL, creatinine 1.0 mg/dL, calcium 9.8 mg/dL, phosphate 1.9 mg/dL, magnesium 1.7 mg/dL, and albumin 4.2 g/dL.

Which of the following symptoms can be associated with her electrolyte abnormalities?

A. Muscle weakness
B. Osteoporosis
C. Osteopenia
D. Osteomalacia
E. Hypertension
F. Hyperparathyroidism

The correct answer is A
Comment: Muscle weakness and osteomalacia (often presenting as bone pain) are classic signs of marked hypophosphatemia. Hypophosphatemia-induced manifestations of muscle dysfunction include a proximal myopathy, affecting skeletal muscle, and dysphasia and ileus, affecting smooth muscle. Metabolic bone disease refers to conditions that produce a diffuse decrease in bone density (osteopenia) and/or strength because of an increase in bone resorption and/or a decrease in bone formation. These conditions include osteoporosis, osteomalacia, and hyperparathyroidism.[1-6]

Case Study 22

Which diagnostic tests should be done first in attempting to distinguish the diagnosis? (Select all that apply)

A. Twenty-four-hour urine phosphate collection
B. Twenty-four-hour urine creatinine collection
C. Twenty-four-hour urine calcium collection
D. Serum calcidiol level
E. Serum calcitriol level

The correct answers are A and B
Comment: The first step in the diagnostic approach to hypophosphatemia is to establish whether or not there is GI loss or urinary loss as the causative factor. This is done by evaluating the appropriateness of urinary phosphate excretion. Thus the 24-hour urinary collection for phosphorus and creatinine is necessary to ensure the adequacy of the collection and to allow estimation of the fractional excretion of phosphate. The 24-hour urine phosphate and creatinine excretion were 800 and 1250 mg, respectively. The fractional phosphate excretion was 43%.[1-6]

Case Study 23

What medical conditions should now be considered in the differential diagnosis? (Select all that apply)

    A. Primary hyperparathyroidism
    B. Poor phosphate intake and diarrhea
    C. Excess ingestion of phosphate-binding antacids
    D. Vitamin D deficiency
    E. Fanconi syndrome
    F. X-linked hypophosphatemic rickets
    G. Oncogenic osteomalacia

The correct answers are E, F, and G
Comment: The fractional phosphate excretion indicated reduced phosphate transport. The causes include hyperparathyroidism and vitamin D deficiency (with secondary hypoparathyroidism).

    The normal calcium concentration is not consistent with primary or secondary hyperparathyroidism. The causes of primary renal phosphate wasting include a generalized defect in proximal tubule transport (Fanconi syndrome), hereditary hypophosphatemic rickets, and oncogenic osteomalacia.[1-6]

Case Study 24

Further evaluation revealed the following: normal blood levels of 25 (OH) Vitamin-D, PTH (3 pg/mL), uric acid (5 mg/dL), and 1,25 (OH) 2 vitamin D level (10 pg/mL). Urine contained no glucose or amino acids with normal uric acid excretion.

What is the most likely diagnosis now?

    A. Fanconi syndrome
    B. Hereditary hypophosphatemic rickets
    C. Oncogenic osteomalacia
    D. Vitamin D deficiency

The correct answer is C
The condition appears to be acquired and the calcitriol level is very low, consistent with this diagnosis.[1,2]

Case Study 25

What is the presumed pathogenesis of this disorder?

    A. Tumor secretion of cyclic adenosine monophosphate (AMP)
    B. Tumor production of the phosphatonin FG23
    C. Tumor production of PTH
    D. Tumor production of calcitonin
    E. None of the above

The correct answer is B
Comment: There are several phosphatonins that have been identified. Overproduction of FG23 appears to be the most common in patients with these tumors. These substances lead to under expression of the cotransporter that is responsible for phosphate reabsorption in the proximal tubule.[1,2]

Case Study 26

What should be done next? (Select all that apply)

    A. Treat with oral phosphate
    B. Treat with 1,25 $(OH)_2$ vitamin D
    C. Total body magnetic resonance imaging (MRI)
    D. Scintigraphy using octreotide labeled with indium-111
    E. Treat with 25 (OH) vitamin D

The correct answers are A, B, C, and D
Comment: Patients with this syndrome require a combination of oral phosphate and calcitriol.[1,2] This is because the use of phosphate alone may lower ionized calcium and lead to secondary hyperparathyroidism. Therapy should continue until the tumor can be identified and removed. Removal of the tumor leads to prompt reversal of the biochemical abnormalities and healing of the bone disease.

Identification of the tumor can involve total body magnetic resonance imaging or scintigraphy using octreotide labeled with indium-111 (since the tumors typically express somastatin receptors).

The patient underwent scanning with indium-11 labeled octreotide. Intense nasopharyngeal uptake was demonstrated indicating an occult octreotide avid hemangiopericytoma. Surgery was recommended.

The patient asks what the likely prognosis is with successful removal of the tumor.

Case Study 27

What do you tell her?

    A. The tumors are typically benign and do not recur; in all likelihood she will be cured.
    B. Tumors often recur.

The correct answer is A
Comment: The tumors are typically benign and do not recur; in all likelihood she will be cured. The patient underwent surgery. Her weakness subsequently improved and her serum phosphate returned to normal. She has been well for 5 years.[1,2]

Case Study 28

A 15-year-old female returns for her annual check-up. When seen last year, physical examination and laboratory studies were within normal limits. Routine bone densitometry revealed low bone density (more than 2.5 standard deviations below normal) and she was placed on alendronate. She now returns for her annual check-up with no complaints. Laboratory studies show hematocrit 46%, BUN 14 mg/dL, serum creatinine 1.1 mg/dL, sodium 140 mmol/L, potassium 3.9 mmol/L, chloride 105 mmol/L, bicarbonate 26 mmol/L, calcium 11.3 mg/dL, phosphate 3.4 mg/dL, magnesium 1.9 mg/dL, and albumin 4.2 g/dL. Urinalysis shows trace protein, glucose negative, no blood, and no casts, RBC, or WBC. The PTH level was 57 pg/mL (normal range 10 to 65 pg/mL).

What is the most likely diagnosis based upon the laboratory studies?

    A. Familial hypocalciuric hypercalcemia
    B. Primary hyperparathyroidism
    C. Malignancy

    D. Granulomatous disease

    E. I am not sure, I would like to order a sestamibi scan for verification

The correct answer is B

Comment: A PTH level in the high normal range is inappropriate in a patient with hypercalcemia, and indicates the presence of primary hyperparathyroidism. This occurs in 15% to 20% of patients with this condition.[1,2]

Case Study 29

What would you like to do now?

    A. Order a sestamibi scan

    B. Call the surgeon

    C. Follow the patient and schedule follow-up in 6 months

    D. Follow-up in 6 months

The correct answer is B

Comment: Surgery is indicated in the following patients:

    Patients with a serum calcium level of 1.0 mg/dL or above the upper limit of normal.

    1. Patients with hypercalciuria (> 400 mg/day) while eating their usual diet

    2.Patients with a creatinine clearance that is 30% or lower than that of age matched normal subjects

    3.Patients with bone density at the hip, lumbar spine, or distal radius that is more than 2.5 standard deviations below peak bone mass (T score <−2.5)

    4.Patients who are less than 50 years old

    5.Patients in whom periodic follow-up will be difficult

    The patient has a serum calcium level, which is more than 1 mg/dL above normal and has a significant decrease in bone density. She is in good health otherwise and should be offered surgery as the first option.[1,2]

Case Study 30

A 14-year-old male presents with nausea, dizziness, weakness, and muscle cramps. His past medical history is significant for hypertension (HTN) and gastroesophageal reflux disease (GERD). His medication regimen includes amlodipine 5 mg daily and hydrochlorothiazide 12.5 mg daily for HTN and pantoprazole 40 mg daily for GERD. He has been taking both medications for 2 years. A chemistry panel was obtained and was significant for potassium 3.3 mEq/L, magnesium 1 mg/dL, Ca 7.7 mg/dL, and albumin 4.1 g/dL.

What is the most likely etiology of his symptoms?

    A. Amlodipine

    B. Pantoprazole

    C. Hydrochlorothiazide

    D. None of the above

The correct answer is B

Comment: He has hypomagnesemia due to chronic use of pantoprazole. Pantoprazole leads to GI Mg loss due to decreased absorption via down regulation of TRPM6 channels. Hypomagnesemia leads to hypokalemia and hypocalcemia.[1,2]

Case Study 31

A 19-year-old man with congestive heart failure (ejection fraction is 20%) presents with serum magnesium of 1.4 mg/dL. He is on lisinopril 40 mg daily, furosemide 40 mg twice daily, and carvedilol 25 mg twice daily. His blood pressure control is optimal, serum creatinine is stable at 0.8 mg/dL, and serum potassium is 3.4 mmol/L.

What is the best approach to his hypokalemia and hypomagnesemia? (Select all that apply)

  A. Discontinue furosemide
  B. Discontinue potassium supplement
  C. Start spironolactone
  D. All of the above

The correct answer is C
Comment: Discontinuation or dose reduction of furosemide may lead to fluid overload. Supplementation with oral potassium and magnesium salts would significantly increase the number and frequency of his medications. Given his diagnosis of congestive heart failure with low ejection fraction, spironolactone 25 mg daily was started to mitigate both hypokalemia and hypomagnesemia resulting from his loop diuretic. Spironolactone decreases morbidity and mortality in patients with severe heart failure.[1]

Case Study 32

A 17-year-old woman with a known history of stage 4 chronic kidney disease (CKD) secondary to diabetic nephropathy presents with nausea, dizziness, muscle cramps, and fasciculations. Her medications include glimepiride 4 mg daily, atorvastatin 40 mg daily, lisinopril 40 mg daily, furosemide 40 mg daily, and patiromer 8.4 daily. Patiromer (a potassium binder) was started due to hyperkalemia resulting from the increase in lisinopril dose. A chemistry panel was ordered, creatinine 3.1 mg/dL, potassium 4.9 mmol/L, magnesium 1 mg/dL.

What should be done next? (Select all that apply)

  A. Discontinue furosemide
  B. Discontinue patiromer
  C. Start magnesium oxide supplement
  D. Start calcium gluconate salt

The correct answers are A and C
Comment: Her symptoms are due to hypomagnesemia. Patiromer binds both potassium and magnesium. In this patient with stage 4 CKD, the use of patiromer allowed her to continue the use of lisinopril at an optimal dose. Furosemide aggravated her hypomagnesemia. In this case patiromer was continued and the patient was supplemented with magnesium oxide 400 mg PO twice daily.[1]

Case Study 33

A 7-year-old girl presents for evaluation of chronic kidney disease (CKD). She is complaining of muscle cramps and fasciculations, polyuria, and polydipsia. Her past medical history is significant for recurrent urinary tract infections and severe myopia. Physical exam revealed that her growth is in the 40th percentile. She is noted to have corneal calcifications. Laboratory evaluation was remarkable for microhematuria, serum creatinine 1 mg/dL, serum magnesium 1.2 mg/dL, serum calcium 9 mg/dL, fractional excretion of magnesium was elevated at 15%, urine calcium was elevated at 12 mg/kg/24 h (normal < 4 mg/kg/24 h). Intact parathyroid hormone level was elevated at 131 pg/mL (normal range 10 to 65 pg/mL). Renal ultrasound revealed nephrocalcinosis.

What is the most likely diagnosis? (Select all that apply)

A. Familial hypomagnesemia type 2
B. Chronic kidney disease
C. Chronic urinary tract infection
D. Diabetes insipidus

The correct answer is A

Comment: This presentation is consistent with familial hypomagnesemia with hypercalciuria and nephrocalcinosis (FHHNC) type 2. Ocular abnormalities are seen only in type 2 FHHNC. This rare genetic disorder is due to a mutation in the tight junction protein claudin 19. A detailed family history is paramount, including inquiring about consanguineous parents. This patient exhibited many of the characteristic features of FHHNC type 2. Genetic testing is required to ascertain the diagnosis.[1]

References

Case Study 1

1. Praga M, Vara J, González-Parra E, et al. Familial hypomagnesemia with hypercalciuria and nephrocalcinosis. *Kidney Int.* 1995;47:1419–1425.
2. Konrad M, Weber S. Recent advances in molecular genetics of hereditary magnesium-losing disorders. *J Am Soc Nephrol.* 2003;14:249–260.
3. Weber S, Schneider L, Peters M, et al. Novel paracellin-1 mutations in 25 families with familial hypomagnesemia with hypercalciuria and nephrocalcinosis. *J Am Soc Nephrol.* 2001;12:1872–1881.
4. Konrad M, Schlingmann KP, Gudermann T. Insights into the molecular nature of magnesium homeostasis. *Am J Physiol Renal Physiol.* 2004;286:F599–F605.
5. Cole DEC, Quamme GA. Inherited disorders of renal magnesium handling. *J Am Soc Nephrol.* 2000;11:1937–1947.
6. Takeuchi K, Kure S, Kato T, et al. Association of a mutation in thiazide-sensitive Na-Cl cotransporter with familial Gitelman's syndrome. *J Clin Endocrinol Metab.* 1996;12:4496–4499.
7. Riveira-Munoz E, Chang Q, Godefroid N, et al. Transcriptional and functional analyses of SLC12A3 mutations: new clues for the pathogenesis of Gitelman syndrome. *J Am Soc Nephrol.* 2007;18:1271–1283.
8. Konrad M, Vollmer M, Lemmink HH, et al. Mutations in the chloride channel gene CLCNKB as a cause of classic Bartter syndrome. *J Am Soc Nephrol.* 2000;11. 1449–1159.

Case Study 2

1. Shah GM, Kirschenbaum MA. Renal magnesium wasting associated with therapeutic agents. *Miner Electrolyte Metab.* 1991;17:58–64.
2. Whang R, Whang DD, Ryan MP. Refractory potassium repletion. A consequence of magnesium deficiency. *Arch Intern Med.* 1992;152:40–45.
3. Geven WB, Monnens LA, Willems HL, et al. Renal magnesium wasting in two families with autosomal dominant inheritance. *Kidney Int.* 1987;31:1140–1144.
4. Assadi F. Hypomagnesemia: an evidence-based approach to clinical cases. *Iran J Kidney Dis.* 2010;4(1):13–19.

Case Study 3

1. Bettinelli A, Bianchetti MG, Girardin E, et al. Use of calcium excretion values to distinguish two forms of primary renal tubular hypokalemic alkalosis: Bartter and Gitelman syndromes. *J Pediatr.* 1992;120:38–43.
2. Assadi F. Disorders of divalent ion metabolism. In: Assadi F, ed. *Clinical Decisions in Pediatric Nephrology: A Problem-Solving Approach to Clinical Cases.* New York: Springer; 2008:97–123.
3. Assadi F. Hypomagnesemia: an evidence-based approach to clinical cases. *Iran J Kidney Dis.* 2010;4(1):13–19.

Case Study 4

1. Assadi F. Hypomagnesemia: an evidence-based approach to clinical cases. *Iran J Kidney Dis.* 2010;4(1):13–19.
2. Elisaf M, Panteli K, Theodorou J, et al. Fractional excretion of magnesium in normal subjects and in patients with hypomagnesemia. *Magnes Res.* 1997;10. 315–230.

Case Study 5

1. Shah GM, Kirschenbaum MA. Renal magnesium wasting associated with therapeutic agents. *Miner Electrolyte Metab.* 1991;17:58–64.
2. Bettinelli A, Bianchetti MG, Girardin E, et al. Use of calcium excretion values to distinguish two forms of primary renal tubular hypokalemic alkalosis: Bartter and Gitelman syndromes. *J Pediatr.* 1992;120:38–43.

Case Study 6

1. Bettinelli A, Bianchetti MG, Girardin E, et al. Use of calcium excretion values to distinguish two forms of primary renal tubular hypokalemic alkalosis: Bartter and Gitelman syndromes. *J Pediatr.* 1992;120:38–43.
2. Takeuchi K, Kure S, Kato T, et al. Association of a mutation in thiazide-sensitive Na-Cl cotransporter with familial Gitelman's syndrome. *J Clin Endocrinol Metab.* 1996;12:4496–4499.
3. Cruz DN, Shaer AJ, Bia MJ, et al. Gitelman's syndrome revisited: an evaluation of symptoms and health-related quality of life. *Kidney Int.* 2001;59:710–717.
4. Assadi F. Hypomagnesemia: an evidence-based approach to clinical cases. *Iran J Kidney Dis.* 2010;4(1):13–19.

Case Study 7

1. Bettinelli A, Bianchetti MG, Girardin E, et al. Use of calcium excretion values to distinguish two forms of primary renal tubular hypokalemic alkalosis: Bartter and Gitelman syndromes. *J Pediatr.* 1992;120:38–43.
2. Takeuchi K, Kure S, Kato T, et al. Association of a mutation in thiazide-sensitive Na-Cl cotransporter with familial Gitelman's syndrome. *J Clin Endocrinol Metab.* 1996;12:4496–4499.
3. Cruz DN, Shaer AJ, Bia MJ, et al. Gitelman's syndrome revisited: an evaluation of symptoms and health-related quality of life. *Kidney Int.* 2001;59:710–717.
4. Assadi F. Hypomagnesemia: an evidence-based approach to clinical cases. *Iran J Kidney Dis.* 2010;4(1):13–19.

Case Study 8

1. Shoback D. Clinical practice. Hypoparathyroidism. *N Engl J Med.* 2008;359:391–403.
2. Assadi F. Hypomagnesemia: an evidence-based approach to clinical cases. *Iran J Kidney Dis.* 2010;4(1):13–19.

Case Study 9

1. Shoback D. Clinical practice. Hypoparathyroidism. *N Engl J Med.* 2008;359:391–403.
2. Epstein M, McGrath S, Law F. Proton-pump inhibitors and hypomagnesemic hypoparathyroidism. *N Engl J Med.* 2006;355:1834–1836.
3. Assadi F. Hypomagnesemia: an evidence-based approach to clinical cases. *Iran J Kidney Dis.* 2010;4(1):13–19.

Case Study 10

1. Shoback D. Clinical practice. Hypoparathyroidism. *N Engl J Med.* 2008;359:391–403.
2. Epstein M, McGrath S, Law F. Proton-pump inhibitors and hypomagnesemic hypoparathyroidism. *N Engl J Med.* 2006;355:1834–1836.
3. Assadi F. Hypomagnesemia: an evidence-based approach to clinical cases. *Iran J Kidney Dis.* 2010;4(1):13–19.

Case Study 11

1. Shoback D. Clinical practice. Hypoparathyroidism. *N Engl J Med.* 2008;359:391–403.
2. Assadi F. Hypomagnesemia: an evidence-based approach to clinical cases. *Iran J Kidney Dis.* 2010;4(1):13–19.

Case Study 12

1. Viering DHHM, de Baaij JHF, Walsh SB, et al. Genetic causes of hypomagnesemia, a clinical overview. *Pediatr Nephrol.* 2017;32:1123–1135.
2. Clissold RL, Hamilton AJ, Hattersley AT, et al. HNF1B-associated renal and extra-renal disease-an expanding clinical spectrum. *Nat Rev Nephrol.* 2015;11:102–112.

Case Study 13

1. Viering DHHM, de Baaij JHF, Walsh SB, et al. Genetic causes of hypomagnesemia, a clinical overview. *Pediatr Nephrol.* 2017;32:1123–1135.
2. Clissold RL, Hamilton AJ, Hattersley AT, et al. HNF1B-associated renal and extra-renal disease-an expanding clinical spectrum. *Nat Rev Nephrol.* 2015;11:102–112.
3. Heidet L, Decramer S, Pawtowski A, et al. Spectrum of HNF1B mutations in a large cohort of patients who harbor renal diseases. *Clin J Am Soc Nephrol.* 2010;5:1079–1090.
4. Faguer S, Decramer S, Chassaing N, et al. Diagnosis, management, and prognosis of HNF1B nephropathy in adulthood. *Kidney Int.* 2011;80:768–776.
5. Clissold RL, Shaw-Smith C, Turnpenny P, et al. Chromosome 17q12 microdeletions but not intragenic HNF1B mutations link developmental kidney disease and psychiatric disorder. *Kidney Int.* 2016;90:203–311.

Case Study 14

1. Visudhiphan P, Visudtibhan A, Chiemchanya S, et al. Neonatal seizures and familial hypomagnesemia with secondary hypocalcemia. *Pediatr Neurol.* 2005;33:202–205.
2. Schlingmann KP, Weber S, Peters M, et al. Hypomagnesemia with secondary hypocalcemia is caused by mutations in TRPM6, a new member of the TRPM gene family. *Nat Genet.* 2002;31:166–170.

Case Study 15

1. Stoll ML, Listman JA. Nephrolithiasis in a neonate with transient renal wasting of calcium and magnesium. *Pediatr Nephrol.* 2002;17:386–389.
2. Dooling EC, Stern L. Hypomagnesemia with convulsions in a newborn infant. Report of a case associated with maternal hypophosphatemia. *Can Med Assoc J.* 1967;97:827–831.
3. Gupta P, Shingla S. Symptomatic transient idiopathic hypomagnesaemia in a neonate. *Singap Med J.* 2011;52:132–133.

Case Study 16

1. Chase LR, Slatopolsky E, Krinski T. Secretion and metabolic efficacy of parathyroid hormone in patients with severe hypomagnesemia. *J Clin Endocrinol Metab.* 1974;38:363–371.
2. Agus ZS. Hypomagnesemia. *J Am Soc Nephrol.* 1999;10:1616–1622.

Case Study 17

1. Chase LR, Slatopolsky E. Secretion and metabolic efficacy of parathyroid hormone in patients with severe hypomagnesemia. *J Clin Endocrinol Metab.* 1974;38:363–371.
2. Agus ZS. Hypomagnesemia. *J Am Soc Nephrol.* 1999;10:1616–1622.

Case Study 18

1. Gardner Jr EC, Hersh T. Primary hyperparathyroidism and the gastrointestinal tract. *South Med J.* 1981;74:197–199.

Case Study 19

1. Wharton B, Bishop N. *Rickets Lancet.* 2003;362:1389–1400.

Case Study 20

1. Jacobson MA, Gambertoglio JG, Aweeka FT, et al. Foscarnet-induced hypocalcemia and effects of foscarnet on calcium metabolism. *J Clin Endocrinol Metab.* 1991;72:1130–1135.

Case Study 21

1. Agus ZS. Hypomagnesemia. *J Am Soc Nephrol.* 1999;10:1616.
2. Clarke BL, Wynne AG, Wilson DM, et al. Osteomalacia associated with adult Fanconi's syndrome: clinical and diagnostic features. *Clin Endocrinol.* 1995;43:479–490.
3. Econs MJ, Samsa GP, Monger M, et al. X-linked hypophosphatemic rickets: a disease often unknown to affected patients. *Bone Miner.* 1994;24:17–24.
4. Lotz M, Zisman E, Bartter FC. Evidence for a phosphorus-depletion syndrome in man. *N Engl J Med.* 1968;278:409–415.
5. Subramanian R, Khardori R. Severe hypophosphatemia. Pathophysiologic implications, clinical presentations, and treatment. *Medicine.* 2000;79:1–8.
6. Wilkins GE, Granleese S, Hegele RG, et al. Oncogenic osteomalacia: evidence for a humoral phosphaturic factor. *J Clin Endocrinol Metab.* 1995;80:1628–1634.

Case Study 22

1. Agus ZS. Hypomagnesemia. *J Am Soc Nephrol.* 1999;10:1616.
2. Clarke BL, Wynne AG, Wilson DM, et al. Osteomalacia associated with adult Fanconi's syndrome: clinical and diagnostic features. *Clin Endocrinol.* 1995;43:479–490.
3. Econs MJ, Samsa GP, Monger M, et al. X-linked hypophosphatemic rickets: a disease often unknown to affected patients. *Bone Miner.* 1994;24:17–24.
4. Lotz M, Zisman E, Bartter FC. Evidence for a phosphorus-depletion syndrome in man. *N Engl J Med.* 1968;278:409–415.
5. Subramanian R, Khardori R. Severe hypophosphatemia. Pathophysiologic implications, clinical presentations, and treatment. *Medicine.* 2000;79:1–8.
6. Wilkins GE, Granleese S, Hegele RG, et al. Oncogenic osteomalacia: evidence for a humoral phosphaturic factor. *J Clin Endocrinol Metab.* 1995;80:1628–1634.

Case Study 23

1. Agus ZS. Hypomagnesemia. *J Am Soc Nephrol.* 1999;10:1616.
2. Clarke BL, Wynne AG, Wilson DM, et al. Osteomalacia associated with adult Fanconi's syndrome: clinical and diagnostic features. *Clin Endocrinol.* 1995;43:479–490.
3. Econs MJ, Samsa GP, Monger M, et al. X-linked hypophosphatemic rickets: a disease often unknown to affected patients. *Bone Miner.* 1994;24:17–24.
4. Lotz M, Zisman E, Bartter FC. Evidence for a phosphorus-depletion syndrome in man. *N Engl J Med.* 1968;278:409–415.
5. Subramanian R, Khardori R. Severe hypophosphatemia. Pathophysiologic implications, clinical presentations, and treatment. *Medicine.* 2000;79:1–8.
6. Wilkins GE, Granleese S, Hegele RG, et al. Oncogenic osteomalacia: evidence for a humoral phosphaturic factor. *J Clin Endocrinol Metab.* 1995;80:1628–1634.

Case Study 24

1. Berenson JR. Treatment of hypercalcemia of malignancy with bisphosphonates. *Semin Oncol.* 2002;29 (6 suppl 21):8–12.
2. Wilkins GE, Granleese S, Hegele RG, et al. Oncogenic osteomalacia: evidence for a humoral phosphaturic factor. *J Clin Endocrinol Metab.* 1995;80:1628–1634.

Case Study 25

1. Berenson JR. Treatment of hypercalcemia of malignancy with bisphosphonates. *Semin Oncol.* 2002;29 (6 suppl 21):8–12.
2. Wilkins GE, Granleese S, Hegele RG, et al. Oncogenic osteomalacia: evidence for a humoral phosphaturic factor. *J Clin Endocrinol Metab.* 1995;80:1628–1634.

Case Study 26

1. Berenson JR. Treatment of hypercalcemia of malignancy with bisphosphonates. *Semin Oncol.* 2002;29 (6 suppl 21):8–12.
2. Wilkins GE, Granleese S, Hegele RG, et al. Oncogenic osteomalacia: evidence for a humoral phosphaturic factor. *J Clin Endocrinol Metab.* 1995;80:1628–1634.

Case Study 27

1. Berenson JR. Treatment of hypercalcemia of malignancy with bisphosphonates. *Semin Oncol.* 2002;29 (6 suppl 21):8–12.
2. Wilkins GE, Granleese S, Hegele RG, et al. Oncogenic osteomalacia: evidence for a humoral phosphaturic factor. *J Clin Endocrinol Metab.* 1995;80:1628–1634.

Case Study 28

1. Heath 3rd H. Clinical spectrum of primary hyperparathyroidism: evolution with changes in medical practice and technology. *J Bone Miner Res.* 1991;6(suppl 2):S63–S70.
2. Siperstein AE, Shen W, Chan AK, et al. Normocalcemic hyperparathyroidism. Biochemical and symptom profiles before and after surgery. *Arch Surg.* 1992;127:1157–1166.

Case Study 29

1. Heath 3rd H. Clinical spectrum of primary hyperparathyroidism: evolution with changes in medical practice and technology. *J Bone Miner Res.* 1991;6(suppl 2):S63–S70.
2. Siperstein AE, Shen W, Chan AK, et al. Normocalcemic hyperparathyroidism. Biochemical and symptom profiles before and after surgery. *Arch Surg.* 1992;127:1157–1166.

Case Study 30

1. Al Alawi AM, Majoni SW, Falhammar H. Magnesium and human health: perspectives and research directions. *Int J Endocrinol.* 2018;2018:9041694. https://doi.org/10.1155/2018/9041694.
2. Tinawi M. Hypokalemia: a practical approach to diagnosis and treatment. *Arch Clin Biomed Res.* 2020;4:48–66.

Case Study 31

1. Pitt B, Zannad F, Remme WJ, et al. The effect of spironolactone on morbidity and mortality in patients with severe heart failure. Randomized aldactone evaluation study investigators. *N Engl J Med.* 1999;341:709–717.

Case Study 32

1. Palmer BF. Potassium binders for hyperkalemia in chronic kidney disease-diet, renin-angiotensin-aldosterone system inhibitor therapy, and hemodialysis. *Mayo Clin Proc.* 2020;95:339–354.

Case Study 33

1. Weber S, Schneider L, Peters M, et al. Novel paracellin-1 mutations in 25 families with familial hypomagnesemia with hypercalciuria and nephrocalcinosis. *J Am Soc Nephrol.* 2001;12:1872–1881.

CHAPTER 12

Hypermagnesemia

Case Study 1

A 12-year-old patient with chronic renal failure developed hypermagnesemia (serum magnesium 3.3 mg/dL) as a result of excess antacid ingestion.

Which of the following electrolyte abnormalities is NOT associated with hypermagnesemia? (Select all that apply)

    A. Causes hyperphosphatemia
    B. Causes hyperkalemia
    C. Causes hypernatremia
    D. Causes hypercalcemia

The correct answers are A and B
Comment: Magnesium helps with skeletal muscle contraction, helps the immune system, adenosine triphosphate (ATP) formation, and cellular growth. Magnesium regulates blood glucose levels and carbohydrate metabolism, and it has a direct relationship with calcium and potassium, not sodium. Magnesium helps with vitamin activation, not minerals.[1–3]

Case Study 2

Which are the causes of hypermagnesemia in this patient? (Select all that apply)

    A. Addison disease
    B. Chronic kidney disease (GFR < 30 mL/min/1.73 m^2)
    C. Tumor lysis syndrome
    D. Hyperthyroidism

The correct answers are A, B, and C
Comment: Hypermagnesemia is commonly caused by kidney failure or drug-induced such as magnesium-containing antacid or laxatives. Less common causes include tumor lysis syndrome, seizure disorders, and prolonged ischemia. Diagnosis is based on a blood level of magnesium greater than 1.1 mmol/L (2.6 mg/dL).[1,2]

Case Study 3

What are the signs and symptoms of hypermagnesemia? (Select all that apply)

    A. Hypertension
    B. Tachycardia
    C. Hyperreflexia
    D. Skeletal muscle weakness

The correct answer is D

Comment: Patients with hypermagnesemia would manifest decreased or absent deep tendon reflexes, bradycardia, hypotension, cardiac arrhythmias, and skeletal muscle weakness.[1,2]

Case Study 4

Which electrocardiogram findings are characteristic of hypermagnesemia? (Select all that apply)

    A. Shortened PR interval
    B. Prolonged PR interval
    C. Widened QRS complex
    D. Shortened QRS complex

The correct answers are B and C

Comment: Typically, electrocardiogram findings for hypermagnesemia patients include prolonged PR intervals and widened QRS complexes. [1]

Case Study 5

Which of the following electrolyte abnormalities would you expect to see with hypermagnesemia? (Select all that apply)

    A. Hyperkalemia
    B. Hyponatremia
    C. Hypophosphatemia
    D. Hypercalcemia

The correct answers are A, C, and D

Comment: Magnesium also has an indirect relationship with phosphorus. If the magnesium is high, the phosphorous will be low. Magnesium has a direct relationship to potassium and calcium. If the magnesium is high, the potassium and calcium will both be high.[1,2]

Case Study 6

How would you treat the elevated serum hypermagnesemia level in this patient? (Select all that apply)

    A. Stop antacid medication
    B. Administer a loop diuretic
    C. Consider hemodialysis
    D. Increased fluid intake

The correct answers are A, B, C, and D

Comment: It is important to discontinue medications that cause hypermagnesemia such as laxatives and antacids. It is important to administer a loop diuretic like furosemide that increases urinary magnesium excretion. Increasing fluid intake and limiting the intake of magnesium-rich foods such as green, leafy vegetables and avocados will also correct hypermagnesemia. Limiting fluid intake will not help with hypermagnesemia.

Hypermagnesemia is defined as a serum magnesium level greater than 2.6 mg/dL. Symptomatic hypermagnesemia is fairly uncommon. It occurs most commonly in patients with renal failure after ingestion of magnesium-containing drugs, such as antacids or purgatives. Hypermagnesemia may also occur in patients with hypothyroidism or Addison disease. Symptoms and signs include hyporeflexia, hypotension, respiratory depression, and cardiac arrest.[1,2]

At serum magnesium concentrations of 6 to 12 mg/dL (2.5 to 5 mmol/L), the ECG shows prolongation of the PR interval, widening of the QRS complex, and increased T-wave amplitude. Deep tendon reflexes disappear as the serum magnesium concentration approaches 12 mg/dL (5.0 mmol/L); hypotension, respiratory depression, and narcosis develop with increasing hypermagnesemia. Cardiac arrest may occur when blood magnesium concentration is greater than 15 mg/dL (6.0 to 7.5 mmol/L).

Treatment of severe magnesium toxicity consists of circulatory and respiratory support and administration of 10% calcium gluconate 10 to 20 mL intravenously (IV). Calcium gluconate may reverse many of the magnesium-induced changes, including respiratory depression. Administration of IV furosemide can increase magnesium excretion when renal function is adequate; volume status should be maintained.[1,2]

Hemodialysis may be valuable in severe hypermagnesemia because a relatively large fraction (about 70%) of blood magnesium is not protein bound and thus is removable with hemodialysis. When hemodynamic compromise occurs and hemodialysis is impractical, peritoneal dialysis is an option.[1,2]

Case Study 7

A 19-year-old woman was diagnosed with severe preeclampsia and noted to have hyperreflexia on the exam. She was started on magnesium sulfate intravenously for seizure prevention. She was given an intravenous loading dose of magnesium (5.0 g) over 30 minutes, followed by a continuous infusion of 3 g/h. Four hours later she became confused, unable to urinate and her deep tendon reflexes were absent.

What would you do next? (Select all that apply)

A. Administer 0.9% saline
B. Give intravenous calcium gluconate
C. Discontinue magnesium sulfate
D. Give intravenous phenobarbital

The correct answers are A, B, and C
Comment: The patient is showing signs of magnesium toxicity. Magnesium infusion was stopped, and she was started on 0.9% normal saline at 125 mL/h and 1.0 g of calcium gluconate intravenously over 5 minutes. Serum magnesium level came back at 7.4 mg/dL and her electrocardiogram (ECG) was unremarkable.[1,2]

Magnesium sulfate is the drug of choice for seizure prophylaxis in preeclampsia. Seizure prevention can be achieved by lowering magnesium doses without inducing magnesium toxicity.[1,2]

Case Study 8

A 16-year-old man with a known history of end-stage kidney disease (ESKD) was brought to the emergency department due to lethargy, confusion, and blurred vision. He has been on hemodialysis (HD) for 5 years. His family reported that he has been using a variety of over-the-counter medications for severe constipation. A neurological exam was remarkable for absent deep tendon reflexes.

How would you manage this patient? (Select all that apply)

A. Acute hemodialysis
B. Continuous renal replacement therapy (CRRT)
C. Peritoneal dialysis
D. Administer intravenous normal saline and calcium gluconate

The correct answers are A and D

Comment: The patient with ESKD developed hypermagnesemia due to ingesting large doses of milk of magnesia (MOM). His serum magnesium level was 8.3 mg/dL. ECG showed no significant abnormalities. He was given 0.9% normal saline and 1.0 g of calcium gluconate. He was urgently dialyzed. After a 4-hour dialytic therapy, his serum magnesium fell to 4.8 mg/dL. He was instructed to avoid magnesium-containing laxatives and antacids.[1]

Case Study 9

A 17-year-old female presented to the emergency department with altered mental status and progressive general weakness. She had a history of chronic constipation. Laboratory tests showed a magnesium level of 6.9 mEq/L. Bradycardia and hypotension developed later. Abdomen computed tomography showed hyper-dense magnesium oxide tablets retained in the colon. A magnesium-free laxative was used for gastrointestinal (GI) decontamination. Despite the use of high-dose inotropic and an elevated trigger for transcutaneous pacing, the cardiac performance improved minimally, and prolonged hypotension and decreased perfusion led to hypoxic encephalopathy.

How would you have treated this patient now?

    A. Initiate peritoneal dialysis
    B. Initiate hemodialysis
    C. Administer intravenous furosemide
    D. Administer intravenous normal saline

The correct answer is B

Comment: In this patient, the magnesium oxide tablets were retained in the GI tract without adequate decontamination resulting in continuous absorption and severe hypermagnesemia. A delay in starting hemodialysis following calcium infusion caused the poor outcome.[1]

Case Study 10

A healthy 20-month-old girl presented to the emergency department with episodes of vomiting and a reduced level of consciousness. The neurological examination showed a symmetric decrease in muscle tone, and the deep tendon reflexes were decreased. On admission, her magnesium (Mg) level was 10.5 mg/dL after receiving magnesium oxide for 4 days because of constipation. She was immediately administered calcium gluconate infusion (3.9 mEq) followed by continuous infusion at a rate of 0.23 mEq/h). She was hydrated with 0.9% sodium chloride to maintain good urine output with furosemide administrating to increase the Mg excretion. The level of the serum Mg decreased to 2.4 mg/dL, enabling her to regain consciousness.

What additional therapeutic measure would you recommend now?

    A. Initiate hemodialysis
    B. Initiate peritoneal dialysis
    C. Administer phenobarbital
    D. Discontinue magnesium-oxide

The correct answer is D

Comment: Prompt administration of intravenous calcium infusion and administration of normal saline and loop diuretic corrected hypermagnesemia without the need for dialysis.[1]

Case Study 11

A 17-year-old male with a known history of type 2 diabetes mellitus presented with fever, cough, shortness of breath, and dysuria. On examination, the patient was semi-conscious, drowsy, and arousable to vocal commands. His vital signs included blood pressure: 120/60 mmHg, pulse: 118 beats/min, temperature: 101°F, PO_2 of 72% in room air, and respiratory rate of 28 breaths/min. Laboratory investigations showed hypercalcemia (13.1 mg/dL), deranged liver functions, and high ammonia levels suggestive of hepatic encephalopathy. Parathyroid hormone levels were within the normal range. The patient was symptomatically managed with antibiotics, lactulose (15 mL), and antacids, and hypercalcemia was managed with calcitonin (100 IU) and aggressive hydration. Three days later, his serum magnesium levels and creatinine levels started to rise. His calculated eGFR was 30 mL/min/1.73 m². Hypermagnesemia persisted despite aggressive treatment with intravenous calcium gluconate and hydration along with loop diuretics and the patient succumbed due to multiorgan dysfunction.

What is the MOST likely cause of hypermagnesemia in this patient?

A. Acute renal failure
B. Hypokalemia
C. Hypocalcemia
D. Hyponatremia

The correct answer is A

Comment: Hypermagnesemia though rarely seen and reported in clinical practice could possibly contribute to increased mortality in critically ill patients. The main reason for hypermagnesemia in critically ill patients is decreased renal function.[1,2]

Case Study 12

An 18-year-old male patient diagnosed with acute appendicitis underwent appendectomy. On day 2 post-surgery he developed coagulopathy and hypotension secondary to sepsis. He was started on vasopressor support, which included noradrenaline and vasopressin. The patient had acute kidney injury with hyponatremia, hypocalcemia, and hypokalemia. Hemodialysis was initiated. Persistent hypermagnesemia (serum magnesium > 5.6 mg/dL) developed despite the above measures and the patient continued to deteriorate leading to death.

What is the MOST likely cause of death in this patient?

A. Hypermagnesemia
B. Hypokalemia
C. Hyponatremia
D. Hypocalcemia

The correct answer is A

Comment: Combination of acute renal failure, hyponatremia, hypokalemia along with persistent hypermagnesemia resulted in death.[1,2]

Case Study 13

A 17-year-old female with a brain tumor underwent surgery. She developed hypotension, hyponatremia, hypokalemia, hypocalcemia, acute kidney injury, and encephalopathy 4 days post-surgery. Dialysis was initiated and electrolyte abnormalities were corrected. The patient developed severe hypermagnesemia (serum magnesium level 8.1 mg/dL), which did not resolve despite treatment with calcium infusion and vasopressin treatment, and died because of multiorgan failure.

What is the MOST likely cause of this patient's hypermagnesemia?

A. Hypocalcemia
B. Hypotension
C. Acute kidney injury
D. Hypokalemia

The correct answer is C

Comment: This patient developed hypermagnesemia in presence of acute kidney disease. Hypermagnesemia persisted after correction of other electrolyte imbalances suggesting acute kidney injury as the underlying cause for hypermagnesemia.

The major etiological factors for hypermagnesemia are decreased renal excretion, increased magnesium intake, and compartment leak or shift. Hypermagnesemia between 7 and 12 mg/dL causes decreased reflexes, confusion, drowsiness, bladder paralysis, flushing, headache, and constipation. A slight reduction in blood pressure and blurred vision caused by diminished accommodation and convergence may manifest. For higher values (> 12.0 mg/dL) muscle paralysis, paralytic ileus, decreased breathing rate, and low blood pressure may occur. Electrocardiogram (ECG) changes included an increase in PR and QRS interval with sinus bradycardia, atrioventricular block, coma, and cardiac arrest (exceeding 15.0 mg/dL) may ensue.[1,2]

Case Study 14

A 19-year-old woman who had been treated for pneumonia a week ago presented with confusion, fever, shortness of breath, and generalized weakness. She had a history of hypertension, which was controlled with amlodipine 10 mg daily and hydrochlorothiazide 12.5 mg daily. She was receiving magnesium-containing laxatives for a week prior to admission. Laboratory investigation showed serum sodium 135 mmol/L, potassium 4.6 mmol/L, chloride 95 mmol/L, bicarbonate 3 mmol/L, blood urea nitrogen 15 mg/dL, creatinine 0.6 mg/L, and estimated glomerular filtration rate (eGFR) 109 mL/min/1.3 m². Serum magnesium level was 5.9 mg/dL, calcium 8.9 mg/dL, and phosphate 3.5 mg/dL. Electrocardiography (ECG) showed a sinus rhythm with a heart rate of 58 beats/min and left bundle branch block (PR, 200 ms; QT interval, 473 ms). Urinary ultrasonography showed normal renal parenchymal echogenicity and thickness. Computed tomography of the abdomen revealed that the rectum was filled with feces and fluid, which suggested the presence of ileus. Intravenous hydration with normal saline, intravenous calcium infusion, and broad-spectrum antibiotics was started. Gastrointestinal decontamination was performed. Twelve hours after the patient's admission, the magnesium level was rechecked, with a result of 7.18 mmol/L. Because of the patient's hemodynamic instability (blood pressure, 60/40 mmHg; heart rate, 60 beats/min) and oliguria, she was transferred to the intensive care unit and was started on vasopressor support with norepinephrine and dopamine, intravenous hydration, and furosemide infusion. Three days after the cessation of magnesium intake and supportive treatment, serum magnesium level decreased (2.16 mg/dL), the patient was weaned from vasopressors, urine output was restored with no need to perform hemodialysis, and the patient was discharged with a full recovery.

Which of the following conditions was responsible for the observed hypermagnesemia in this patient? (Select all that apply)

A. Excessive magnesium intake
B. Bowel disorders
C. Pneumonia
D. Hypertension

The correct answer is A

Comment: This patient developed severe hypermagnesemia after taking magnesium-containing laxatives without preexisting renal dysfunction and was treated successfully. This case suggests that severe hypermagnesemia can occur in the absence of preexisting renal dysfunction, especially in patients with bowel disorders.[1-3]

Case Study 15

A 15-year-old girl was admitted with acute pyelonephritis. During her hospital stay, she received magnesium-containing laxatives for chronic constipation. She became confused and lethargic on the seventh day of medication, although inflammatory markers were decreasing. Her blood pressure was 85/44 mmHg and her pulse was 65 beats/min. The physical and neurological examinations were unremarkable. The serum magnesium level was elevated to 6.11 mg/dL and peaked at 7.04 mg/dL. Concurrent laboratory studies showed serum creatinine 0.89 mg/dL, blood urea nitrogen 44 mg/dL, and serum calcium 7.1 mg/dL. Results of arterial blood gas analysis in room air was pH, 7.52; PO_2, 84.9 mmHg; PCO_2, 42 mmHg; bicarbonate, 34.4 mmol/L; and base excess, 10.8 mmol/L). Serum lactate level was 1.6 mmol/L. An electrocardiogram (ECG) showed a sinus rhythm with a heart rate of 62 beats/min. Intravenous hydration with normal saline, loop diuretics, and intravenous calcium administration was promptly initiated. Blood pressure improved with intravenous hydration (110/67 mmHg), and urine output was 3 L/day. Subsequently, the serum magnesium level decreased and was 2.12 mg/dL after three days. The patient was diagnosed with irritable bowel syndrome, and her treatment was planned with dietary modification and other laxatives.

What additional therapeutic measure would you consider?

A. Initiate hemodialysis
B. Initiate peritoneal dialysis
C. Initiate continuous renal replacement therapy
D. None of the above

The correct answer is D

Comment: This patient developed severe hypermagnesemia after receiving magnesium-containing laxatives in the absence of renal dysfunction and was treated successfully without dialysis intervention.

Hypermagnesemia is an uncommon but serious clinical condition that can be fatal. Magnesium-containing products are widely used as antacids or laxatives. This patient demonstrates that excessive use of magnesium-containing laxatives can cause severe hypermagnesemia even in patients with normal renal function. Physicians should be aware of the effects of these medications in constipated patients.[1-3]

Case Study 16

What caused severe hypermagnesemia? (Select all that apply)

A. Acute kidney injury
B. Excessive use of magnesium-containing laxatives
C. Hypokalemia
D. Hypocalcemia

The correct answers are A and B

Comment: Severe symptomatic hypermagnesemia may result from unsupervised use of magnesium-containing over-the-counter laxatives, which are often considered benign. In the setting of renal insufficiency, severe magnesium toxicity can develop especially in the elderly.

The presentation can mimic various medical conditions such as sepsis or respiratory failure and hence the clinician should have a high degree of suspicion to order further testing to successfully diagnose this potentially life-threatening electrolyte disturbance. Once diagnosed, treatment with rapid supportive measures—intravenous calcium, fluids, loop diuretics, and urgent hemodialysis are highly effective in preventing significant morbidity and mortality.[1-4]

Case Study 17

This 1.6 kg male patient was born at 29 weeks gestation to a 19-year-old Gravida 1, Para 0 mother. Pregnancy was complicated by preterm labor, tobacco use, and marijuana abuse. Two doses of betamethasone were administered before delivery. The infant was delivered by spontaneous vaginal delivery with Apgar scores of 9 at 1 and 5 minutes. Resuscitation consisted of bulb suction and bagmask ventilation. The infant required 5 cm of nasal continuous positive airway pressure and was weaned to room air within 24 hours. Intravenous fluids were started at birth. On the second day of life, nasogastric feeding with breast milk was initiated, and intravenous fluids were changed to total parenteral nutrition (TPN). On the 10th day of life, while on nasogastric feedings of 120 mL/kg/day and TPN of 40 mL/kg/day, the infant was noted to have hypotonia, temperature instability, and lethargy. Blood was drawn for a complete blood count and blood culture, spinal tap and urine culture were collected, and intravenous antibiotics were started. Initial arterial blood gases were consistent with severe metabolic acidosis; the infant developed hypotension, bradycardia, and apnea. He was intubated and received multiple boluses of Ringer lactate with dopamine, dobutamine, and epinephrine infusions. Acidosis was corrected with bicarbonate without any improvement in hypotension and bradycardia. On admission, he had refractory bradycardia with a heart rate of 80 to 100 beats/min, systolic blood pressure of 42 to 48 mmHg by Doppler, serum creatinine of 0.9 mg/dL, ionized calcium of 1.6 mmol/L, and total calcium of 11.2 mg/dL. The patient received multiple doses of epinephrine through the endotracheal tube and intravenously and continued on intravenous infusions of epinephrine, dopamine, and dobutamine for hypotension. Serum magnesium was 7.4 mmol/L after the episode. Liver enzymes, serum osmolality, and urine osmolality were within normal limits. The infant was stabilized with mechanical ventilation. An electrocardiogram (ECG) was consistent with sinus bradycardia, a head ultrasound was negative for hemorrhage, and the initial electroencephalogram (EEG) was consistent with diffuse encephalopathy. Echocardiography revealed a patent foramen oval without any structural anomalies. Nerve conduction studies showed neuromuscular junction blockade. The infant was given an infusion of calcium, normal saline along with furosemide. The serum magnesium level was monitored closely along with serum electrolytes. The patient weaned quickly from the ventilator, as serum magnesium level returned to normal, and he was intubated to room air on the 15th day after admission. Nasogastric feeding was started on the seventh day after admission when serum magnesium level was within normal limits and repeat EEG and nerve conduction velocity was normal. The infant continued to do well, and he was discharged on the 53rd day of life with an adjusted gestational age of 36 weeks. On discharge, he weighed 2680 g, was on room air, and was taking feedings well.

What is the MOST likely cause of hypermagnesemia in this patient?

    A. Excessive magnesium intake through TPN
    B. Sepsis
    C. Acute kidney injury
    D. Hyperparathyroidism

The correct answer is A
Comment: Hypermagnesemia in newborns causes parasympathetic blockade, including cutaneous flushing, hypotension, prolonged QT-interval, delayed intraventricular conduction, respiratory depression, neuromuscular blockade, and coma and clinically mimics a central brainstem

herniation syndrome. In this case, the infant received erroneously prepared total parenteral nutrition (TPN), which contained excess amounts of magnesium sulfate.

Unexplained sudden onset of apnea, refractory bradycardia, and refractory hypotension should raise suspicion of hypermagnesemia, which is reversible if identified and treated early. Iatrogenic hypermagnesemia has been reported from the administration of parenteral magnesium, excessive magnesium in dialysate solution, and multiple doses of cathartic therapy given in conjunction with charcoal. Early recognition and treatment of hypermagnesemia may prevent or minimize life-threatening events; however, the vast majority of mild hypermagnesemia patients may be missed. Hypotension, electrocardiographic changes, and evidence of sedation appear at serum magnesium concentrations of 3 to 8 mEq/L. The disappearance of deep tendon reflexes, respiratory depression, weakness, and coma are reported at magnesium levels of 5 to 15 mEq/L; cardiac arrest is reported at serum magnesium levels of 20 to 30 mEq/L.

Appropriate initial treatment of hypermagnesemia involves removal of exogenous magnesium source, and the use of intravenous calcium. The exact mechanism of action of calcium is not known, but it causes displacement of magnesium from the cell membrane, which results in transient reversal of symptoms of hypermagnesemia. Intravenous infusion of glucose and saline are also conservative treatment modalities, but renal dialysis, either peritoneal or hemodialysis is the treatment of choice in refractory hypermagnesemia.[1–4]

References

Case Study 1

1. Lerma EV, Nissenson R. *Nephrology Secrets.* Elsevier Health Sciences; 2011:568. ISBN:9780323081276.
2. Felsenfeld AJ, Levine BS, Rodriguez M. Pathophysiology of calcium, phosphorus, and magnesium dysregulation in chronic kidney disease. *Semin Dial.* 2015;28(6):564–577.
3. Cheungpasitporn W, Thongprayoon C, Qian Q. Dysmagnesemia in hospitalized patients: prevalence and prognostic importance. *Mayo Clin Proc.* 2015;90(8):1001–1010.

Case Study 2

1. Ronco C, Bellomo R, Kellum JA, Ricci Z. *Critical Care Nephrology.* Elsevier Health Sciences; 2017:344. ISBN:9780323449427.
2. Lerma EV, Nissenson R. *Nephrology Secrets.* Elsevier Health Sciences; 2011:568. ISBN:9780323081276.

Case Study 3

1. Felsenfeld AJ, Levine BS, Rodriguez M. Pathophysiology of calcium, phosphorus, and magnesium dysregulation in chronic kidney disease. *Semin Dial.* 2015;28(6):564–757.
2. Cheungpasitporn W, Thongprayoon C, Qian Q. Dysmagnesemia in hospitalized patients: prevalence and prognostic importance. *Mayo Clin Proc.* 2015;90(8):1001–1010.

Case Study 4

1. van den Bergh WM, Algra A, Rinkel GJ. Electrocardiographic abnormalities and serum magnesium in patients with subarachnoid hemorrhage. *Stroke.* 2004;35(3):644–648. https://doi.org/10.1161/01.STR.0000117092.38460.4F.

Case Study 5

1. Felsenfeld AJ, Levine BS, Rodriguez M. Pathophysiology of calcium, phosphorus, and magnesium dysregulation in chronic kidney disease. *Semin Dial.* 2015;28(6):564–577.
2. Cheungpasitporn W, Thongprayoon C, Qian Q. Dysmagnesemia in hospitalized patients: prevalence and prognostic importance. *Mayo Clin Proc.* 2015;90(8):1001–1010.

Case Study 6

1. Felsenfeld AJ, Levine BS, Rodriguez M. Pathophysiology of calcium, phosphorus, and magnesium dysregulation in chronic kidney disease. *Semin Dial.* 2015;28(6):564–577.

2. Cheungpasitporn W, Thongprayoon C, Qian Q. Dysmagnesemia in hospitalized patients: prevalence and prognostic importance. *Mayo Clin Proc.* 2015;90(8):1001–1010.

Case Study 7

1. Tinawi M. Hypertension in pregnancy. *Arch Intern Med Res.* 2020;3:10–17.
2. Okusanya B, Oladapo O, Long Q, et al. Clinical pharmacokinetic properties of magnesium sulphate in women with pre-eclampsia and eclampsia. *Br J Obstet Gynaecol.* 2016;123:356–366.

Case Study 8

1. Guerrera M, Volpe S, James J. Therapeutic uses of magnesium. *Am Fam Physician.* 2009;80:157–162.

Case Study 9

1. Weng YM, Chen SY, Chen SC, et al. Hypermagnesemia in a constipated female. *J Emerg Med.* 2013;44:e57–e60.

Case Study 10

1. Araki K, Kawashima Y, Magota M, et al. Hypermagnesemia in a 20-month-old healthy girl caused by the use of a laxative: a case report. *J Med Case Reports.* 2021;15:129. https://doi.org/10.1186/s13256-021-02686-9.

Case Study 11

1. Deheinzelin D, Negri EM, Tucci MR, et al. Hypomagnesemia in critically ill cancer patients: a prospective study of predictive factors. *Braz J Med Biol Res.* 2000;33:1443–1448.
2. Quamme GA, Schlingmann KP, Konra MS. Mechanisms and disorders of magnesium metabolism. In: 4th ed. Cambridge, MA: Academic Press; 2008:1747–1767. Alpern RJ, Herbert SC, eds. Seldin and Giebisch's The Kidney; Vol. 2.

Case Study 12

1. Deheinzelin D, Negri EM, Tucci MR, et al. Hypomagnesemia in critically ill cancer patients: a prospective study of predictive factors. *Braz J Med Biol Res.* 2000;33:1443–1448.
2. Quamme GA, Schlingmann KP, Konra MS. Mechanisms and disorders of magnesium metabolism. In: 4th ed. Cambridge, MA: Academic Press; 2008:1747–1767. Alpern RJ, Herbert SC, eds. Seldin and Giebisch's The Kidney; Vol. 2.

Case Study 13

1. Deheinzelin D, Negri EM, Tucci MR, et al. Hypomagnesemia in critically ill cancer patients: a prospective study of predictive factors. *Braz J Med Biol Res.* 2000;33:1443–1448.
2. Quamme GA, Schlingmann KP, Konra MS. Mechanisms and disorders of magnesium metabolism. In: 4th ed. Cambridge, MA: Academic Press; 2008:1747–1767. Alpern RJ, Herbert SC, eds. Seldin and Giebisch's The Kidney; Vol. 2.

Case Study 14

1. Smogorzewski MJ, Stubbs JR, Yu ASL. Disorders of calcium, magnesium, and phosphate balance. In: Skorecki K, Chertow G, Marsden P, Yu A, Taal M, eds. *Brenner & Rector's the Kidney.* 10th ed. Philadelphia: Elsevier Inc.; 2016:625–626.
2. Bokhari SR, Siriki R, Teran FJ, et al. Fatal hypermagnesemia due to laxative use: case report and review of the literature. *Am J Med Sci.* 2017;355:390–395.
3. Weng YM, Chen SY, Chen HC, et al. Hypermagnesemia in a constipated female. *J Emerg Med.* 2013;44:e57–e60.

Case Study 15

1. Smogorzewski MJ, Stubbs JR, Yu ASL. Disorders of calcium, magnesium, and phosphate balance. In: Skorecki K, Chertow G, Mars-den P, Yu A, Taal M, eds. *Brenner & Rector's the Kidney.* 10th ed. Philadelphia: Elsevier Inc.; 2016:625–626.

2. Bokhari SR, Siriki R, Teran FJ, et al. Fatal hypermagnesemia due to laxative use: case report and review of the literature. *Am J Med Sci.* 2017;355:390–395.
3. Weng YM, Chen SY, Chen HC, et al. Hypermagnesemia in a constipated female. *J Emerg Med.* 2013;44:e57–e60.

Case Study 16

1. Jhang WK, Lee YJ, Kim AY, et al. Severe hypermagnesemia presenting with abnormal electrocardiographic findings similar to those of hyperkalemia in a child undergoing peritoneal dialysis. *Korean J Pediatr.* 2013;56(7):308–311.
2. Smogorzewski MJ, Stubbs JR, Yu ASL. Disorders of calcium, magnesium, and phosphate balance. In: Skorecki K, Chertow G, Mars-den P, Yu A, Taal M, eds. *Brenner & Rector's the Kidney.* 10th ed. Philadelphia: Elsevier Inc.; 2016:625–626.
3. Bokhari SR, Siriki R, Teran FJ, et al. Fatal hypermagnesemia due to laxative use: case report and review of the literature. *Am J Med Sci.* 2017;355:390–395.
4. Weng YM, Chen SY, Chen HC, et al. Hypermagnesemia in a constipated female. *J Emerg Med.* 2013;44:e57–e60.

Case Study 17

1. Sullivan JE, Berman BW. The pediatric forum: hypermagnesemia with lethargy and hypotonia due to administration of magnesium hydroxide to a 4-week-old infant. *Arch Pediatr Adolesc Med.* 2000;154(12):1272–1274.
2. Donovan EF, Tsang RC, Steichen JJ, et al. Neonatal hypermagnesemia: effect on parathyroid hormone and calcium homeostasis. *J Pediatr.* 1980;96:305–310.
3. Donovan EF, Tsang RC, Steichen JJ, et al. Neonatal hypermagnesemia: effect on parathyroid hormone and calcium homeostasis. *J Pediatr.* 1980;96:305–310.
4. Herschel M, Mittendorf R. Tocolytic magnesium sulphate toxicity and unexpected neonatal death—clinical perinatal case presentation. *J Perinatol.* 2001;21:261–262.